BY JENNIFER VANDERBES

Easter Island

The Secret of Raven Point

Strangers at the Feast

Wonder Drug

Wonder Drug

WONDER DRUG

The Secret History
of Thalidomide in America
and Its Hidden Victims

JENNIFER VANDERBES

Random House
New York

Published in the United States by Random House, an imprint and
division of Penguin Random House LLC, New York.

RANDOM HOUSE and the HOUSE colophon are registered trademarks of
Penguin Random House LLC.

Grateful acknowledgment is made to the following to reprint previously published material:
British Medical Journal c/o Copyright Clearance Center: Letter by A. Leslie Florence to
the *British Medical Journal* entitled "Is Thalidomide to Blame?" published December 31,
1960. Reprinted with permission from the *British Medical Journal.*
Elsevier c/o Copyright Clearance Center: Excerpt reprinted from *The Lancet,* vol. 278,
issue 7205, "Iatrogenic Diseases of the Newborn," pages no. 753–754, copyright 1961.
Reprinted with permission from Elsevier.

Library of Congress Cataloging-in-Publication Data
Names: Vanderbes, Jennifer, author.
Title: Wonder drug: the secret history of thalidomide in America and its hidden victims /
by Jennifer Vanderbes.
Other titles: Secret history of thalidomide in America and its hidden victims
Description: First edition. | New York: Random House, [2023] |
Includes bibliographical references and index.
Identifiers: LCCN 2022049196 (print) | LCCN 2022049197 (ebook) |
ISBN 9780525512264 (hardcover) | ISBN 9780525512271 (ebook)
Subjects: LCSH: Thalidomide—United States—History. | Thalidomide—Side effects—
United States. | Pharmaceutical industry—Moral and ethical aspects.
Classification: LCC RA1242.T5 V36 2023 (print) | LCC RA1242.T5 (ebook) |
DDC 615/.78209409046—dc23/eng/20230228
LC record available at https://lccn.loc.gov/2022049196
LC ebook record available at https://lccn.loc.gov/2022049197

Printed in the United States of America on acid-free paper

randomhousebooks.com

2 4 6 8 9 7 5 3 1

First Edition

Book design by Fritz Metsch

For Annika and Ellery

and for all those who were not counted

Contents

Cast of Characters

United States

FRANCES OLDHAM KELSEY—pharmacologist and physician hired by the Food and Drug Administration in 1960 as a medical reviewer

FREMONT ELLIS KELSEY ("KELSE" OR ELLIS)—Frances's husband, a pharmacologist

GEORGE LARRICK—FDA commissioner, 1954–1965

EUGENE M. K. GEILING (E. M. K.)—Frances's mentor, South African–born pharmacologist at the University of Chicago

JOSEPH MURRAY—Merrell's FDA liaison

EVERT FLORUS VAN MAANEN ("FLOR")—doctor, Merrell's head of biological sciences, who oversaw animal research

RAYMOND POGGE—doctor, Merrell's director of medical research

THOMAS JONES—Merrell's director of medical science, promoted to oversee the Kevadon trials after Raymond Pogge's departure

RALPH SMITH—Frances's immediate supervisor at the FDA

RAY O. NULSEN—Cincinnati-based ob-gyn who delivered multiple babies with phocomelia while running Kevadon trials for Merrell

ESTES KEFAUVER—U.S. senator from Tennessee who led the subcommittee investigation into the drug industry

BARBARA MOULTON—former FDA medical reviewer and whistle-blower

EPPES WAYLES BROWNE, JR.—Moulton's husband and staff economist for Senator Kefauver

HELEN BROOKE TAUSSIG—pediatric heart surgeon at Johns Hopkins University, traveled to Germany to investigate babies harmed by thalidomide

JOHN NESTOR—FDA medical reviewer, Frances's ally

MORTON MINTZ—American journalist, broke the thalidomide story for
The Washington Post in 1962

Germany

HERMANN WIRTZ—Nazi Party member, co-founded Chemie Grünenthal

HEINRICH MÜCKTER—former Wehrmacht doctor hired as chief scientific
officer of Chemie Grünenthal

HANS-WERNER VON SCHRADER-BEIELSTEIN—doctor, head of Chemie
Grünenthal's research department

AUGUSTIN BLASIU—German doctor whose research on post-partum
women using thalidomide was used to suggest the drug was safe during
pregnancy

RALF VOSS—Düsseldorf-based nerve specialist, raised the alarm about thalidomide's link to peripheral neuritis

KARL-HERMANN SCHULTE-HILLEN—German lawyer and father of thalidomide survivor Jan

LINDE SCHULTE-HILLEN—Karl's wife, mother of thalidomide survivor Jan

WIDUKIND LENZ—German pediatrician and geneticist, alerted the German medical community to thalidomide's link to birth deformities

ELINOR KAMATH—American journalist based in Germany who alerted
her fellow foreign correspondents and the U.S. embassy to the news of
thalidomide's dangers

United Kingdom

GEORGE SOMERS—pharmacologist for Distillers UK

DENIS BURLEY—medical adviser at Distillers, London

A. LESLIE FLORENCE—Scotland-based doctor who alerted Distillers of
thalidomide's peripheral neuritis side effects, which he publicized in
the *British Medical Journal*

WILLIAM MCBRIDE—Australian ob-gyn at Crown Street Women's Hospital, delivered multiple babies harmed by thalidomide and led the charge
to prove the drug's dangers

HAROLD EVANS—journalist, helmed the *Sunday Times* (London) exposé
of thalidomide

Prologue

On a hot August night in 1962, Ann Morris felt her first contraction. Her husband, Doug, guided her out of their small Cincinnati apartment, where a gleaming crib and piles of hand-sewn baby quilts had been arranged. Settling into their new Chevrolet—in anticipation of the baby, Doug had surrendered his beloved Corvette—the couple drove five minutes through the quiet, dark city streets to the Jewish Hospital.

In the labor ward, Ann's pain intensified, and her contractions continued into the next day. At thirty-one, Ann—who had married Doug just a year earlier—was a little old to be having her first baby. But labor was progressing normally, and Ann, raised on a Kentucky farm where she picked tobacco and slaughtered chickens, was not one to wilt at discomfort. Her only complaint, in an otherwise easy pregnancy, had been morning sickness, and her doctor had given her a small white bottle of vitamins, which eased her nausea.

When Ann awoke in the hospital after the baby's delivery, Doug entered the room grim-faced. He told her that their newborn—a girl—was missing arms and legs. She was not expected to live long. The couple had a list of baby names, but now their first choice—Gale Elizabeth—seemed wrong. In fact, the whole list seemed off. They scrambled to come up with something and landed on "Carolyn Jean."

While Ann was sedated, the hospital arranged to place the girl in foster care and urged Doug and Ann not to even see her. Doug went home to destroy the photos he had taken of Ann gleefully preparing for the baby. Meanwhile, Ann remained alone in a private hospital room, away from other new mothers, until, finally, the delivering doctor appeared with an odd question: Had Ann gone to Canada and bought *thalidomide?*

Ann had first read about thalidomide a week earlier in *Life* magazine. An article called "The Drug That Left a Trail of Heartbreak" showed page after page of photographs of armless infants in Europe. Ann had shuddered at the German tragedy but felt no connection to it. She had never been overseas and told the doctor she certainly hadn't gone to Canada to get a drug. She gave the matter no more thought.

Ann was never contacted by the FDA or by the Ohio or Cincinnati health authorities. No doctor or nurse from the Jewish Hospital ever told her that within the past year at least four other babies had been born at the same hospital with the same deformity—phocomelia—a birth defect so rare that most doctors would never encounter a single case. And no one would tell her that the Cincinnati-based William S. Merrell Company, located at 110 East Amity Road, just fifteen minutes across town from her home, had sent millions of thalidomide "samples" to more than twelve hundred doctors across the country, including two hundred obstetricians. For three years these pills, in various colors and dosages, without proper labels, had been casually handed out for everything from insomnia to headaches to morning sickness.

The baby, Carolyn Jean, survived. She spent almost a year in foster care until she was finally reclaimed by her parents. Despite all predictions, she thrived—becoming a professional artist and a mother of four. Over the years, when people asked Ann what had caused her daughter's disfigurement, Ann would say, "It's just one of those things that happens."

In July of 1962, a sleeping pill billed as "the safest thing since water" was revealed to have killed or disfigured more than ten thousand babies worldwide in the "single largest holocaust" in medical history.

Sensational images of legless, armless infants filled newspapers. Politicians admonished pharmaceutical firms. Pills of every kind fell under suspicion. At the peak of the baby boom, the bliss of impending motherhood became fraught with dread. Women unfortunate enough to have taken thalidomide—often consuming only a single tablet, at the behest of their doctor—were cast as wayward druggies. And thousands of parents were left to raise children with such extreme and unprecedented physical malformations that the medical profession lacked any knowledge to assist.

The question emerged: Who should have protected the world from this catastrophe? What bureaucratic safeguards could have foreseen it? Was it an unavoidable accident of the era's chemical wizardry, or had some negligence, some deliberate disregard fueled by greed, maimed those thousands of babies?

As government agencies and courts scrambled to investigate the disaster, a sinister story came to light. Thalidomide had been created by a Nazi-founded German pharmaceutical firm that apparently bullied doctors and buried documents. For four years the company had sold and licensed the drug across the globe, hailing it as completely atoxic, safe for everyone, children and pregnant women included, with scant data to back the claims. Expectant mothers in almost fifty countries had innocently taken the toxic sedative, and the shock of their maimed babies struck a huge blow to public confidence in the booming postwar pharmaceuticals industry.

Since World War II, when the manufacture of antibiotics and antimalarials bolstered drug firms, pharmaceuticals had become a multibillion-dollar business. By 1960, drugs were the most profitable industry in the United States. Pills promising to ease every ache, pain, and worry became a trusted part of daily life. Thalidomide in particular held an unprecedented, glittering promise: It was billed as a one-size-fits-all drug free of risk—no addiction, no side effects, no chance of overdose. It looked like the pharmaceutical world's unsinkable ship. But no one—not the chemists who patented it, the doctors who prescribed it, or the firms that sold it—knew how the drug worked inside the human body. The research had been shoddy, the safety claims imprudent. By the time thalidomide had been consumed by millions around the world and the drug's trail of damage came to light, the public asked: What drove the creation of wonder drugs—wellness or profit? And if something went wildly wrong, who would be held accountable?

Behind the tale of slapdash science and corporate callousness lay an equally compelling, heartening story of quiet heroism. Around the globe, a few lone doctors, parents, and journalists had, over a grueling year, detected the birth defects—sometimes in their own children—and collectively sounded the alarm, forcing the drug firms disavowing thalidomide's dangers to recall the product. No government agency or health authority had done what this loosely knit group of concerned citizens had: expose and stop the largest pharmaceutical scandal of the twentieth century.

When I first came across records of their extraordinary feat, I wanted to honor these renegades. A German pediatrician, trying to escape the shame of his father's Nazi past, risked his career to battle a powerful drug firm. A young German lawyer, seeking justice for his limbless son, launched the largest criminal trial in Germany since Nuremberg. A cocksure Australian obstetrician, devastated to learn that the drug he had given to his pregnant patients had maimed their babies, cobbled together his own animal research lab in a parking lot shed to prove the drug's dangers.

But my primary focus in this book is the relatively unknown story of thalidomide in America. As the only country in the world that refused to put thalidomide on the market during its initial launch, the United States brought its own valiant cast to the tale: Elinor Kamath, a young American reporter stationed in Germany, fought to make the drug's dangers international news; Helen Taussig, a deaf female pediatric heart surgeon, flew to Germany to gather evidence; Barbara Moulton, a Food and Drug Administration official and the first female whistle-blower in American history, risked her career to reform the agency; Morton Mintz, an upstart *Washington Post* reporter with a disabled child, broke the chilling news; Estes Kefauver, a rogue U.S. senator from Tennessee, used the thalidomide episode to force Congress to overhaul the drug industry. But chief among the heroes of this saga is Frances Kelsey—the only doctor in the world to recognize danger in thalidomide's scientific paperwork.

As an FDA medical reviewer, Kelsey single-handedly kept thalidomide off the American market—a bureaucratic battle that consumed nearly a year and a half of her life. For this, the demure married mother of two earned the media spotlight in 1962 and became a national hero. President John F. Kennedy awarded her a medal. Her photograph graced *Life* magazine. At a time when every safeguard around the world had failed, so powerful was the appeal of Frances Kelsey's incorruptibility that her story came to obscure a disturbing footnote in the American thalidomide story—namely that the drug *had* been widely circulated within the United States. While awaiting FDA approval, the William S. Merrell Company had launched clinical trials so vast and informal that the FDA would eventually beg the Justice Department to bring criminal charges against the firm.

This book involved 283 interviews with victims, scientists, lawyers, doctors, and journalists across the globe, as well as visits to public and private archives and various courthouses. I probed thousands of decades-old documents and spoke to many people who had never before discussed their role in these events. Frances Kelsey's life had never been written about, and many of the other key women who fought this battle had been—unsurprisingly—sidelined in early accounts. My research uncovered key elements buried for over sixty years: Trial transcripts revealed that the William S. Merrell Company withheld toxic animal data from the FDA. Multiple obstetricians who conducted thalidomide trials for Merrell had, in fact, witnessed birth malformations at least a year before the firm asked physicians to stop using the drug. Most important, details of an FDA investigation showed staggering finds: one thousand thalidomide pills stashed in the medicine cabinet of a Virginia doctor months after the drug's dangers had made headlines; official "trial" doctors missing records of which patients had received the drug; physicians falsifying patient charts to erase any record that thalidomide had been given. Pills had been handed off, in bulk, from doctor to doctor. Heaps of the drug went to charities. A mysterious shipment of thalidomide arrived at a mission in Taiwan, from an American church, a year *after* the drug's recall. Further, another American drug company had run secret thalidomide trials years before and purportedly buried evidence of the drug's teratogenic effects. It became clear that most pregnant women in the United States who'd taken thalidomide had no idea what the drug had been. And when their babies were born with phocomelia, no doctor copped to the cause.

This de facto cover-up allowed a false narrative—that America had been spared the thalidomide catastrophe—to become national legend, a blazing FDA success story. In fact, dozens of victims harmed by corporate greed, medical incompetence, and widespread lying would have to wait almost sixty years to find out what happened. This is that story.

Part I

THE
ROOKIE

The human being who would not harm you on an individual, face-to-face basis, who is charitable, civic-minded, loving and devout, will wound or kill you from behind the corporate veil.

—Morton Mintz

One

Rain pounded the hood of Frances Kelsey's car as she inched through the downtown Washington, D.C., traffic. She'd be late, again. For the past five weeks, every morning had been a struggle to get to work on time. Because she was not a woman short on accomplishment—she had two advanced degrees and a scientific textbook to her name—her lateness had become a family joke. Even though Mom had won national research prizes and harpooned sperm whales, she was being bested by traffic, unable to make it from the family's new house in Chevy Chase to the National Mall in under an hour.

Today Frances was driving through the fringes of Hurricane Donna, with rain dousing the Northeast. High-speed winds bent and rustled trees along the road. Excitement was in the air, if not in Frances's life.

It was September 12, 1960, and the forty-six-year-old married mother of two had just moved halfway across the country for a position at the Food and Drug Administration. After decades of hands-on lab research with beavers and armadillos and summer boating trips to collect massive whale gland specimens, Frances was now an FDA medical reviewer: a doctor who assessed paperwork, not patients. A bureaucrat. It was not the profession she'd trained for, but she knew it was important work, and a necessary concession to her husband's new job.

Three years before the publication of *The Feminine Mystique* launched the feminist revolution, Frances was an oddity of her day: She held both an MD and a PhD and had forged a career in the hard sciences while married with children. She wasn't emotive. She wasn't frilly. She relegated makeup to special occasions and ignored the gray in her blunt-cut chin-length hair. Born in rural Canada, Frances—a solid five foot seven—

remained tomboyish well into adulthood, fishing, clam digging, lugging her stick out to a field for a game of hockey whenever the air was crisp. She neither cooked nor cleaned house, but she knew that to keep her family running smoothly she had to relinquish some professional ground to Ellis. In seventeen years of marriage, Frances had moved states, shifted careers, earned degrees, and secured freelance work a half dozen times to oblige his career.

But this nine-to-five FDA desk job was a jolt for the normally bustling Frances. For the past seven years, living in South Dakota, where Ellis had chaired the university's pharmacology department, Frances had juggled a host of on-the-go jobs. In addition to her university lab research with beaver thyroids, she had regularly hopped the overnight train to Chicago to secure her radioisotope diagnostics license. She had spent a full year commuting to Yankton for a hospital medical internship, leaving Ellis to cook dinners and put the girls to bed. Frances also zipped across the state for weeks at a time to fill in for vacationing small-town physicians. Often the first female doctor to grace the Badlands outposts, Frances made headlines: "Lemmon Patients Are Treated by Lady Physician," boasted a local newspaper. So remote was the town of Lemmon that Frances had been dropped there by a chartered prop plane.

Frances had loved juggling emergencies in these remote South Dakota communities. Births, burst appendixes. Any "hectic series of crises" fascinated her, and she proudly embraced the grisly. One story she often recounted was of the hunter she tended upon her arrival in Lemmon—a man blasted in the abdomen by an antelope rifle in a hunting accident.

Back at home with daughters Susan and Christine, Phillip the Siamese cat, and their Saint Bernard, George, Frances tried to make the most of university-town life. She and Ellis, a hulking charmer of a man, socialized at the Vermillion Eagles Club and religiously played bridge. Brilliant, fun-loving, and quick-witted, the duo shared a zest for life that earned them a reputation as bon vivants. "Frankie and Kelse" were known for their well-stocked bar and the lively parties around the fireplace of their white clapboard colonial home. The parties were so lively that, before they began, the whole family laughingly tugged closed the "Weeks curtains"—thick drapes the couple had installed on their dining room windows after discovering that the dour man living next door was university president I. D.

Weeks. Frankie and Kelse had "borrowed" a reel-to-reel audio device from the university and set it up behind the couch to record the gatherings. The girls spent the night crisscrossing the crowd of adults, carrying platters of olives and soda crackers and bacon-wrapped chicken livers.

But by 1956, three years into their South Dakota stint, Frankie and Ellis had overstayed their welcome. "This is a desolate area," Ellis wrote to a friend, "from the standpoint of professional colleagues." In Vermillion, egos were fragile and résumés flimsy, and the couple became the target of spiteful gossip. A university dean advised colleagues to shun the Kelseys, warning that anyone foolish enough to collaborate with them would be "left out in the cold" when they made off with "all of the data." Frances — who, as a woman, had been sidelined her whole career — shrugged off the drama. Having just become a U.S. citizen, she toyed with a career move — and Washington, D.C., where their former graduate school adviser had just moved, brimmed with scientific government jobs. Every night, she and Kelse ogled D.C. real estate listings. They planned their South Dakota exit with the patience and intensity of a small prison break.

After a three-year bureaucratic slog, mailing applications across the country, Ellis had finally secured a National Institutes of Health job when a man at the Food and Drug Administration contacted him. Ralph Smith, who had met Ellis at a pharmacology conference, now helmed the FDA's New Drug Branch. He wanted to hire "a man with a PhD as well as an MD" as an FDA medical officer.

Ellis, who merely held a PhD, confessed his limits. But he offered the name of a brilliant MD *and* PhD — his wife, Dr. Frances Kelsey.

At the National Mall, at Jefferson Drive and Seventh Street, Frances finally pulled into the parking lot of the shabby, unmarked FDA building, a deteriorating, prefab army structure from World War II. Compared to the Capitol's marble grandeur, this agency looked like the government's armpit.

The Food and Drug Administration had earned its name in 1930. It was a rebranding of the Bureau of Chemistry, a Civil War–era creation that had monitored the nation's food, chemicals, and medicine for over seventy years. When the FDA was initially christened, food was its chief focus; the drug sector at that time — composed of small, regional apothecaries–

turned–pharmaceutical firms—barely dented the nation's gross domestic product. But wartime subsidies had expanded those firms into national corporations. By 1960—the year Frances arrived in Washington, D.C.— drugs were the country's most profitable industry, to the tune of $2.7 billion in annual sales. The Goliath sector was overseen by one very underfunded federal agency: Frances's new employer, the Food and Drug Administration.

Tasked with monitoring all food, drugs, cosmetics, and medical devices throughout the United States, the FDA Washington headquarters coordinated eighteen regional offices and inspectors in forty-one cities. But budget cuts under the Truman and early Eisenhower administrations had crippled the bureau so that by the mid-1950s, fewer than nine hundred employees struggled to keep pace with its massive mandate. When American drug firms submitted a staggering 369 applications to market new products in 1959—essentially proposing a patented drug each day—the agency scrambled to find more doctors to review all the scientific paperwork. Enter Frances.

Frances worked out of room 2605, a run-down office on the second floor. The green paint was peeling, the wooden floor was bare, and a long metal table pushed against the wall had been anointed her "desk" by some government furniture provisioner wrestling with the agency's shoestring budget. Frances was highly credentialed but unpretentious, so the setting didn't trouble her. And this morning she was giddy. After a monthlong orientation of slideshows and lectures, today she would dive into actual work. On the table sat her assignment: New Drug Application (NDA) 12-611—a few phone books' worth of data, letters, and reports, bound in blue folders, submitted by a Cincinnati pharmaceutical company for a new sedative called Kevadon.

The cover page described the drug as an unusually safe, nonbarbiturate hypnotic already sold in over forty-six countries. The application, submitted by the William S. Merrell Company, brimmed with praise from American doctors who had used Kevadon in clinical trials, hailing it as "highly encouraging" and "superior to other sleep-inducing agents." Drafts of research papers—soon to be published—indicated similarly rave conclusions. It seemed her bosses had lobbed her an easy one.

A few hundred pages of the application, in German, came from Chemie Grünenthal, the overseas firm that had invented the drug. Frances could read only rudimentary German, but Merrell—which had licensed the product from Chemie Grünenthal—had summarized the European research, which also seemed to celebrate the sedative as effective and harmless.

Per agency regulations, Frances had sixty days to review the materials on her desk and to decide if the drug was safe for national distribution. Unless she found a specific problem, the product would then automatically be approved for sale. The situation looked simple; the drug, known generically as thalidomide, had already passed medical review boards in scores of countries.

Still, Frances loved data analysis. She'd spent years conducting research and had even worked for *The Journal of the American Medical Association* (*JAMA*), assessing which studies merited publication. As coauthor of the leading American graduate pharmacology textbook, she was supremely well versed in drug research. Even though this application seemed a rubber-stamper, the work ethic that had earned Frances scientific prizes and allowed her to flourish in a male field dictated that she scrutinize every last line. She turned back to the first pages and began.

Frances "Frankie" Kathleen Oldham was home-birthed in 1914 in a vast wooden house on Vancouver Island.

The house, called Balgonie, on the island's southern side, was hand-built by her father, Frank Trevor Oldham. The Australian-born colonel had served for decades in the Royal Field Artillery of the British army, stationed in India and China. By 1911, the wiry, handsome colonel was ready to start a new life on his military pension with his young Scottish bride. They moved to the Pacific coast of Canada and had four children.

Where Colonel Oldham was easygoing, fond of reading and tending his vegetable garden, his wife, Katherine Booth Stuart, was tempestuous. An amateur actress, "Kitty" loved horses, golfing, and swimming, though she would eventually drown under mysterious circumstances. Kitty came from a family of well-educated Scottish women, and, tasked with raising children in the Canadian wilderness, she let them manage themselves. Frances, or "Frankie"—the second born—regularly hiked through the towering evergreens and rolling meadows beyond Balgonie. The family owned thirty acres, including a stream where Frankie swam and fished for trout. At a pond in the woods, Frankie collected frogs, snakes, and bugs, hauling them up to her small second-floor bedroom for study.

From an early age, Frankie displayed a fearsome intellect, determinedly eavesdropping when her mother taught her older brother to read. Her parents arranged painting, piano, and dancing lessons for her and strong-armed a local Irish schoolmaster named Canon Barrie to admit their pre-cocious daughter to the small school he had started for boys.

There Frankie studied Latin, algebra, and geometry at her own level, fostering her intellectual independence. The school also toughened her: Regularly tripped and kicked by her male classmates, Frankie learned to retaliate. At night, back home, she boasted to her family of her counter-attacks. Determined not to lag boys in any skill, Frankie also enlisted a male friend to teach her to shoot and give her secret driving lessons. (Her family, who lived modestly, traveled the town's narrow roads by horse and buggy.)

Frankie's feral tendencies did not go unnoticed, and when the boys' school foundered at the start of the Depression, her parents opted to find her a gentler environment. After a year of private tutoring, fourteen-year-old Frankie was sent to the prim St. George's School for Girls in Victoria, British Columbia.

But by that point, her overseers also worried. "Frankie's conduct leaves much to be desired," Miss Suttie, the principal, wrote. "I should like to feel that Frankie could be relied upon to keep the few rules of the school when I am not there. Her record of order marks & fines is disgraceful for a high school girl."

At Frankie's next prep school, the St. Margaret's School for Girls, the principal noted some progress: "Frankie has improved greatly in manner and appearance during this year." Nonetheless, Frankie "must endeavor to correct her awkward gait." She was also faulted for being discourteous to her elders.

But Frankie thrived academically, and at high school graduation, she made the bold choice to attend college. On her mother's side, Frankie had two Scottish aunts—a lawyer and a doctor—whose lives struck her as "greatly enriched." In Scotland, education was second only to religion. And her father had already deemed his daughter a wunderkind.

In 1934, Frances received a BS in biology from McGill, but Depression-era unemployment allocated the few available jobs to men. When her father couldn't even finagle her a position at Vancouver's Departure Bay Biological Station, Frankie decided to summer in the British Isles with her mother and return in the fall for even more school.

Enrolling in a master's program at McGill, Frances hoped to study the newly popular pituitary gland, the "master gland" or "conductor of the endocrine orchestra." But all the spots in endocrinology were taken. The chair suggested she try the fledgling pharmacology department, where a notoriously crabby professor was researching the posterior lobe of the pituitary. The less popular department, it seemed, might accommodate a woman. So Frances trudged one flight up to Raymond Stehle, a bald, bespectacled researcher who immediately made clear his distaste for graduate students. But Frances pressed him for a position.

Within two years, Frances had her master's degree, but the raging Depression still curbed the job market. Stehle, who had warmed to Frances, offered her a fifty-dollars-a-month grant to stay on as his research assistant. But soon Stehle suggested a better plan: The chairman of the University of Chicago's brand-new pharmacology department was researching the posterior pituitary gland—now Frances's specialty. Stehle urged Frances to apply for a job.

Hopes in check, Frances dashed off a résumé and letter. Within a week, an airmail special delivery from the University of Chicago's Department of Pharmacology offered her one hundred dollars a month—double her McGill salary—to assist in research. Frances was ecstatic.

One trouble: The letter had been addressed to "Mr. Oldham." The department clearly expected a man, and Frances, morally scrupulous, intended to clarify.

"Don't be ridiculous," Stehle protested. "Accept the job, sign your name, put Miss in brackets afterwards, and go!"

Frances telegrammed her parents:

Leaving for Chicago Saturday . . . Excellent prospects. Very thrilled. Address International House. University of Chicago. Very well. Hope same with you all. Love Frankie.

Within the week, Frances—now twenty-one—had packed her things and boarded a series of southbound trains that took her to the United States for the first time.

It was March 1936, Chicago sparkled with wintry frost, and Frankie settled into her small dormitory room at the International House. She unpacked her beloved hockey stick, her notebooks, her journals. A short, chilly walk away was the pharmacology department and her new boss, the mysterious Professor Eugene Maximilian Karl Geiling.

E. M. K. Geiling, South African born, was a meticulous scientist with a theatrical flair. A charismatic bachelor, he traveled with two valets and a pet bulldog. Two tracks of silver hair flanked his wide bald crown. Wire-rimmed spectacles and a nearly lipless mouth lent his face a scholar's intensity. But Geiling's meaty hands and broad sloped shoulders hinted at the football player he'd once been. He often regaled students with a harrowing tale: As a young man, he was on a passenger ship off the coast of Cape Town when a mine exploded underwater. He scrambled onto a lifeboat and for five grueling hours watched nineteen fellow passengers die. As a result, Professor Geiling—"Pete" to his students—claimed to despise water. Yet he boasted of annual whaling trips off the Queen Charlotte Islands where he sawed and hacked at sperm whales to gather giant endocrine glands in gallon-sized specimen jars.

(In the spring of 1941, Geiling would make the "Screwy News" column of newspapers across the country when, to test the plausibility of the biblical story of the whale swallowing Jonah, he crawled the entire length of a sperm whale's gullet. "It was a pretty slimy trip," he boasted to reporters upon exiting the dead whale, "but there was plenty of room.")

Geiling's educational lineage ran back to Germany, via his mentor John Jacob Abel, an American who had trained in Strasbourg with Oswald Schmiedeberg, considered the father of modern pharmacology. On Abel's return to the states, he founded the Johns Hopkins Department of Pharmacology, where Geiling arrived at age thirty. For fifteen years, Geiling honed his research skills, transitioning from Abel's graduate student to colleague and then friend. Together the two men pioneered the discovery of crystallized insulin. As Abel shot to fame with epinephrine discoveries, Geiling began to crusade against the era's quack medicine. In 1932, he made headlines testifying in a high-profile government trial for the new FDA.

Potions and "proprietary medicine" had been a staple of American life since colonial times, but it had taken until 1906 for legislation to address such products. The new law had been spearheaded by a preacher's son named Harvey Washington Wiley. While teaching chemistry at Purdue University, Wiley was recruited by the Indiana state government to investigate possible adulterations of commercial honey and maple syrup. When 90 percent of Wiley's samples proved fake, he gave a fiery speech that drew the attention of the U.S. Department of Agriculture and earned him an appointment as the very first head of the Bureau of Chemistry (the FDA's precursor). In his new post, Wiley soon discovered a rampant, nationwide food crisis: black pepper cut with soil; coffee grounds thickened with charcoal; candy containing lead. His exposé of milk revealed a thinned, chalk-whitened product swimming with worms.

"The comparison of turning over a log and watching the bugs scamper to cover is too tame," Wiley moaned. It was more like "removing a huge brush pile to uncover a nest of hornets."

Wiley traveled the country to share his findings. The press dubbed him the "Crusading Chemist." Housewives deemed him a guardian of family safety.

But it took eight years for lawmakers to act on Wiley's discoveries. Not until 1890 was legislation put forth to regulate food production. Even so, journalist Morton Mintz would later write, the bill was "defeated by a durable alliance of quacks, ruthless crooks, pious frauds, scoundrels, high-priced lawyer-lobbyists, vested interests, liars, corrupt members of Congress, venal publishers, cowards in high office, the stupid, the apathetic, and the duped."

A scandal—rancid "embalmed beef" shipped to American soldiers fighting the Spanish-American War—briefly moved the needle on public opinion, but Congress still dragged its feet. So Wiley set out to prove that toxicity lurked *everywhere*.

In 1902, with a $5,000 congressional grant "to investigate the character of food preservatives, coloring matters, and other substances added to food" in "hygienic table trials," Wiley served his first experimental dinner to government workers he'd recruited as volunteer subjects. For weeks, he fed them three meals a day, incrementally sneaking borax, salicylic acid, sulfuric acid, saltpeter, formaldehyde, and copper sulfate into the food. He noted the health changes in his subjects—which were dismal. When newspapers got wind of the study, they dubbed his diners the "Poison Squad." The public was riveted. Wiley's long crusade at last came to fruition with the 1906 Food and Drug Act, the first legislation of its kind in the United States.

The new law curbed hidden ingredients in food and enacted stricter oversight of proprietary medicine. The government could now ban products such as "Cureforhedake BraneFude," whose chief active ingredient, acetanilide, was toxic. Or "Dr. Johnson's Mild Combination Treatment for Cancer," which did not, in fact, treat cancer. But the 1906 act had limits. When interpreting the law, the Supreme Court cared only that product ingredients be listed accurately. "Radithor"—a pricey radioactive water sold as a cure for male impotence, venereal disease, and 160 other medical problems—contained radium particles that could erode bone. When the potion killed a prominent steel magnate—the radium ate away at his skull—the courts essentially shrugged. Because the package had disclosed "Radium and Mesothorium in Triple Distilled Water," it was the man's bad luck for not grasping radium's bone-eating tendencies.

An amendment in 1912 supposedly aimed at expanding government powers inadvertently worsened matters. By forbidding "false *and* fraudulent" labeling (italics added), the law now forced prosecutors to *prove* fraud. The government slogged on. But the few court victories came at staggering prices. A $50,000 trial might render a verdict with a $50 fine.

One of the FDA's highest-profile targets of the time was B&M Balm, a rank goo, originally fed to horses, of turpentine, ammonia, water, and egg. A stable owner and a bookie had together decided to market the product as a human cure for, well, everything—rheumatism, tuberculosis, pneumonia, cancer, whooping cough, scarlet fever. In fact, it did nothing. But at trial, the defense argued that the company owner's *lack* of medical education proved that he genuinely believed his claims—ergo, no fraud. The jury agreed. B&M then smugly repurposed the verdict as a marketing point:

"Since B&M has been tested in these trials," a new round of ads read, "each of these testimonials has been submitted to the court under oath."

The FDA took a second swing at B&M a few years later, with concrete proof of B&M's intent to deceive: The company had pilfered letterhead from the Massachusetts College of Pharmacy to forge claims that the balm changed blood hydrogen-ion concentrations. In addition, the company had shelled out seventy-five dollars a month to physicians to reassure worried customers. The FDA's case was so strong that a doctor who had been paid $15,000 to attest to B&M's scientific properties fled before testifying.

The trial brimmed with gasp-worthy revelations, but its most dramatic moment was the entrance of E. M. K. Geiling. Strutting to the stand in a jacket and tie, Geiling carried two suitcases. "I have brought my authorities," he announced in his South African accent, producing paperwork to show the "total nonsense" of the balm's claims. After decades of government trials mired in "he said, she said" disputes, Geiling had brought a new gold standard to the courtroom: a scientific discussion of how medicine acted on the body. This time, the jury sided with the FDA.

In 1936, Geiling joined the faculty of the University of Chicago, determined to find a methodical way to discuss *how* drugs behaved in the human body. He wanted animal studies to guide medical practice. If you could see how a drug operated inside a rabbit or chicken, for example, it could inform how the substance was tested and used in humans. He mapped out a fledgling interdisciplinary field called clinical pharmacology.

As he set up his lab on the sun-drenched fifth floor of the biochemistry building, he posted notices around the medical school, hoping to lure medical students. But even basic pharmacology was a nascent field in the 1930s, a specialty shadowing the developing drug industry. Initially, Geiling had no takers. So for the time being, the hardy young woman from Canada was his sole research assistant.

Frances, knowing Geiling doubted her abilities, worked feverishly to prove him wrong. Geiling had recently determined that in whales, porpoises, seals, and armadillos, the anterior and posterior lobes of the pituitary gland were entirely separated, allowing for isolated study of each lobe. Frances commenced research on the posterior pituitary gland of the nine-banded armadillo, and when the new university quarter began, she enrolled as his first PhD student.

But Frances never lost the urge to roam and explore. She traveled to a Texas farm to catch her armadillo specimens among the yucca and prickly pear. In the summer, she signed on for Geiling's Kunghit Island expedition to collect massive whale pituitaries. She spent days gathering specimens at the whaling station, wandering the butchering sheds and carcass platform, where Japanese workers flensed blubber from whales like banana peels. At night, she dined in the bunkhouse, where the cook served visitors whale meat. Frances thought it tasted like steak.

Having grown up by the water, Frances yearned to join the Norwegian crews who set out daily on ninety-foot boats to harpoon whales—blue whales, right whales, sperm whales, fin whales, and humpbacks. But every excuse was given to keep her on land: It was a bad day; the seas were rough. The Norwegians, it turned out, thought women at sea brought bad luck. But she prodded the son of the station manager and he finally snuck her out. Not only did Frances spot a whale and direct the boat's harpooner, but she was the sole scientist on the entire island to survive an expedition without vomiting.

When one summer Geiling wanted lingcod tissue (thought to produce insulin), Frances pulled on her waders and, for months, thudded across the decks of Japanese commercial fishing boats, sorting the oozing entrails of hundreds of massive lingcods. At the summer's end, she returned to the lab with an impressive collection of bottles full of tissue. She resumed her research that fall, but in October, Geiling halted all work in his lab. He had received an urgent call from the American Medical Association, a pharmaceutical watchdog group, about a slew of deaths linked to a new liquid medicine: Elixir Sulfanilamide.

Inspired by powdered sulfanilamide, a drug used to treat infections during World War I, a Tennessee-based drug company named Massengill had decided that a liquid version might sell well—especially for children. Massengill's chemist whipped up a mixture of sulfanilamide, water, and diethylene glycol—a component of antifreeze. He added pink raspberry extract for color and saccharin and caramel for sweetness, and by September 1937, the company had distributed 240 gallons of its elixir nationwide, recommending it for everything from gonorrhea to sore throats. Within a month, seventy-one adults and thirty-four children were dead.

After Geiling's powerful testimony at the B&M trial, he had joined the

American Medical Association's Council on Drugs. The AMA now begged him to figure out why, exactly, the elixir was lethal. Frances, who had at last earned her stripes in the lab, was appointed to his investigative team. She recalled:

> Dr. Geiling immediately set up animal studies for acute and chronic toxicity. . . . My particular task was to watch the rats. . . . In no time at all, it was perfectly apparent that it was the diethylene glycol that was at fault. . . . The rats soon died, just as the kids did.

Antifreeze was the culprit, and in an unprecedented nationwide effort, the AMA and FDA fanned out across the country to seize all elixir shipments.

Massengill, it turned out, had never run animal tests on its liquid concoction. Nonetheless, according to the Food and Drug Act of 1906, Massengill had fulfilled its legal duty by listing the product's ingredients. The fact that no one—not even the Massengill chemist—grasped the danger of drinking antifreeze was a legally pardonable "whoops." Only a minor technicality rendered Massengill culpable: The word "elixir" was reserved for drugs containing ethanol. For this linguistic misstep, Massengill was fined.

Presaging the defense of almost every drug firm in every subsequent pharmaceutical disaster, Massengill's owner, Samuel Evans Massengill, insisted that the company "not once could have foreseen the unlooked-for results." How could you be blamed for overlooking a danger you hadn't even imagined? Massengill's owner was adamant that he did not feel "any responsibility on our part."

The firm's chemist, otherwise inclined, committed suicide before trial.

The fatalities caused by liquid sulfanilamide proved a legislative tipping point. For five years, a bill had been kicking around Congress to remedy gaps in the 1906 law. On the heels of a 1933 book called *100,000,000 Guinea Pigs: Dangers in Everyday Foods, Drugs, and Cosmetics*, Senator Royal S. Copeland of New York, a former doctor and health commissioner, had introduced a measure to prohibit misleading advertising and grant the FDA greater regulatory powers. In support, the FDA assembled an exhibit of posters and dioramas to showcase the greatest hits of dangerous quackery—a young woman blinded by eyelash dye, three Rhode Island sisters dead from using B&M Balm, and, of course, the steel magnate whose skull was eaten away by Radithor. Many people, including Eleanor Roosevelt, recoiled at this "Chamber of Horrors," but Copeland couldn't rally Congress. The press—whose relentless muckraking exposés had helped Wiley stir public support for the original 1906 bill—now depended heavily on drug advertising income and stayed mute. Everyone knew murky medicine was being sold; no one was ready to act.

But Massengill's legal pardon for the deaths of so many children outraged the nation. A grieving mother's letter to President Franklin D. Roosevelt, which ran in newspapers, prompted action.

> All that is left to us is the caring for her little grave. Even the memory of her is mixed with sorrow for we can see her little body tossing to and fro and hear that little voice screaming with pain. . . . It is my plea that you will take steps to prevent such sales of drugs that will take little lives and leave such suffering behind.

Roosevelt—long a supporter of the Copeland bill—complied, and E. M. K. Geiling was once again summoned, this time to map out the standards needed in the new law to ensure the safety of drugs. Among other things, Geiling suggested that companies be required to submit animal safety data to the FDA before marketing products, essentially necessitating FDA "approval" to sell a drug.

The 1938 Food, Drug, and Cosmetic Act, signed by President Roosevelt on June 25, marked the nation's biggest overhaul of drug regulations since 1906—and Geiling's upstart Chicago pharmacology lab, including his protégé, Frankie Oldham, had been at the center.

At age twenty-four, she became Dr. Oldham—she would henceforth shed "Frankie" and ask to regularly be addressed as "Doctor"—the University of Chicago's first PhD in pharmacology. Not only had she knuckled down to investigate a national drug disaster, but she had also watched the U.S. government strike a legislative blow against a powerful industry. And yet it was an industry that, on the eve of World War II, was about to become exponentially more formidable.

1. The voluntary consent of the human subject is absolutely essential.

—Nuremberg Code (1947),
"Permissible Medical Experiments"

Two

There are essentially two eras in medicine—nature made and lab made. Most of human history existed in the former, in which "medicine" or "drugs" referred to mortar-and-pestle concoctions of herbs, fruits, vines, and fungi. Neanderthals used poplar to ease tooth abscesses. Antibiotic-producing molds served as their primal Pepto Bismol. The Kahun Papyrus of approximately 1850 B.C., one of the oldest records of human medicine, details a variety of vaginal pastes and potions made of milk, oil, dates, herbs, and beer. The 108-page Ebers Papyrus describes remedies for stiffened limbs, eye diseases, fractures, burns, worms, gangrene, dropsy, and liver disease about three hundred years later. Among the hundreds of treatments, willow bark (aspirin's precursor) is suggested for pain relief. Shamans, healers, medicine men, and medicine women plied this trade. And eventually apothecary shops formalized the business, bottling potions, sticking on labels. But these storefronts still peddled backyard brews; the apothecary practiced something akin to "mixology"—not chemistry.

In 1832, a visionary German, Justus von Liebig, upended that. Liebig, arguably the grandfather of modern pharmaceuticals, was born in 1803 in the town of Darmstadt. The son of a chemical manufacturer who compounded paints, varnishes, and pigments, Liebig tinkered in his father's workshop and eventually apprenticed under a local apothecary. Justus formalized his training with a chemistry degree from the Prussian University of Bonn—the preeminent chemistry program in Europe—and a doctorate from the University of Erlangen in Bavaria.

He eventually secured a post as a professor at the University of Giessen, but Liebig was more scientific visionary than academic. Everywhere he looked, he imagined how chemicals might be put to new use, and he liked working in a laboratory with an array of unexplored materials. Discovering that nitrogen and trace minerals were key plant nutrients, Liebig kick-started the fertilizer industry. His beef extract spawned Liebig's Extract of Meat Company. From seaweed and fungi, he isolated liquid chloroform (think kidnappers and white cloth), a general anesthetic integral to nineteenth-century medicine.

But Liebig's crowning accomplishment was chloral hydrate. In 1832, he poured ethanol (grain alcohol) into a flask with sulfuric acid and bubbled pungent green chlorine gas through the solution; this somehow exchanged the atoms in the chlorine and ethanol molecules, creating white crystals, which Liebig initially called "chloral"—an amalgamation of "chlor" and "alcohol." Neither ethanol nor chlorine on its own had any medicinal application, but Liebig's new white crystals—$C_2H_3Cl_3O_2$—were eventually found to depress the nervous system. His new molecule marked a dramatic departure from previous medicine. Man made and lab made, chloral hydrate became the world's first synthetic drug.

Within thirty years, chloral hydrate (a powder that you could swallow rather than inject) came to trump morphine as the go-to sedative in asylums and posh households. Because molecular creations could be patented, an inventor stood to reap all profits. Two existing industries rushed to cash in on this new lucrative venture.

Apothecaries, long in the business of peddling opium-laced syrups with names like "Hoopers Anodyne, the Infant's Friend," pivoted to synthetic drugs. Merck, an apothecary in Liebig's hometown, became the world's first pharmaceutical firm in 1890, followed by Hoffmann–La Roche in Switzerland; Burroughs Wellcome in England; Poulenc Frères in France; and Smith, Kline & French in Philadelphia.

European textile manufacturers also seized the moment. These firms, already extracting chemicals from coal tar to produce synthetic dyes, had the framework for research and manufacture. After Liebig's success with chloral hydrate, these companies pored over their sticky dye by-products to see which atoms might be retooled as the next wonder drug.

This was the Bayer story. In 1887, the German dye company invented the fever and pain reliever Phenacetin, followed a decade later by acetylsalicylic acid—a one-size-fits-all tablet for aches, pains, and fevers. Branded as "Aspirin," it became the world's first blockbuster drug. Next, the firm introduced a new class of drugs made from barbituric acid: barbiturates. Rather than targeting physical pain alone, these drugs also aimed to ease *mental* anguish. Veronal (barbital) in 1903 was followed nine years later by the more potent Luminal (phenobarbital). Popular as sleep aids, anesthetics, and anticonvulsants, barbiturates became immensely popular as daily mood remedies.

Soon opioids—cheap, synthetic versions of morphine and codeine—hit the market: oxycodone (1917), hydrocodone (1924), pethidine (1939), and methadone (1939). And as molecular tinkering was perfected, drugs with tailor-made applications emerged. In 1939, Parke-Davis's Dilantin became the first successful nonbarbiturate epilepsy treatment.

By World War II, pharmaceuticals—both nature made and lab made—emerged as chief military assets. In the Pacific campaign, forces with Atabrine and quinine had the edge in curing malaria-ravaged soldiers. To prepare for the invasion of Normandy, the U.S. government underwrote private-sector production of sulfa and penicillin to treat wounded soldiers. Synthetic feel-good drugs, too, found combat uses: Before suicide missions, Japanese kamikaze pilots received injections of methamphetamines. Allied soldiers popped Benzedrine to stave off fatigue. Field hospitals fed barbiturates to shell-shocked soldiers. Wehrmacht troops fortified themselves with *Stuka-Tablette*—a methamphetamine—before the blitzkrieg in France. And Hitler himself, a pharmaceutical connoisseur, received some eight hundred drug injections throughout the war, including frequent shots of oxycodone. When Luminal—one of the newer barbiturates—proved toxic in large doses, it became Hitler's chosen method for mass euthanasia.

The war's acceleration of pharmaceutical production meant that when the Axis powers fell, American drug firms were poised to expand. In addition, the Allies sent military-civilian T-Force teams behind invading troops, storming German factories, laboratories, and libraries to confiscate military, scientific, and industrial records. In one instance, two Allied soldiers located a concrete dugout in the mountains marked "Achtung! Minen!" After a coin toss, the loser hitched the jeep to the dugout door, held his breath, and stepped on the gas. There was no explosion. Instead, the door tore loose to reveal a 1,600-foot-deep mine shaft, at the bottom of which, beneath cylinders of liquid oxygen, lay the entire cache of German patent records.

At the end of World War I, the Treaty of Versailles had forced Germany to surrender intellectual assets such as Bayer's American trademark registration for "Aspirin" (which is why Duane Reade and CVS can sell their own "aspirin"). The 1917 Trading with the Enemy Act had even allowed the U.S. government to seize German chemical patents to relicense cheaply to American firms. But the Second World War's pillaging occurred absent a treaty or congressional act or public discussion.

The biggest postwar windfall came from IG Farben, a conglomerate of six German firms, including Bayer, which had ranked for decades as the world's largest chemical and pharmaceutical firm. The Farben spoils had everything: instructions for making solid fuels, synthetic rubber, textiles, chemicals, plastics, drugs, and over fifty thousand dyes. The pharmaceutical records held exceptional value; as the fertile crescent of modern pharmaceuticals, Germany's chemical output had dwarfed those of all other nations for over a century. The total value of the plunder of its postwar intellectual property was estimated to be in the billions of dollars. On August 25, 1945, President Harry S. Truman quietly decreed Germany's one million proprietary documents available to American firms. Germany bemoaned these reparations, but American compassion for the largest company, IG Farben, dwindled, especially as details of its wartime misdeeds came to light.

On May 3, 1947, the United States indicted twenty-four directors of IG Farben for war crimes. Not only had IG Farben been the chief donor to Hitler's election campaign, but it had also built the Auschwitz-Monowitz chemical factory, where at least thirty thousand prisoners had died. It held a significant stake in Degesch, which had made the infamous Zyklon B gas used to exterminate over one million prisoners.

U.S.A. v. Carl Krauch et al. was the sixth of the thirteen famous Nuremberg trials. Among the defendants was senior IG Farben researcher Dr. Otto Ambros. The charismatic and dapper Ambros had been Hitler's adviser and chief chemical weapons engineer. (The *a* in "sarin"—a toxic nerve gas developed by the Nazis—is for "Ambros.") In addition to helping establish the Auschwitz-Monowitz plant, he had set up a forced labor camp at Dyhernfurth to produce nerve gas. At Auschwitz, he allegedly arranged experiments on prisoners with Bayer chemicals and poisons. The camps offered Bayer an unlimited supply of human test subjects.

Correspondence between the Auschwitz camp commander and Bayer headquarters showed a request for women to test a "new sleep-inducing drug":

Please prepare for us 150 women in the best health possible.

Received the order for 150 women. Despite their macerated condition they were considered satisfactory. We will keep you informed of the developments regarding the experiments.

All 150 women died.

Another 200 women with strep throat were injected—via their lungs—with a Bayer antibacterial. It killed every one of them, slowly and painfully. A Ukrainian girl at Auschwitz would later recall how for three years a Nazi doctor frequently had her bound naked to a bed while pills from bottles marked "Bayer" were shoved down her throat. At the war's end, she discovered she was sterile.

Ambros and the other Farben executives on trial claimed they had merely served as middle management, overseeing paperwork, unaware of what was happening at the camps. "I am only a chemist," Ambros protested. Though named as a manager on projects that killed tens of thousands, he dismissed his title as "honorary." But Nuremberg prosecutor Telford Taylor saw unique peril in these white-collar medical masterminds—and unique guilt. "These IG Farben criminals, not the lunatic Nazi fanatics," he said, "are the main war criminals." After all, Farben had given the Nazis Zyklon B and Luminal—sanitized methods to kill millions. These executives killed from afar, in masses, protected by a veneer of professionalism. What would happen if they were allowed to go out in the world and resume their careers?

"If the guilt of these criminals is not brought to light and if they are not punished," Taylor's team worried, "they will represent a much greater threat to the future peace of the world than Hitler if he were still alive."

On July 30, 1948, thirteen defendants received prison terms of up to eight years for their "disregard of basic human rights." The longest sentence was reserved for Ambros. By 1951, IG Farben, felled by the verdicts, collapsed into pieces. Since the Allied patent plunder had decimated most other German drug giants, there was, suddenly, an unexpected opening for industry newcomers.

Two brothers, ardent Nazi enthusiasts and owners of a small soap firm called Dalli-Werke, Mäurer & Wirtz, launched a drug branch to capitalize on the recent surfeit of unemployed Nazi researchers. They called the subsidiary Chemie Grünenthal and eventually hired Otto Ambros to lead their advisory committee.

The quaint town of Stolberg sits in the hills of Germany near the Belgian border. Once a vital mecca of brass production, by the midnineteenth century the town's manufacturers had diversified into glass, textiles, and haberdashery.

In 1845, however, Michael Mäurer and his stepson Andreas August Wirtz built a factory in Stolberg to fashion soaps from animal fats. The products soon appeared in shops throughout Germany and neighboring countries, and by the turn of the century, Mäurer & Wirtz—prestigious and profitable—began trademarking its items.

World War II was good for the company, which was run by Andreas's grandsons, Hermann and Alfred Wirtz. The Wirtz brothers were Nazi Party members, and an Aryanization program reportedly let them commandeer two Jewish-owned firms—Doering Werke in Berlin and Riva in Vienna—to expand their operations, and they were granted several hundred slave laborers.

But at the war's end, Nazi subsidies vanished, the country was occupied, cities had been leveled, and food was scarce. The brothers sought new revenue streams. According to company lore, during bombing raids at the war's end, the soap factory manager, a Belgian named Jakob Chauvristé, had taken shelter with a pharmacist who anticipated massive postwar demand for antibiotics—which were cheap to make and highly profitable. Thus in 1946, Alfred and Hermann designated an abandoned eighteenth-century copper foundry in Stolberg as the headquarters of their start-up drug firm. Glistening ivy climbed the three-story stone building topped with onion-domed roofs. White-trimmed windows overlooked a rhododendron-filled courtyard. For its fairy-tale surroundings, the brothers named the company Grünenthal—"Green Valley."

On December 23, 1946, Chauvristé and Hermann Wirtz officially registered as the firm's directors. Since no one running the company had any training in pharmacology or medicine, they quickly hired a chief scientific officer: thirty-two-year-old Heinrich Mückter. Though he was only partway through his pharmacology degree, Mückter had made a name for himself during the war as a Wehrmacht medical officer researching typhus. To study vaccines, he had arranged for typhus to be injected into prisoners at Auschwitz and Buchenwald. His research killed hundreds, and after the war, as Polish authorities pursued him, he fled to Germany and enrolled in the University of Bonn, where Grünenthal recruited him. Mückter, known to be arrogant and self-important, would become the chief villain in the thalidomide story.

The fledgling drug company offered many other former SS officers professional sanctuary. Martin Staemmler, a "racial hygiene" advocate who had helped forge Nazi population-control policy, became head of pathology. A former SS nutrition inspector, Dr. Ernst-Günther Schenck, also joined the firm—a choice opportunity since he had been barred from practicing medicine in Germany, on account of killing hundreds of prisoners with "protein sausage" experiments. In 1956, the firm would also hire Heinz Baumkötter, former chief medical officer of the Sachsenhausen camp. Released early despite a life sentence from a Soviet military tribunal, he would again be found guilty of mass murder by a West German court. His time served in the USSR, however, negated the sentence, so, twice convicted of murder, Baumkötter traveled around Germany selling Grünenthal products.

The crowning act of Grünenthal's SS revival was the hire of Otto Ambros. Released early from his Nuremberg sentence, Ambros was eventually granted a plum seat on Chemie Grünenthal's board of directors.

Grünenthal made its first foray into pharmaceuticals with antibiotics, a decision described in official company history as a humanitarian gesture: Since the Aachen border region was "completely cut off from any supply of medicines," the firm purportedly wanted to help. These first products were American antibiotics, manufactured under license, which meant royalties were paid to the American creators and profits were limited. The big money would come from *inventing* drugs, but competition with uni-

versities and international pharmaceutical firms was fierce. And Mückter
was assisted by an even less experienced pharmacist, Wilhelm Kunz.

Nonetheless, the duo rapidly created two new antibiotics: xanthocillin
and tyrothricin. So wildly serendipitous were these discoveries that they
verged on unbelievable. (When it emerged years later that Mückter hadn't
filed patents for either, some would accuse Grünenthal of simply bringing
to market wartime inventions that had escaped the Allied plunder.)

By 1948, Grünenthal was selling its own antibiotics and the firm's investment grew sixfold. Next, the firm added a Danish antibiotic named
Pulmo 500 to its product line. The drug—used to treat meningitis and
pneumonia—sold well in Germany, but by 1954, German physicians had
begun reporting severe reactions to the product; it was also killing people
over a hundred times more often than basic penicillin. Doctors prescribing the drug suspected that Grünenthal had cut corners; safety research
was missing. The drug had been "used in man," they claimed, "before
thorough experiments on animals had been published." Three West German scientists went so far as to accuse Grünenthal of negligence. But Grünenthal continued to sell the drug with no warning to doctors.

Antibiotics were a competitive international market, however. Large
British and American firms churned out the products quickly and cheaply.
Revenues stalling, Grünenthal needed a new molecule it could license to
overseas firms.

In the spring of 1954, Mückter directed his researchers to begin tinkering in search of a diuretic for obesity. He told Kunz to create peptides
(small protein-like molecules) from carbon-based compounds (organic,
living things) and study the by-products. It was a broad directive for the
unskilled pharmacist. But Kunz was now overseen by an actual pharmacologist, Herbert Keller from the University of Bonn, who quickly fixated
on one of Kunz's creations: a white, tasteless molecule, phthalimodoglutarimide. The substance showed no diuretic potential—instead, it bore a
strong structural resemblance to barbiturates—formally known as gluteth-
imides. This was exciting. Hypnotics and sedatives, first introduced in asylums to treat psychiatric and neurological disorders, had recently found
broad appeal in the general population. Everyone seemed to want help
relaxing and going to sleep, and barbiturates, a soaring drug class, were
fattening the coffers of pharmaceutical firms. Mückter, whose contract

with Grünenthal granted him a bonus of 1 percent of the profits on any discovery, directed Kunz and Keller to concentrate on the white powder, K-17 (Kunz's seventeenth by-product). (Its formal laboratory name, phthalimodoglutarimide, would eventually be shortened to the more pronounceable "thalidomide.")

Traditionally, the first lab experiment to test a compound's sedative-hypnotic properties was to give some to a rat, then tip over the drugged rat to see if it could right itself. Hypnotics muddle an animal's "righting reflex." But there is no record of Grünenthal conducting this test. (Interestingly, thalidomide doesn't compromise the righting reflex.) The company instead fast-tracked to a more complex experiment: It put rats on a treadmill. A normal hypnotic will slow a rat's speed—generally in proportion to dosage. Here, thalidomide failed.

Many researchers would have given up. The firm's new molecule resembled a barbiturate but didn't seem to act as one—a chemical sibling with a dramatically different personality. Also, the thalidomide molecule, unlike known sedatives, was asymmetrical, which meant it might behave in different ways in different configurations. Yet Mückter pressed on. This molecule seemed the firm's moon shot. But to market thalidomide as a hypnotic, Mückter would have to ditch the premise that "sleep is distinguished by loss of co-coordination capacity." He would have to redefine sleep and devise an unprecedented lab experiment.

The "jiggle cage" was elaborate: The contraption consisted of a cage, levers, a bath of sulfuric acid, platinum wires, and a device to measure the release of hydrogen gas. When the mice jiggled, the wires plunged into the acid bath and electrolyzed the water to release hydrogen. When Grünenthal's researchers gave mice thalidomide, they noted a 50 percent reduction in hydrogen gas production, meaning less jiggling. The mice were not asleep, but the firm *interpreted* this as sleep and anointed the drug hypnotic.

There was good reason to want the new substance to qualify as a hypnotic. Barbiturates all suffered one fatal flaw—too much could kill you. Experiments with thalidomide, however, showed that *no* amount would kill a lab mouse. A non-lethal hypnotic could easily become a blockbuster.

Between May of 1954 and May of 1955, Kunz and Keller raced to file five patents for thalidomide and thalidomide-related substances. The paperwork covered every possible production process—the German patents listed seven methods, and subsequent overseas filings in the United States, the UK, Switzerland, and France noted an additional six. But in the haste of patent filing, the actual product created by these six methods underwent no animal safety tests. And of the original five production processes in the German patents, only one generated the drug the firm would eventually sell—and that version had not been used to prove thalidomide's safety. In fact, no paperwork from Grünenthal's initial animal safety testing of the drug would survive. A decade later, when German authorities demanded to see the drug's experimental data, Grünenthal would claim the paperwork had been lost in a company move.

In time, even Grünenthal's "discovery" of thalidomide would come under scrutiny. The U.S. and UK patents filed in the spring of 1955 mysteriously describe the drug's sedative effects in *humans*—before any human trials were recorded:

> The products of the invention possess valuable therapeutic properties. They cause a strongly pronounced lowering of the motility, i.e., the phenomenon of motion, and have a very low toxicity. They may generally be employed for "central attenuation" (vegetative dystonia). The products of the invention do not have any peripherally paralyzing curare-like effects.
>
> In addition, the compounds have certain spasmolytic and antihistamine effects. Dispensed in larger quantities, the products of the invention and particularly 3-phthalimido-2, 6-dioxopiperidine [i.e., pure thalidomide] are effective as soporifics.

How could the firm detail how the drug acted in people in early 1955, when Grünenthal had barely completed a few mice studies? Where had this clinical data come from? Had humans been given the drug before long-term animal safety tests were completed? For decades, this question would haunt the company: How had Mückter's team known—in the face of the drug's failure to sedate mice—that it would sedate *humans*? Did someone at the firm have previous experience with the substance? Given Grünenthal's ties with SS doctors, had thalidomide been tested in the camps?

The company's official human trials—for which it reported paperwork— began in the spring of 1955. Grünenthal sent the drug to nine German physicians ostensibly to gather clinical data. This did not go well. On December 16, 1955, the investigating doctors—an array of dermatologists, psychiatrists, and neurologists—reported their results to Grünenthal at a symposium.

Four doctors liked the drug, but their methodology was shoddy. Dr. Herman Jung had used thalidomide at his Cologne clinic on only twenty patients for a mere four weeks and was on a retainer from Grünenthal, paid two hundred deutsche marks per month. Jung seemed dazzled by his rapid results—four male youths had overcome the urge to masturbate, and several married men, to the delight of their wives, ceased ejaculating prematurely. The drug had "no undesirable side effect," Jung declared, predicting it would be a moneymaker. Dr. Heinz Esser of Düsseldorf, who tested it on 350 patients, likewise praised the sedative. But Esser had tested it for only twelve weeks, and when he later noted side effects of dizziness, shivering, and ear buzzing, he ceased prescribing the drug. The other two positive reports at the symposium also stemmed from rushed or poorly documented trials. One doctor had used the drug on patients with brain injuries and described thalidomide's effects—high praise, it seems—as comparable to a lobotomy.

Of the remaining five doctors, four had mixed feelings. Dr. Karl Vorlaender of Münster had noted nausea, giddiness, and wakefulness in his patients. Plus, addiction after three weeks. But when he asked Grünenthal for more time to run a longer, larger trial, Grünenthal refused. Dr. Gerhard Kloos in Göttingen didn't need more time. Three of his colleagues had tried the pills themselves and wound up nauseated and dizzy. He loathed the drug.

Most important, not a single doctor had gathered data on long-term human use. Also lacking at the symposium was any discussion of how thalidomide was absorbed, metabolized, or excreted. No one seemed to know what the drug did inside the human body. Grünenthal's managing director, Chauvristé, acknowledged that more work was needed before thalidomide went to market. So the company sent the drug to another round of physicians—with even worse results.

Three Berlin-based doctors relayed serious concerns. Dr. Ferdinand

Piacenza observed side effects so worrisome—a full body rash in all his patients and "paresthesia" in one participant after small doses—that he stopped his trial. On March 25, 1956, Piacenza wrote to Mückter of thalidomide's "absolute intolerability" in humans. Mückter feigned astonishment: "We have never had such a negative report as yours," he wrote back, explaining that the company had been testing thalidomide in clinics and sanatoriums for about two years (indicating that Grünenthal unofficially began human testing in 1954, before long-term animal experiments were complete). Mückter dismissed Piacenza's concerns, suggesting that he had likely administered improperly high doses. "K17 is such a strong sedative," Mückter cautioned, "that in general small doses are sufficient."

The year 1956 would also mark the emergence of a more pronounced side effect. In December, a baby girl was born to the wife of a Chemie Grünenthal employee in Aachen, near Stolberg. Months earlier, the man had eagerly brought home samples of his firm's new wonder sedative for his pregnant wife. On Christmas Day, their daughter was born without ears.

The better known thalidomide becomes, the more people ask questions. Mostly they ask about its metabolism and breakdown in the body. This also interests Merrell in the USA. Unfortunately we have practically nothing on this.

—Chemie Grünenthal memo,

March 1960

Three

In 1940, the broad-shouldered, twenty-eight-year-old Fremont Ellis Kelsey arrived at Geiling's University of Chicago lab as an instructor of pharmacology and researcher. The six-foot-tall biochemist—who went by "Kelse"—was a scientific prodigy with a wild side. In high school he boasted a reputation as a truant, and in college he'd mysteriously vanished "somewhere north" for two years to manage a band.

Fun-loving and laid-back, Kelse entered rooms with boisterous thunder. An outspoken idealist who loathed pretense or hypocrisy, Kelse was the sole child of a Pennsylvania master bricklayer. His mother, who worked the soda fountain at Kresge's department store and catered church weddings, was deemed "coarse" by some and "confident" by others. This direct, jolly woman had shaped Ellis's gender expectations. He liked his women strong.

Fortunately, Frances was still working as a research associate in Geiling's lab. In the four years since her arrival, the pharmacology department had seen an influx of new students and researchers. Frances, however, remained the sole woman. She spent long hours on her lab stool, but in her free time, she played field hockey on the university commons and at night, in her dorm room, devoured the great tomes of literature: *Travels in Arabia Deserta, Man and the State, The History of British Civilization, Seven Pillars of Wisdom, Woodrow Wilson: Life & Letters*. Always meticulous, she kept a detailed reading log. In the evenings, she eagerly went to see theater.

In the lab, Frances and Kelse spent days researching side by side, and Ellis—with his loud voice and charming laugh—soon grew fascinated by

the no-nonsense twenty-six-year-old. She sat working all day at her micro-
scope with bobby-pinned chestnut hair. After several months, he mustered
the courage to invite the elusive "Dr. Oldham" to the Civic Opera, where
Frances sat transfixed by the performance—until she suddenly checked
her watch and excused herself. Returning with her bulging purse mysteriously clutched to her chest, Frances matter-of-factly told Kelse that she
had just peed into a jar for a pharmacology department experiment. Kelse,
warm but direct, was not a man who ruffled easily: In a gesture foreshad-
owing a lifetime of devotion, he offered to hold Frances's jar of urine for
the night.

The war abroad reshaped Chicago as the city's industries churned out
billions in munitions. After Pearl Harbor, Geiling's lab pivoted to government work, and at the request of the National Defense Research Committee, Geiling helmed a Toxicity Laboratory to study chemical warfare
agents. Several small buildings between Fifty-seventh and Fifty-eighth
streets hosted the top-secret project, where sixty researchers evaluated
more than two thousand chemicals. Frances, as a woman, was banned
from the research.

She was, however, included in another wartime project—the search
for a new antimalarial. As malaria felled troops worldwide, supplies of quinine, the traditional remedy, had plunged. American drug firms, chemists,
and pharmacists had been summoned to scour shelves for any potential
alternate treatment, and soon thousands of "vials" arrived at Geiling's lab.
Even basement and backyard tinkerers submitted candidates: Dried fish
soaked in milk. An ink bottle full of a strange, dark liquid from a veterinar-
ian who bragged that he'd successfully tested the substance—first on his
secretary, then on his cattle.

Geiling's lab fed the chemicals first to chickens and ducks, and anything promising was then given to rats, dogs, and monkeys. Frances rel-
ished the research—a chance to probe the metabolic process of drugs.
One study, in particular, fascinated her: While she and Ellis were testing
how rabbits broke down quinine in their livers, the duo discovered that
pregnant rabbits had difficulty processing quinine. And embryonic rabbits
totally failed to metabolize the drug. While embryology was still a young

field—it would be a decade before ultrasounds revealed the developmental chronology of a human fetus—by the 1930s the embryo was understood as a separate, independent creature from the mother. Their Chicago quinine experiment advanced the field, showing that embryos, with their less-developed enzyme systems, could react to a drug quite differently from their mothers. Frances and Ellis, who kept their romance under wraps, co-authored the lab's noteworthy paper.

But this research didn't quite satisfy Frances's itch to get in on the war action. Still banned from the toxicity lab, Frances penned a frustrated letter to a childhood friend, Roger Stanier, asking about her chances of getting a job in gas warfare research in Canada, where he was working. "I don't think a woman would have much of a chance," Roger confessed. "Canadians are so damned prejudiced about women scientists that even Marie Curie would never have risen above a lab."

Roger and Frances had by that point been corresponding for months, and eventually Roger—who knew nothing of Frances's relationship with Ellis—proposed, on paper. "I'm very fond of you," he wrote in July of 1943, "and think we could get along quite well together."

Frances went about her lab work distracted and unhappy for weeks—confusing colleagues, especially Ellis. And when she returned to Canada for her annual summer vacation, Kelse wrote affectionately, and a little urgently. By the time Frances returned to Chicago, Kelse—who sensed another man in the picture—also proposed. Frances immediately accepted, and their surprised lab mates rejoiced.

On a drizzly Monday in December 1943, at Chicago's Church of the Redeemer, Frances Kathleen Oldham married Fremont Ellis Kelsey. Geiling hosted a reception at his lavish home for a group that included Ellis's mother and Frances's sister and parents. The couple soon set up house on South Maryland Avenue. With university colleagues, they now owned a thirty-nine-foot gaff-rigged yawl called *The Owl*, and Frances loved the chance to get out on the water. The newlyweds now worked, lived, and sailed together.

As the war escalated, the government ramped up its antimalarial project. Geiling's team was directed at last to test quinine substitutes in people. The question was—which people?

In 1944, no protocol existed to recruit human subjects for drug experiments. But a controlled setting was ideal, and the government thought a prison might do. The University of Chicago was contracted to enlist inmates at nearby Stateville Penitentiary in Joliet, Illinois. An initial call for 200 prisoners to assist the war effort yielded 487 volunteers, with the inmates not only serving as research subjects (exposed to malaria via mosquitoes, then given treatments) but also conducting lab work and reporting their results.

Geiling forbade Frances from entering the penitentiary, but Ellis protested and drove her to the prison himself. At long last, Frances got her wished-for excitement, especially when she met Nathan Leopold, half of the infamous Leopold and Loeb murderer duo. Leopold, who had volunteered as a subject, impressed Frances with his industriousness—he organized classes for non-English-speaking inmates and oversaw the prison laboratory.

But Frances's work at Stateville was cut short when her father fell ill in the summer of 1944. Returning to Canada for several months (Ellis ceded her his vacation days), she left a lovesick Ellis to pen daily letters:

> I forgot to tell you I love you. I love you. I love you very much. I love you very very much. I love you too goddamned much . . . E

> I don't understand such an empty feeling or being quite so lonesome—after all I got on well for 30 years.

Frances wrote less frequently, less effusively—and Kelse complained of staring into an empty mailbox. Keen on starting a family, Kelse wanted her back. "Remember the offspring we must get ordered this winter . . . ," he nudged. When she returned in October, the couple playfully used code words to track her ovulation, but their attempts at conception failed.

They were further frustrated when Frances, who had just been promoted to associate professor of pharmacology, had to surrender her post. The war had popularized pharmacology. With troops returning to reclaim jobs, the University of Chicago invoked an old antinepotism rule forbidding husbands and wives from working in the same department. Even though Frances and Kelse had been married three years, one of them now had to quit. Frances—knowing that as a woman she'd need more credentials than Ellis to run the professional gauntlet ahead—said goodbye to Geiling's lab after almost a decade and enrolled in the University of Chicago Medical School. Midway through her degree, Frances, now thirty-three, entered Chicago's Lying-In Hospital and gave birth to her first daughter, Susan. Before graduating, she would give birth to a second girl, named Christine.

I was my mother's seventh child. She claims she knew

something was wrong before I was born, because she

didn't feel the kicks. Then I was born missing legs.

—*Eileen Cronin,*

born September 1960,

Cincinnati, Ohio

Four

It was the fall of 1960, and Frances was finally warming up to Washington, D.C. There was an energizing bustle to the city, and she wrote to friends of an "opulent" life in which she attended National Cathedral concerts. For a belated birthday celebration, Ellis and the girls took her to Harrison's Seafood—their new favorite haunt.

Frances even embraced her American citizenship, taking the family to a three-hour Democratic rally one Saturday. Later they all watched the first-ever televised debate, between presidential nominees Nixon and Kennedy.

Their two-story brick and white clapboard house was starting to feel cozy. Ellis had been sawing and hammering for weeks, building bookshelves for the living room, while Frances organized her backyard garden, where her beans, squash, and tomatoes miraculously survived the vigorous investigations of their dog, George. Frances and Ellis had even hosted a few dinner guests, including E. M. K. Geiling, who now lived and worked in D.C. as an official consultant for the FDA.

Work, however, was going less well.

The New Drug Application for Kevadon (thalidomide) irked Frances. The firm behind it—the William S. Merrell Company—was a Cincinnati-based subsidiary of Richardson-Merrell. The firm was no Merck or Pfizer, but it regularly ranked around number three hundred on *Fortune* magazine's list of the country's largest industrial companies. Merrell had a few successful drugs under its belt, notably a cholesterol pill, triparanol (MER/29), which had recently hit the market as the company's bestselling prescription product. As for thalidomide, Frances had data on her desk from Merrell as well as two overseas companies—Chemie Grünenthal and Distillers—that had been selling the sedative for several years.

And yet Frances found the documents . . . murky.

The law spelled out what Merrell had to show the FDA to put a product on the market. The requirements stemmed from the 1938 law E. M. K. Geiling had helped codify. Drug firms had to present (1) the drug's basic chemistry: purity assurances, shelf life and stability information, etc.; (2) the drug's pharmacology: this came from animal studies showing the drug's safety; and (3) clinical data from human trials, arranged by the drugmakers, in which outside physicians recorded their findings.

Part 1 of the application—the chemistry—worried Frances. She saw right away that thalidomide was asymmetrical. Thalidomide contained a "chiral" carbon—a carbon bonded to four different groups, in this case a hydrogen, a nitrogen, a carbonyl (a carbon double-bonded to an oxygen), and a methylene (a carbon bonded to two hydrogens). This configuration meant that the mirror image of a three-dimensional drawing of thalidomide was not a replica. Thalidomide could therefore exist in two forms—a right-handed and a left-handed configuration—each potentially behaving differently. Further, the actual drug manufactured would be a compounded mass of molecules, with any given dose theoretically having all right-handed molecules, all left-handed molecules, or a mixture.

A drug's action rarely differed wildly in different forms, but nothing in the Kevadon application even mentioned the molecule's asymmetry. Which form of the drug had been used in experiments? Had differing results been looked for?

At first glance, the animal data appeared more promising. All three companies—Merrell, Grünenthal, and Distillers—had tested the drug in mice, rats, and dogs for both forms of toxicity: acute (one dose will kill you) and chronic (long term). The conclusions looked good. At massive doses, rats were mildly slowed for about six hours but fine afterward. Dogs fed megadoses recovered from sluggishness within four hours. And mice administered high levels of the drug showed "no significant symptoms of toxicity or overt changes in behavior."

"In the various species of experimental animals," the brochure for doctors read, "it was not possible to determine an acute LD50 of Kevadon."

That was stunning. "LD50" referred to the lethal dose of any drug that would kill half (50 percent) of one's experimental animals. If *no* LD50 existed, thalidomide's unprecedented safety could render it a bestseller.

But as Frances studied the pages, she saw that the animal data came mostly from Germany. And what tripped her up was a set of Chemie Grünenthal data explaining a "jiggle cage." The drug didn't put animals to sleep. Instead, caged mice would "jiggle less" after being dosed with thalidomide. In twenty years as a pharmacologist, Frances had never heard of such an experiment. But its implication rattled her: If a drug that put humans to sleep didn't put animals to sleep, the drug might not be absorbed at all by animals. That could account for the lack of an LD50. More crucial: If humans were put to sleep by thalidomide, suggesting human bodies absorbed the compound, was the drug still safe?

Merrell's own animal data was sparse. The firm had not tested different doses for long periods. Instead, extremely high doses were given to verify that the drug couldn't kill an animal. But even those studies woefully lacked detail. Where was the weight and condition of each animal subject? The dates and dosages? Frances bristled when she saw that the animal data in the brochure for doctors contradicted what was presented in the application.

By far the worst, however, were the human studies.

Before receiving FDA approval, drug companies were allowed to run clinical trials. Merrell listed thirty-seven "investigators"—doctors who had started testing Kevadon a year earlier on 1,589 patients. But after poring over the four-tome NDA for weeks, Frances couldn't find data corresponding to these trials. Nothing detailed the experience of the human subjects. There were no patient reports to show what condition had been treated, or the drug's level of effectiveness. Nothing indicated the age or sex of the subjects. And where was the dosage, frequency of administration, duration of administration? What about results of clinical and laboratory examinations, or the description of any adverse effects? The omissions floored her.

The doctors' reports read, to Frances, like wildly enthusiastic testimonials from a bygone era, absent any scientific observation. Rather than presenting their own data, physicians referenced other doctors' findings, citing unpublished studies in a self-referential web. Merrell's investigators referenced Grünenthal's research from the 1950s to justify their own gusto. But could they read German?

Further, Frances found no explanation of how the drug behaved in the body or how the chemical was absorbed. This was the specialty she'd studied for years, the key tenet of clinical pharmacology—how drugs acted on the body.

And not a single double-blind placebo study had been conducted to prove the drug sedated humans. If the drug failed in its stated purpose, no side effect would be acceptable.

Yet none of the trial doctors seemed to have looked for side effects, certainly not long term—problems that fell under the umbrella of "chronic toxicity." Despite the thousand-plus patients using the drug, nothing suggested these subjects had been monitored. It was as if the doctors running the trials assumed the drug to be so harmless that they had decided to sidestep safety research.

This wasn't the first time Frances recoiled at shoddy "studies."

While in medical school, she had worked for *The Journal of the American Medical Association* (JAMA). From its bullpen-style Chicago office, she fielded pharmacological questions from doctors around the country, penned editorials, and helped decide which studies deserved publication. When she moved to South Dakota, she kept up the job, moonlighting "at large" after her long hours filling in for traveling doctors.

Frances loved the JAMA job, largely because her editorials and evaluations were unsigned, her womanhood thus a secret. Her ability, for once, went unquestioned.

Also, her JAMA writing was entirely her own. Frances had published dozens of scientific papers, but with the exception of her very first—"The Actions of the Preparations from the Posterior Lobe of the Pituitary Gland upon the Imbibition of Water by Frogs"—they had been co-authored. Her textbook, too, shared a credit with E. M. K. Geiling and Ellis. When the words were hers alone, she used them sharply:

> The objections raised by the authors of this letter are not only poorly presented but are carelessly documented. . . . In view of its many inaccuracies, publication of this letter is definitely not recommended.

This stridency might have surprised those who knew Frances casually. At a party, drink in hand, she was a fun-loving hostess. She could veer toward soft-spoken, understated, the fierceness of her mind masked by her subdued voice. It was Ellis, a burly six feet tall, who boomed opinions across rooms, quick to argue. Frances instead let her brown eyes drift away if she disapproved of a conversation, or simply refreshed her drink. Her wry smile suggested a private joke, not scorn. On the page, however, Frances ranted—particularly against sloppy science. The rigor required of her, as a woman, to get three advanced degrees had left her intolerant of anything but precision.

She churned out letters of correction, harping on errors, typos. So heavily referenced and footnoted were her own editorials that her boss, Austin Smith, pleaded with her to halve her citations. She had an opinion on her editor, too: She did not like him.

After long days diagnosing gout or tending rattlesnake bites, as Frances sat at her desk, fingers on her black Remington typewriter, she'd grown wary of Smith and the AMA. Something was amiss with the papers published in the journal. As industry profits soared, it seemed that drug research was getting progressively more rushed.

Frances sounded her first alarm in 1956, when she told Smith that Nepera Chemical was reprinting *JAMA* articles in its ads as promotional props. Worse, a recent spate of half-baked papers submitted to the journal seemed puppeteered by drug firms themselves. In October of 1957, Frances again noted the "aggressive selling" and "downright deception" in the industry. As a licensed physician, almost daily she received boxes of sample pills from drug firms, plus brass plaques or artwork. But her concerns fell on deaf ears.

The reason for Smith's ambivalence soon became clear. In 1958, after a decade as the editor of *JAMA*, Smith defected to Washington for a job with the Pharmaceutical Manufacturers Association (PMA)—the country's oldest drug industry lobby. The 140-company alliance, which sold over 90 percent of the country's drugs, had tapped Smith to be its first full-time, salaried president. The increasingly aggressive industry was recruiting its former overseers.

Even the FDA had cozied up to the industry. Shortly after Smith took the job, he presented an award to FDA commissioner George Larrick on behalf of the PMA for Larrick's "understanding of mutual problems." Where former commissioners had used the agency as an iron fist, Larrick treated it more like a velvet glove.

The commissioner—a short man with a fondness for bow ties—was an odd choice to oversee the country's most powerful sector. Born in Springfield, Ohio, George Larrick had once dreamed of being a medical doctor. But after two years at Wittenberg College and a single premed course at Ohio State, in 1923 he abandoned university life for a food inspector job at the Bureau of Chemistry—the small basement division of the Department of Agriculture that would later become the FDA. As he advanced from senior food and drug inspector to chief inspector, he even played a hand, at age thirty-six, in the Elixir Sulfanilamide recall.

By the end of World War II, Larrick had vaulted to the agency's administrative side, anointed assistant commissioner, associate commissioner, and then deputy commissioner. By that point, he was a father of four who spent weekends on his Virginia farm by the Potomac, enjoying his orchard, vegetable garden, and sheep. Then, in 1954—after thirty years at the agency—the man who had never completed his undergraduate degree, the man who knew nothing about the science of how drugs were made or worked, the man who fled the capital each weekend to run crab lines into the Potomac, became FDA commissioner.

The drug sector exulted. Gone were the crusading chemists and nitpicky medical doctors who had formerly held the post. Larrick—whose appointment the pharmaceutical firms had openly orchestrated—seemed like a reliable ally. His tenure, in fact, became "one of sweetness and light, togetherness, of loving one's neighbor," noted a trade journal of the day. A later deputy commissioner who worked with him described the "very warm spot in [Larrick's] heart for the responsible members of the drug industry." Unsurprisingly, fraternization became the rule at Larrick's FDA. Medical reviewers, wooed with lavish lunches, granted bureaucratic favors. Questionable drug applications received friendly support. The agency essentially helped pharmaceutical firms circumvent its own regulatory hurdles.

This put Frances in a bind. The Kevadon application was a wreck. Nothing she'd seen suggested the drug should go on sale, but she lacked clear medical grounds on which to reject it. Absent a nameable safety problem—for example, data indicating dangerous side effects—she would have no choice but to green-light the product at the end of sixty days. The burden of proof fell on her. But Frances couldn't conduct a proper assessment without real human data, which Merrell had seemingly withheld.

Per agency protocol, two other reviewers had been assigned sections of the application: a chemist, Lee Geismar, and a pharmacologist, Jiro Oyama. Geismar told Frances that she was equally troubled by the paperwork. She had fled Germany with her parents in 1938 and still spoke German fluently, so she'd been able to plow through the original German research. She told Frances that Merrell's English translations and summaries were filled with errors.

Oyama took a sunnier view. He agreed that the long-term safety data was paltry and that the drug's safety seemed to hinge on its level of absorption. But he didn't think this warranted a holdup. The FDA should deem Kevadon ready for sale, he thought, but restrict it to short-term use pending long-term human data.

Frances wasn't swayed. After two decades building her reputation as an impeccable researcher, she would not rubber-stamp a scientific mess. Once this drug went on the market, she was responsible for what it did. But the sixty-day clock was ticking. Each day she stared at the paperwork brought the drug one day closer to automatic approval.

Then she remembered that one person had recently defied Commissioner Larrick, had in fact stood up to the entire FDA. Barbara Moulton, a former medical reviewer, had appeared before Congress to decry the agency's rushed approvals and coziness with pharmaceutical firms. For this, Moulton had been fired, smeared, and blacklisted, her failed crusade wrecking her career. Frances decided to find her.

We have sufficient raw material for 15,000,000 tablets . . . we are ready for plant production. . . . I do not feel . . . that we should wait for final approval of our New Drug Application.

—*William S. Merrell Company memo,*
October 1960

My parents were dairy farmers, and my mother was trying to keep working the farm when she was pregnant. But she got morning sickness, so her doctor gave her these pills.

Then I was born all messed up. My right hand is just a stub, the arm and elbow fused together. And my left is like a seal-paw, all the fingers fused and crooked. My legs are bad, too.

One is missing a knee, and my upper leg is pretty much not there.

Years later, I asked her why I was different from everyone else. She said, "Because of a drug called thalidomide."

—Eric Barrett,

born November 1960,

Punxsutawney, Pennsylvania

Five

On June 2, 1960, almost two months before Frances began work at the FDA, a forty-four-year-old chain-smoking tornado of a woman strode into the Caucus Room of the Old Senate Office Building to testify before Tennessee senator Estes Kefauver's Subcommittee on Antitrust and Monopoly.

Few American women had ever testified before Congress. In 1866, Clara Barton told a government committee of the horrific conditions in prisons. Five years later, Victoria Woodhull and Susan B. Anthony sat before Congress to argue for women's suffrage, followed by Belva Ann Lockwood in 1904. But now Dr. Barbara Moulton was blowing the whistle on the corrupt federal agency at which she had worked for five years.

Barbara was born in 1915 in Chicago, the second child of Harold Glenn Moulton and Frances Christine Rawlins Moulton. Her father, a professor of economics at the University of Chicago, had once roamed the Michigan wilderness as one of eight barefoot farm children—a life described in a 1924 book by his mother called *True Stories of Pioneer Life*. Nine-year-old Barbara, gifted her grandmother's book, devoured these tales of "hardships, hopes, pleasures, and modest triumphs."

All eight of the Moulton Michigan homestead children graduated from college, and Barbara's father earned a doctorate in economics. When hired by the Brookings Institution, one of the earliest American think tanks, he moved his family to Washington, D.C. There, Barbara graduated from the Madeira School in Virginia, and majored in astronomy at Smith College.

Barbara spent her second two years of college in Vienna, Austria, where she dabbled in psychoanalysis and attended concerts. She returned to the States to complete her bachelor's degree in 1937 and then, like Frances,

embarked upon a decade of advanced study. She received an MA in bacteriology and an MD from George Washington University. She followed
this with internships in general medicine and surgery and several university appointments, until in February of 1955, Barbara joined the Food and
Drug Administration.

Barbara—a highly opinionated, unmarried woman who could drive a
car with one hand while striking a match and lighting a cigarette with the
other—was an odd fit for a civil servant. Barbara loved Lucky Strikes and
pearls and extravagant hats, and the birthday parties she threw herself were
legendary. But she also craved the wilderness of her grandmother's tales,
so on weekends she drove to her family's West Virginia farm, where she
canoed or commandeered her niece and nephew for campouts along the
Appalachian Trail. She passed many afternoons drawing the patterns of
each of her Holstein calves. (Years later, during her late-in-life wedding at
the farm, Barbara, in her wedding gown and waders, rushed away from her
guests to assist a cow in labor.)

It was only a matter of time before the free-spirited Barbara Moulton
butted heads with the FDA's old-boy bureaucracy. The agency assigned
her to review a morass of New Drug Applications on which she had no
authority to act. Pharmaceutical firms meddled. Superiors undermined
her. Any attempt to reject a questionable drug landed her in a bureaucratic
labyrinth. Larrick seemingly wanted all new drugs on sale, fast. When Barbara pushed for new safeguards, colleagues stonewalled her. Her request
that Wyeth Laboratories add a written warning about addiction risk to a
product earned her a reprimand from a superior for undermining his "policy of friendliness with industry." When four pharmaceutical representatives swarmed her office to protest her delay of a drug application lacking
long-term safety data, the chief of the New Drug Branch stepped in to approve the application. In February of 1960, Barbara resigned.

But Barbara Moulton was not one to go quietly into the night. She
promptly sought out Leonor Sullivan, a Missouri congresswoman and
consumer safety advocate. Having served as campaign manager for her
congressman husband for five elections, Sullivan had been sidelined by
Missouri's Democratic leaders after his death in 1951. When they refused
to nominate her for the special election in the tradition of widow's succession, Sullivan nonetheless ran, defeating all seven Democratic primary

contenders and crushing the Republican incumbent by a ratio of two to one. She finally took her seat in the Eighty-third Congress, the first woman ever elected from Missouri, and went on to win landslide victories in her next eleven elections. Moulton's tale of FDA corruption roused Sullivan, and she directed her to the man in Washington best poised to assist: the legendary Senator Estes Kefauver.

The lanky six-foot-three freshman senator from Tennessee had become a household name in the early 1950s for his national probe of organized crime. In televised government hearings, Kefauver had grilled a parade of underworld characters under klieg lights. The folksy senator faced off against bookies and mobsters for eleven months, introducing a riveted American public to the "mafia." For this, the Tennessee progressive became a "non-partisan" national hero, graced the cover of *Time* magazine, and was voted one of America's "ten most admired men."

But there was a personal edge to Kefauver's political ambitions. Estes's older brother, Robert, had been the family's golden boy growing up. Estes was Robert's less scholarly sidekick who occasionally showed "flashes of promise." But the brothers, two years apart, were inseparable, adventuring around Madisonville, Tennessee, "like twins." Then, when Estes was eleven, tragedy struck. During an outing to the Tellico River, Estes jumped in and swam to the other side, only to hear a commotion as he climbed out on the opposite bank: Robert had drowned.

For nearly a year, the eleven-year-old Estes burrowed into his grief, reading biographies of Abraham Lincoln, Robert E. Lee, and other powerful leaders. When he emerged from his depression, it was with a fierce determination to make up for his brother's lost future.

By the time Kefauver entered politics (after a brief stint as a lawyer), personal humility and an obsession with justice defined his career. Brilliant and passionately unpretentious, Kefauver solicited advice from senators and cabdrivers alike. To playfully embrace his "Davy Crockett" Tennessee roots, the Yale-educated lawyer donned a racoon cap and stopped campaign cars en route to major speeches to shake hands with field-workers. Once, when several supporters eagerly wandered into his hotel room for an autograph, Kefauver graciously signed from the shower, the curtain wrapped around his drenched body.

Kefauver believed fervently in a government for and of the people. And the people were *for* him—Kefauver pulled off landslide after landslide in his Tennessee races, despite risky civil rights stances. He had notably defied other Dixie states by refusing to sign the 1956 Southern Manifesto, a denouncement of the *Brown v. Board of Education* ruling.

By age fifty-six, the political maverick had made two powerful bids for the Democratic presidential nomination. In 1956, he won the party's formal vice presidential nomination in a dramatic vote by convention delegates (besting an upstart JFK).

But politicians—even within Kefauver's party—came to fear him. His righteousness made them look crooked. Deemed "liberal" by southern conservatives and "conservative" by northern liberals, Kefauver grew increasingly isolated in Washington: respected but cast out. Around the Capitol it was said that Kefauver was going to be "one of the finest men who never got elected President."

By 1957, he had surrendered his White House dreams and pivoted to legislative goals. He assumed leadership of the Subcommittee on Antitrust and Monopoly to fight the economic exploitation of the many by the few. Kefauver announced plans to investigate, industry by industry, the effects of concentrated economic power. Were small bands of manufacturers fixing prices?

Steel and automobile companies came first, and then an economist on Kefauver's staff, Dr. Irene Till, suggested "drugs" as his next target. Till's husband had been prescribed an antibiotic for strep throat that cost fifty cents a pill—eight dollars for a four-day supply. When the doctor offered to swap it for another brand, it turned out *every* company sold its antibiotic for the exact same price. It looked like price collusion.

An informal survey by Kefauver's team quickly turned up reports of reckless advertising and outlandish prices. But to prove price-fixing, they needed to know what the drugs cost to make, data the manufacturers deftly concealed. When John Blair, Kefauver's chief economist, chanced upon an FTC quarterly financial report that for the first time detailed pharmaceuticals as an independent industry, he saw that the net revenues of drug firms reached nearly 19 percent of invested capital—more than double the average profit of other industries.

"My God, just look at those profits," Blair marveled to his colleagues.

Drug companies were raking it in. The question was: How?

Kefauver's seasoned team began its official probe of the pharmaceutical world. The work was overseen by eight firecracker minds, one of whom was economist Eppes Wayles Browne, Jr. (who would later marry Barbara Moulton).

As the group dug deeper, astonishing figures emerged: Wholesale pharmaceuticals had raked in between $2 billion and $2.25 billion in sales in 1957. Thirteen pharmaceutical firms ranked among the country's top fifty companies, with the three front-runners making 33 to 38 percent in net profits—after taxes.

But drugmakers weren't car or steel manufacturers; they were ostensibly supplying a public necessity. Shouldn't lowering prices be a goal when it came to health? Blair was distraught to meet an elderly man in line at a prescription counter who said that on his four-dollar daily income he spent one dollar a day on Deltasone (prednisone) for his arthritis. Worse—he stopped taking the drug at the end of every month so he could pay for the Orinase tablets his wife needed for her diabetes.

"How in the world can poor people afford to stay alive these days?" Kefauver asked Blair.

But to argue that drug prices were outlandish, the team needed to nail down the manufacturing costs. The industry was threatening a Supreme Court battle to guard those figures.

Kefauver's crew got a break when they found paperwork showing that drug firms were selling drugs to one another. Those contracts gave Kefauver grounds for subpoenas, and in the sea of documents that arrived, they pinpointed data on the cost of making prednisone: $2.37 per gram. From that they knew that a five-milligram pill cost about a penny in raw material. Kefauver's team added in a half cent for tableting to arrive at a manufacture cost of 1.567 cents per pill. Druggists were charged 18 cents, and the consumer 30 cents. Americans were buying medicine at an almost 2,000 percent markup.

Kefauver was floored. He pored over the documents to make sure there was no error. The figures laid bare industry abuse. Drug firms, already trying to derail his upcoming Senate bid, would be enraged if he went public with these numbers. Nonetheless, in September 1959, Kefauver announced he would soon begin official hearings on the drug industry.

The public cheered—it seemed everyone had been growing incensed

at the cost of medicine. Fifty to a hundred fan letters a day urged Kefauver
to "clean out the rats." Doctors, too, wanted to shake Kefauver's hand. One
physician sent along five days' worth of promotional materials he'd received from drug firms—a huge carton overflowing with brochures, letters, and drug samples—what the firms called "starter doses." Other
doctors offered probe tips: Look into Merck's Decadron, they urged. The
top-selling cortical steroid, marketed as having "no worrisome side effects,"
in fact caused blood problems.

Kefauver soon realized that price-fixing was only the tip of the iceberg.
Like Harvey Wiley a century earlier, Kefauver turned up a hornet's nest
everywhere he looked. Drug firms, it turned out, planted promotional "articles" in newspapers and magazines. Pfizer had even fabricated the names
of eight supporting doctors in its antibiotic Sigmamycin's sales materials.

On the eve of the hearings, the drug industry braced for attack. The
Pharmaceutical Manufacturers Association sent President Austin Smith—
former editor of JAMA—to ask Kefauver to discuss drugs by their generic,
not trade, names. Drug firms had long used deliberately convoluted mon-
ikers like *piperidolate hydrochloride* or *chlordiazepoxide* for their cheap
generics—making zingy trade names like Dactil or Librium easier for doctors and patients to recall—and thus demand. But Kefauver refused to
sidestep trade names. And when the PMA asked that Smith be called as
the first witness, Kefauver refused.

On December 7, 1959, just before 10:00 A.M., Kefauver stepped into the
marble-walled committee room of the Senate for his anticipated hearings.
At a long wooden table, a glass of water and research papers at hand, Kefauver got to work. Several hundred people sat with eyes trained on the
renegade senator—sixteen members of Kefauver's subcommittee staff, as
well as reporters, television crews, tourists, and anxious drug industry representatives. Kefauver had made clear he would study every nook and
cranny of the trade. The charges at play? Possible violation of antitrust
laws, price-fixing that led to overpricing, and dangerously misleading advertising.

Kefauver kicked things off with a series of charts to show that the Scher-
ing Corp. of New Jersey marked up drugs as much as 7,000 percent. When
the president of the firm blamed high drug prices on the dearth of ill customers, bemoaning the inability to "put two sick people in every bed when

there is only one person sick," a disgusted member of the drug industry actually stormed out.

Five firms, Kefauver then showed, were "fixing" the price of tetracycline—the market's most popular antibiotic. Upjohn was selling a fourteen-cent drug for fifteen dollars, and a former Pfizer doctor explained that he had quit due to the firm's "perverted marketing attitudes." Diabinese, an antidiabetic marketed for its "almost complete absence of unfavorable side effects," actually harmed over a quarter of patients.

A key eye-opener was the vast role of pharmaceutical marketing. Drug firms now spent a quarter of their income on promotion, turning out more than 3.7 billion pages of paid journal advertising and 740 million direct mailers in a single year. One doctor testified that "it would take two railroad cars, one hundred and ten large mail trucks, and eight hundred postmen to deliver the daily load of drug circulars and samples to doctors if mailed to a single city."

The industry did not placidly take the beating. Austin Smith of the Pharmaceutical Manufacturers Association defended the high price of drugs by asking: "I wonder if any member of the subcommittee knows how much it costs to die?" Smith, recently ill, argued that the $15.30 he had paid for eight days of an antibiotic was cheap compared to the $900-plus in doctors' and lawyers' fees it would have cost him to perish. He also noted that people saved by drugs contributed an additional billion in taxes each year.

After six months exposing the outlandish profits of the drug companies, Kefauver's probe shifted to the FDA.

The agency, under Larrick, had initially shunned Kefauver's subcommittee investigation. But a *Saturday Review* article about Dr. Henry Welch, head of the FDA's antibiotics division, had placed the agency squarely in Kefauver's crosshairs. Welch, it turned out, was double-dipping: While working at the FDA he was also a paid editor for two medical journals—*Antibiotics and Chemotherapy* and *Antibiotic Medicine & Clinical Therapy*—both heavily underwritten by pharmaceutical advertising.

When a witness appeared before Kefauver's committee to show that Welch's "honorariums" between 1953 and 1960 had totaled a jaw-dropping $287,142 (over $2 million in today's dollars), Welch filed for retirement from the FDA. Claiming a heart condition, he never took the stand. Commissioner Larrick quickly painted Welch—who was his close friend—as a lone bad apple in a virtuous agency.

But in June 1960, a witness argued that FDA corruption ran far *deeper* than Welch.

Barbara Moulton, who had never submitted her resignation letter to the FDA, decided to read it all into congressional testimony. She arrived at the subcommittee meeting in early June, sparklingly bejeweled. With her red lipstick perfectly penciled, she was a stunning contrast to the parade of pale men in starched-collared shirts who had sat before Kefauver's team. When she began to speak, her moral heft silenced the crowd.

Moulton, it turned out, had been onto Henry Welch's shenanigans as far back as 1956. She grew leery when Welch showed up at an antibiotics conference at the posh Willard Hotel to give a blustery speech about a "third great new era of antibiotics" and the "blessings" of "synergistic combinations" of drugs, a speech so obviously scripted to promote Pfizer's Sigmamycin that foreign symposium participants were stunned—did the U.S. drug industry have that much influence over government regulators? Moulton took a look at the Sigmamycin paperwork and quickly noticed a lack of well-controlled studies. But when she alerted her bosses, they argued that Welch "added luster to the Food and Drug Administration." They wanted nothing "done against him."

Sigmamycin wasn't the only drug Welch had shadily promoted, and Welch, Moulton explained, had built a "little dynasty" of FDA lackeys. The whole agency was crooked, with drug firms wining and dining medical reviewers. If a lone medical reviewer—such as herself—resisted a firm's efforts? A half dozen representatives could swoop in to "argue the case" or lobby an agency superior. In the end, for her refusal to be "sufficiently polite" to the drug industry, Moulton was transferred out of her position.

Moulton warned Kefauver's subcommittee that the FDA had become "a mere service bureau for industry." And then she sought to cut the head off the beast—with a takedown of the commissioner.

While the agency dealt with exceedingly complex medical matters, Moulton explained, Larrick was "a man with neither legal nor scientific training." He lacked "intellectual integrity" and was merely a "civil servant with no particular background in the field, other than years of association with it." In short, a woman with two advanced degrees stood before Congress to say her boss wasn't smart enough. She demanded Larrick's resignation.

But Moulton did more than throw punches. Intent on improving product safety, she mapped out the danger of the current drug-approval process: A sole medical officer could swiftly put a drug on the market, but blocking a questionable drug required elaborate intra-agency support. She also proposed an amendment to the 1938 Food, Drug, and Cosmetic Act: that drug manufacturers must prove efficacy. "No drug is 'safe,'" she argued, "if it fails to cure a serious disease for which a cure is available."

Intrigued by Moulton's accusations, the Department of Health, Education and Welfare (the FDA's parent organization) launched an inquiry: A group of scientists would probe FDA procedures while another group would investigate individual behavior within the agency. Moulton's "lady doctor" testimony received minor newspaper coverage.

And yet Moulton paid a vast price. "I have jeopardized, perhaps irreparably, my own opportunities for future Government employment," Moulton predicted at the time, and her fear proved well founded. She was quickly blacklisted and her attempts, years later, to rejoin the FDA were spurned.

When Frances Kelsey tracked her down in the autumn of 1960, Moulton had resumed some private-practice hours as a physician, but she was effectively out of work, lolling around her West Virginia farm. Larrick, of course, remained FDA commissioner. But Moulton had aired the FDA's dirty laundry, laying bare its failings in the official government record. It was a historic moment lost to the public consciousness, but never to her. Upon her death in 1997, a family friend would find hundreds of dusty copies of her congressional testimony piled throughout her farmhouse.

In 1960, though, she still believed she could win the fight. And when Frances asked for help with the Kevadon application, Moulton was ready to roll up her sleeves.

KEVADON

A New Hypnotic

Composition

Chemically, Kevadon (brand of thalidomide) is an entirely new and molecularly different hypnotic. It is a non-barbiturate alpha (N-phthalimido) glutarimide, represented by the following:

Indication:

Kevadon is indicated in the symptomatic treatment of insomnia . . .

SAFETY DATA:

Kevadon is unique among potent sleep-inducing agents because of its tremendous margin of safety. . . . The compound is so non-toxic that the Ld50 could not be determined.

A dog weighing 6.5 Kg tolerated well a single dose of 10,000 mg. of thalidomide administered orally by means of a tube. . . .

Nulsen administered 100 mg. of Kevadon to 81 expectant mothers and Blasiu to 160 nursing mothers. In both instances, all of the babies were born or nursed without any abnormalities or harmful effects from the medication.

—William S. Merrell Co.,

Kevadon preliminary medical brochure,

November 1960

Six

Frances set aside her paperwork for an evening to watch the 1960 presidential election returns with Ellis and the girls. The next day, they listened to Kennedy's acceptance speech. But when Frances returned to work later that week, her stress resumed: It was mid-November, and the sixty-day clock on the thalidomide application was about to lapse.

Fortunately, Barbara Moulton, now a friend, tipped Frances off to an agency loophole: Invoking section 505(b) of the Federal Food, Drug, and Cosmetic Act, Frances could deem the Kevadon application "incomplete" and ask Merrell for more data, restarting the sixty-day clock. It was a delay, not a denial, but it would keep the drug off the market while Frances gathered more information. Frances mailed her decision to the William S. Merrell Company under the wire, spelling out her position and the company's problematic gaps in data.

Joseph Murray—Merrell's liaison with the FDA—immediately called to protest. But Frances stood firm.

Almost overnight, Merrell regrouped. Its affiliate National Drug Company (another subsidiary of Richardson-Merrell) submitted its own NDA for thalidomide, but under the German trade name "Contergan." Merrell then submitted new paperwork on absorption studies, with a chemical description showing the advantage of thalidomide over Doriden, another nonbarbiturate sedative. Certain the drug would be approved, Merrell announced an additional plant for manufacturing Kevadon in Pennsylvania.

By mid-December, Joseph Murray had arrived in Washington, D.C., with new data. Jiro Oyama, the pharmacologist, and Lee Geismar, the German-born chemist, both sat with Frances and a few other members of the FDA as Murray walked them through a presentation highlighting new isotope studies showing that only 40 percent of thalidomide was absorbed by the human body—suggesting high safety.

But Frances balked: If the drug was so poorly absorbed, did it even work? What evidence did the firm have that sedation wasn't a placebo effect? The company's fundamental claim for thalidomide's safety could, after all, come down to its poor absorption. Also, where was any clear data from radioactive studies? (Frances had studied radioisotope diagnostics in her South Dakota days.) Plus, the drug's asymmetry—and what that might mean for differing forms—had still not been addressed.

Frances sent the men packing, insisting on more long-term data. Within a few weeks, a Merrell detail man hand-delivered yet another round of paperwork. But it was addressed only to Frances, absent a copy for the application. Frances immediately called Murray, collect—his error would be on his own dime—and Murray explained that the new materials were for her "personal information." Frances knew from Barbara Moulton all about drug firm reps trying to cozy up to medical reviewers, and she made it clear to Murray that she wasn't having "personal" discussions.

That evening, Frances showed Ellis the new Kevadon paperwork. The couple had been lab partners for years, they had written a pharmacology textbook together, and for months Frances had been updating Ellis at night about the weird NDA. Now Frances wanted his official scientific assessment.

Ellis thought the whole thing was a suspicious mess.

"None of these data is of any value whatsoever," Ellis wrote, "except to demonstrate that all of the drug is not excreted unchanged in the feces!" One section of the NDA seemed "an interesting collection of meaningless pseudoscientific jargon apparently intended to impress chemically unsophisticated readers." In another section, "the data are completely meaningless as presented." Experimental procedures, he pointed out, were either not described or sloppy. And he cringed at the "very unusual claim that thalidomide has no LD_{50}. No other substance can make that claim!!!" Ellis didn't buy a word of it. And some of the safety claims were based on such abuses of elementary concepts of pharmacology that he couldn't believe it was "honest incompetence."

Frances had known the data was sloppy, but Ellis had thrown suspicion on what she had imagined was ineptitude.

Were the gaps in the application more than accidental errors?

Part II

THE
DRUG

I want to emphasize that the patients took Contergan for at most most eight to ten days. Never was this drug prescribed for pregnant women. It is my absolute principle never to give sleeping pills or tranquilizers to mothers-to-be. . . . I would most emphatically have resisted the circulation of such a letter using my name and referring to my report. I consider that this letter from the firm to the medical profession is unfair, misleading and irresponsible.

—Dr. Augustin Peter Blasiu,
statement to German authorities,
June 5, 1964

Seven

Hans-Werner von Schrader-Beielstein, head of Chemie Grünenthal's research department, was a wiry, soft-spoken doctor with crystal-blue eyes and pockmarked skin. In 1957, newly hired at Grünenthal, he was concerned about its new wonder drug, set to hit the German market in two months. The young father had recently seen his wife through two insomnia-ridden pregnancies, and he took a conservative and nature-first approach to remedies in pregnancy. If a tableted drug was needed, von Schrader-Beielstein wanted to ensure it was "non-hazardous."

So, von Schrader-Beielstein wrote to Harold Siebke, a gynecology professor: Would Siebke "examine" thalidomide in his pregnant patients to ensure the drug was safe and effective? Over a year earlier, Siebke's clinic had published a paper called "The Effect of Medication on the Unborn Child." Siebke seemed the man for the job. But he did not respond, and von Schrader-Beielstein dropped the matter.

By late summer, when Grünenthal learned that a flu epidemic was forecast for the fall, the firm moved swiftly to roll out its new products. On October 1, Grünenthal launched two over-the-counter versions of thalidomide: "Grippex"—a cold and flu treatment that was a mixture of thalidomide, quinine, phenacetin (a synthetic fever reducer), vitamin C, and salicylamide (akin to aspirin)—and a tablet form of pure thalidomide sold as "Contergan." The firm knew that side effects—tingling, numbness, dizziness—had been noted in trial patients and that several doctors had panned the drug. The firm also lacked data suggesting the drug was safe during pregnancy. Nonetheless, fifty advertisements in German medical journals and two hundred thousand physician mailings hailed the drug as "completely non-poisonous" and "astonishingly safe." Considering that

West Germany was about the size of Michigan, it was a staggeringly aggressive campaign. A marketing memo emphasized "the atoxicity proved in animal experiments." Doctors were assured that the drug was so benign it could even be taken in higher-than-recommended dosages.

It wasn't until the following year, once the drug had gained a wide audience, that Grünenthal gathered pregnancy data. This time, the firm asked obstetrician and gynecologist Augustin Blasiu to test the new sedative. On May 2, 1958, Blasiu published "Experiences with Contergan in Gynecology," detailing the response of 370 female patients. To Grünenthal's delight, Blasiu reported that "side effects were not observed either with mothers or babies."

Almost overnight, Grünenthal trumpeted Blasiu's findings throughout the medical community. More than forty thousand doctors received a promotional mailing celebrating the ob-gyn's use of Contergan to alleviate the "sleeplessness, unrest and tension" of pregnancy.

> Blasiu has given many patients in his gynecological department and in his obstetrical practice Contergan and Contergan Forte. Depth and length of sleep were good and patients could be easily awakened from deep sleep. Contergan had no effect on the nursing baby.

Grünenthal, however, failed to share Blasiu's specific data and omitted a crucial clarification: Blasiu had never administered the drug to a single pregnant patient. He had given Contergan to postpartum women only, and the nursing mothers—who accounted for about half of his subjects— took the drug for approximately one week.

Nonetheless, like a game of telephone, Blasiu's report begat a cascade of assurances about thalidomide's safety in pregnant women. The erroneous belief took hold even within Grünenthal. Thalidomide's international distributors parroted the pregnancy safety claim. Firms in thirty-five countries throughout Europe, Africa, Asia, and the Americas received a copy of Blasiu's full report from the company—but no one, it seems, bothered to translate the data from the original German. Grünenthal's spin on the Blasiu study became a key tenet of its marketing, and the myth of thalidomide's prenatal safety spread swiftly across the globe.

One of Grünenthal's chief international partners was Distillers Bio-chemicals (DCBL), a British spirits and liquor company. Having manu-factured penicillin during World War II at the request of the British government, at the war's end Distillers launched a proper pharmaceutical branch. But by the mid-1950s, research and development was proving un-expectedly costly, and the firm sought to license foreign drugs.

Thalidomide seemed a prime candidate. Hearing the pitch on a visit to Grünenthal in 1956, Dr. Walter Kennedy, Distillers' German-speaking medical adviser, immediately alerted company director E. G. Gross. "If all the details about this are true," an astonished Kennedy wrote, "then it is a most remarkable drug. In short it is impossible to give a toxic dose; it has no narcotic effect; it has no influence on breathing or circulation."

Britain was in the midst of a sedative craze—one million Britons took sleeping pills nightly, accounting for 12 percent of all National Health pre-scriptions. Eager to capitalize on this, Gross flew to Germany to persuade Grünenthal that his upstart company could handle distribution. But Gross paid for his enthusiasm. After nearly a year of negotiations, Grünenthal wrested royalties from the British firm for a whopping sixteen years and mandated that Distillers put the drug on sale within nine months.

This meant that once the contract was signed in July 1957, DCBL faced an impossibly short window for safety research.

But Kennedy—who had already secured raw thalidomide for animals and thousands of tablets for humans—was eager to jump-start testing. The firm hired a pharmacologist, George Somers, who immediately began ad-ministering thalidomide to mice. But Somers delivered bad news: His lab mice weren't slowed down; he didn't think the drug was a "sedative."

Kennedy, convinced Grünenthal had already done the key animal test-ing and that his firm's own work was just pro forma, brushed off Somers's concern. Having already sent thalidomide to a "large number" of doctors in England in "pilot scale trials" meant to "arouse interest," Kennedy re-solved to move forward.

In August 1957, however, a thornier problem arose: James Murdoch at Edinburgh University, an acquaintance of Kennedy's who had agreed to test the drug in humans, reported to Kennedy that thalidomide blocked thyroid action. Murdoch shared a draft of his paper, which described it as "unjustifiable" to suggest anyone use the drug long term without "the results of a more detailed study of its long-term effects in a larger series of patients." Murdoch was essentially stating that the drug was far from ready to go on sale.

Kennedy panicked—the nine-month clock with Grünenthal was ticking—and begged Murdoch to delete the demand for more detailed studies. Murdoch conceded.

But members of Distillers began grumbling that thalidomide was falling short of its shimmering promise. Had Grünenthal misled them? Meanwhile, Somers couldn't replicate safety data on another Grünenthal product—Supracillin. The antibiotic was known to harm hearing, but Grünenthal had promised that its own version eliminated this danger. Somers's experimental cats, however, were going deaf.

Within Distillers, objections now arose to using the phrase "no known toxicity" in their thalidomide promotion, since the company's own lab tests hadn't proven this. "Exceptionally *low* toxicity" seemed more accurate. But the decision-makers at Distillers felt that if Grünenthal, the drug's creator, claimed "no known toxicity," they had a right to parrot it.

In January of 1958, the *British Medical Journal* finally published the Murdoch study, which, while tempered, still asserted that thalidomide disrupted thyroid action. This rattled George Somers, the Distillers pharmacologist, who recommended lowering dosages and "avoiding prolonged administration . . . until we have more experience with the drug."

Rather than heed his warning, Kennedy prevailed upon another researcher testing the antithyroid effects of thalidomide to send a letter to the *BMJ* supporting long-term use of the drug. It was a win for Distillers. But Murdoch's paper, essentially undermining the "no known toxicity" claim, remained at large.

On April 14, 1958—just under the nine-month deadline set by Grünenthal—Distillers launched Distaval and Distaval Forte throughout the United Kingdom, hailing the sedative as "super-safe."

Distillers had proved an exceptionally compliant partner for Grünenthal, but finding an American licensee proved challenging. In 1956—two years after Grünenthal filed its first thalidomide patent—the German firm signed a deal with Smith, Kline & French in the United States. SKF quickly started animal testing on the drug, followed by "limited clinical trials" in humans, shipping supplies to sixty-seven physicians around the country, primarily in New Jersey and California. But within a year, SKF shocked Grünenthal by rejecting the drug. Citing an apparent "lack of efficacy," in January 1958, SKF completely withdrew its license paperwork. "The material was not of interest," the firm determined, closing out the project. But the yearlong delay in deeming the drug ineffective—a determination usually made quickly for a sedative—would later prompt suspicions.

Next, Grünenthal approached the American firm Lederle about thalidomide distribution in the United States. The companies were already in business together, with Grünenthal selling Lederle's cancer drug, aminopterin, since 1953. (Aminopterin had been known, since 1952, to cause miscarriages and birth defects.)

Lederle, for reasons unknown, declined thalidomide.

Then in March 1958, two representatives from Vick Chemical visited Grünenthal's Stolberg offices. Vick—a hundred-year-old American firm known for its VapoRub—had recently acquired several smaller drug firms, including the William S. Merrell Company in Cincinnati, and was about to rename itself Richardson-Merrell. Dr. Evert Florus Van Maanen, head of the biological sciences division at Merrell, was so intrigued by thalidomide that he and his colleague immediately relayed the news to Merrell's director of medical research, Raymond Pogge.

If there is a shadowy, inscrutable figure in the American story of thalidomide, it is Raymond Pogge. Little is known about Pogge beyond his key role in bringing to market two Merrell drugs that would be linked to birth defects and prompt a blizzard of lawsuits. But Pogge was an audaciously lucky man. In 1961, he would walk away, unharmed, from a Denver plane crash that killed seventeen people. And for the rest of his life he would walk away from any public accountability for the twentieth century's biggest drug scandal.

Pogge was a medical doctor. And while he had no training in pharmacy or pharmacology, creating drugs was his secret passion. At the end of World War II, the twentysomething-year-old Pogge had lived in Louisiana, treating leprosy patients at Carville prison. When Promin, the standard leprosy treatment, nauseated prison volunteers, Pogge sought a way to make the drug go down easier. He added glucose, calcium, vitamin D, and penicillin to the Promin and—voilà—the "Pogge Cure-All Cocktail" worked wonders—leprous nodules vanished and mouth lesions healed.

Pogge then took a job in the Merck medical department, setting up human studies for drugs, then started work at Merrell in 1950, where he resumed pharmaceutical tinkering.

A three-month residency after medical school marked the extent of Pogge's training in obstetrics, but for some reason, he grew fascinated with the idea of a drug for morning sickness. At the time, no such product existed. Recalling that about half the pregnant patients he had tended in his residency complained of nausea, Pogge envisioned a vast, untapped market given the three to four million pregnancies per year in the United States. As Merrell's director of medical research, Pogge proposed a delayed-release nausea drug. If women took the tablet at bedtime, a multilayered coating would dissolve through the night to release the active ingredients before morning sickness.

In the spirit of his cure-all cocktail, Pogge combined several existing pharmaceuticals—pyridoxine, dicyclomine hydrochloride, and doxylamine succinate. Because the three ingredients already had FDA approval, he bypassed animal tests to assess the drug's effect on the fetus, even though pharmacologists knew that, in combination, ingredients could behave differently. But Pogge was seemingly not a nitpicker. Even the drug's human trials were expedited: In fact, only one clinical study assessed the new product in humans: 277 pregnant women, children, and women with motion sickness were administered Pogge's creation to assess its ability to quell nausea. The trial did not track side effects and did not follow up with pregnant patients to determine the drug's effects on the fetus. The study focused on efficacy, not safety. Yet the FDA seemed fine with this. In July 1956, Pogge's Bendectin was allowed to hit the American market—to huge commercial success.

When Pogge heard about Grünenthal's new product, he recognized an even greater gold mine. Anxiety was emerging as a vast market. The recent success of Miltown, launched in 1955, had laid bare America's appetite for sedatives. In just six months, the drug had garnered sales of $2 million, with Milton Berle, Lauren Bacall, and Lucille Ball singing its praises. Every pharmaceutical company now wanted in on the tranquilizer action.

Thalidomide, a licensed drug from overseas for which the key work had already been done, fit the bill.

Vick negotiated a thalidomide contract with Grünenthal, arranging to pay the German firm $25,000 for the first-year license and $30,000 for the second year, indefinitely renewable at that rate. When the deal closed in October 1958, all of Merrell rejoiced.

At that point, Pogge began setting up clinical trials. Since thalidomide was not a combination of previously sold products, Pogge knew the FDA would demand human testing.

Pogge approached Frank Ayd, chief of psychiatry at Baltimore's Franklin Square Hospital, suggesting thalidomide might help Ayd's obsessive-compulsive patients. Soon Ayd was dispensing the drug to roughly one hundred patients and asking for resupplies. Pogge also enlisted Drs. William Hollander, Louis Lasagna, and Sidney Cohen, an LSD enthusiast. Pogge wrangled a few other physicians—all paid for their work—then reached out to his friend and golf partner Dr. Ray O. Nulsen.

A Cincinnati-based ob-gyn, Nulsen had been fraternity brothers at the University of Cincinnati with the great-grandson of Merrell's founder, William Stanley Merrell. Since 1940, Nulsen had helped the local drug firm with its clinical research and was instrumental in helping Pogge to launch Bendectin. Nulsen's 1957 rave in *The Ohio Medical Journal*— "Bendectin in the Treatment of Nausea in Pregnancy"—had, in fact, been penned by Pogge. Nulsen proved equally willing to help his pal with thalidomide—agreeing to dispense it to his patients. On the attending staff at both the Jewish Hospital and Deaconess, Nulsen tended about 350 pregnant women a year.

Pogge asked Nulsen to give out thalidomide for nervous tension at night, and Nulsen began dispensing twenty-five-milligram doses to his patients. Nulsen loved the drug, using it himself for power naps, even giving it to his wife. Pretty soon, he scaled his patients up to fifty milligrams and one hundred milligrams and requested resupplies from Merrell in the thousands. But his "results" trickled into the firm informally. His office did not track how many pills it received or gave out. Only when Nulsen lunched with Pogge did he purportedly pull informal notes from his billfold to relay his "impressions" of how patients responded to the drug. Nulsen's secretary eventually assembled his patient cards to provide more formal data to Pogge—who wanted a publishable paper from the obstetrician. Pogge, grateful, mailed her a one-hundred-dollar check.

By the spring of 1960, Pogge had deputized his own secretary, Margaret Higgins, to help him spin Nulsen's data into a research paper focusing on third-trimester use. Pogge assembled the footnotes and sent the draft to Nulsen. On April 13, 1960, Nulsen submitted it, under his own name, to the *Journal of Obstetrics and Gynecology.*

The editor promptly wrote back: Did the drug cross the placenta or appear in breast milk?

Nulsen forwarded the question to Pogge, who, along with his secretary, added: "There is no danger to the baby if some of it appears in the milk or passes the placental barrier." The new version was returned to Nulsen, who signed off on it. The revised paper was scheduled for publication the following summer.

Pogge then summoned Nulsen for more work. Pogge wanted to know if thalidomide could be turbocharged. APC—a combination of aspirin, phenacetin, and caffeine—was a popular over-the-counter medicine. Could thalidomide boost aspirin and vice versa? Pogge asked Nulsen to test MRD-640—a four-part pill that combined thalidomide with APC, and Nulsen began giving it to patients complaining of headaches.

Pogge then asked Nulsen one more favor, under the table. Bendectin was now a top-selling drug for morning sickness, that hallmark first-trimester symptom. Could Nulsen swap thalidomide for Bendectin in patients with nausea to see if thalidomide was also effective? Nulsen was happy to accommodate.

But then on April 25, 1960, after Pogge had enlisted thirty-seven doctors to "investigate" the German sedative, just weeks after he'd added a sweeping safety claim about pregnancy to Nulsen's paper, he did something odd. He wrote to Merrell's vice president, "There is a difference of professional opinion on the adequacy of presently available support for claims that Kevadon is safe." This was just a few months before they would submit their FDA application. He did not elaborate. And after ten years at the William S. Merrell Company, Pogge quit.

RAYMOND POGGE: The Nulsen studies were conducted in the city of Cincinnati, and I had possession of individual case reports in which the effect on the mother and the lack of effect on the baby was described.

LAWYER: You did have information concerning the effect on the baby?

RAYMOND POGGE: I had information indicating that there was no effect on the baby.

LAWYER: But there was information of observations made of the babies?

—*Diamond v. William Merrell Co.*

and Richardson-Merrell,

1969

I was reassured by the people

at Merrell that the drug was innocuous.

—*Dr. Ray O. Nulsen*

Eight

The weather in Cincinnati was pleasant for midfall, but the men—forty-five of them—were stuck in the hotel ballroom. They'd traveled from across the country for the two-day "Kevadon Hospital Clinical Program" seminar hosted by the William S. Merrell Company. Kevadon was the brand name for thalidomide in the United States.

It was October 1960.

The attendees were mostly division managers, Merrell's top-ranking sales representatives who oversaw dozens of "detail men"—door-to-door or, more aptly, doctor-to-doctor, salesmen—precursors to today's pharmaceutical sales reps. A few of the company's top detail men milled about the room that day, as well as eight hospital representatives. Most of these sales reps had worked for Merrell for years, ascending the ranks, having started as detail men themselves. For weeks at a stretch they lived out of their cars, using their briefcases as desks as they drove throughout their territory, physician to physician, touting the latest Merrell pill, gifting doctors monogrammed golf balls and desk calendars.

The goal was to motivate doctors to write prescriptions. To that end, the firm gave detail men talking points called a "structured detail" for each new drug. Detail men knew little about pharmacology or medicine. Some had college degrees, but that was generally the limit of their education. Yet physicians depended on these friendly emissaries as their chief source of information on new drugs.

Behind the broad grins and solid handshakes, however, the detail men were shrewd. Appraising their marks according to Merrell's three categories—"Dr. Snob," "Dr. Resistant," or "Dr. Backslapper"—detail men reported back on each doctor's approachability, size of practice, and volume of prescriptions—sometimes dropping in on local pharmacies to gauge how often a doctor wrote prescriptions. Since they earned commissions on top of their salaries, Dr. Backslapper—the jovial physician who frequently prescribed new products—was their prime target.

There was a very predictable pattern to new-product promotion, which made the detail men realize something was dramatically different about this Cincinnati seminar, and it wasn't just the throng of division reps crammed into the hotel conference room.

A significant lineup of Merrell bigwigs graced the room: Phillip Ritter, the newly promoted vice president who came from the New York advertising world, kicked off the conference at 9:00 A.M. as keynote speaker and was slated to speak again at a fancy dinner that evening. Dr. Evert Florus Van Maanen, director of biological sciences, and Thomas Jones—the brand-new director of medical science—were also scheduled to take the podium.

At the day's start, the detail men had been handed faux-leather three-ring binders with pages to review. Kevadon, they were told, was safer than barbiturates and just as effective. A sleeping pill with no hangover. Since every doctor dispensed sedatives to every kind of patient, the prescription promise was massive.

But there was a kink. The drug lacked FDA approval, so doctors couldn't prescribe it and the detail men couldn't work their usual charms. Instead, they'd have to do something totally unprecedented—enlist doctors as clinical investigators.

But it wasn't entirely clear exactly what that meant. Throughout the morning, Merrell executives had been confusingly referring to a "Hospital Clinical Program of this type." Finally, Charles Gill, Merrell's hospital manager, spoke to clarify. He said the men would each be given an American Hospital Association directory to locate large teaching hospitals. The bigger, the better. They would target hospitals with a staff of residents and interns. Since detail men usually visited only private-practice physicians, they would have to pore over hospital staff lists and annual reports. Start with the department chiefs, Gill told the men. Hit up the heads of medicine, surgery, anesthesiology, and obstetrics-gynecology. And once they secured a meeting? "Appeal to the doctor's ego," Gill emphasized, and tell him "we think he is important enough to be selected as one of the first to use Kevadon in that section of the country."

To highlight the significance of these meetings, the detail men were to request fifteen-minute appointment slots—roughly double the usual time—and call themselves "Special Kevadon Representatives."

As for the lack of FDA approval, they should spin that fact as a perk. Doctors would be getting advance news of an important product! Gill directed the men to a form letter to doctors: "I feel that you would be interested in obtaining information on Kevadon *before* it becomes commercially available."

The next part of the assignment got trickier. Since the detail men couldn't urge doctors to prescribe the product, they would ask the doctors to run "clinical trials." But a clinical trial was a formal human study, intended to gather data on a drug's efficacy and side effects. This was a huge ask. So if doctors were reluctant, Gill cautioned, the detail men should downplay the work.

He directed the men to a key section of their "script" in the leather binders:

> Bear in mind that these are not basic clinical research studies. We have firmly established the safety, dosage and usefulness of Kevadon by both foreign and U.S. laboratory and clinical studies. . . . If your work yields case reports, personal communication or published work, all well and good. But the main purpose is to establish local studies whose results will be spread among hospital staff members.

Merrell, in essence, wanted buzz.

As the plan was laid out, the rash of hiring in early summer suddenly made sense to the sales managers. In June, they'd been told to double their detailing staffs, an ambitious target that resulted in a suboptimal workforce. This large, inexperienced team would now have two months to set up nearly eight hundred studies. Each detail man and division manager would establish at least fifteen "trials," with the hospital reps assigned twenty-five. Given that even the most experienced detail man in the industry had never enlisted a single clinical investigator, the proposal was radical.

The detail men were to focus exclusively on this project. "Only emergency requirements should take precedence over establishing your Kevadon studies," they were told. Once Kevadon secured national release, the detailing blitz would end. On that prickly point, Gill said the doctors should be told FDA approval was expected in 1961, perhaps by February. Approval, they must emphasize in conversation with doctors, was imminent.

At that, Gill turned the podium over to Dr. Evert Florus Van Maanen, who would explain the science of the drug. Because if Merrell was going to such unprecedented lengths to promote Kevadon, the men in the room were dying to know: What was this thing?

Dr. Van Maanen had been a beloved professor of pharmacology at the University of Cincinnati before he came to work at Merrell. Born in the Netherlands, the gregarious blue-eyed Dutchman had served in the Royal Dutch Artillery during World War II and the Dutch underground resistance. When the conflict ended, "Flor" struck out for a fresh start in the United States. Having studied chemistry as an undergraduate, he enrolled in the pharmacology PhD program at Harvard. From there, he accepted a teaching post at the University of Cincinnati as an instructor and then assistant professor of pharmacology.

Flor loved teaching, but the private sector soon enticed him, and he joined William S. Merrell Company as an associate director of research. He still dropped in on his university lab on Saturdays—enjoying the company of his students and university colleagues, many of whom had become like family. Essentially, though, Van Maanen's work was his life.

And his career was on the upswing. In October 1960, as Flor addressed the Cincinnati conference room, the forty-two-year-old had just been promoted to Merrell's director of biological sciences, overseeing five departments—endocrinology, pharmacology, biochemistry, microbiology, and toxicology-pathology—and all of Merrell's animal research. So it fell to him to explain to the sales force the physiology, pharmacology, and toxicology of Kevadon.

The headline for Kevadon was, of course, its spectacular safety. To hammer that home, Van Maanen had to explain the "LD50"—the dose of a drug that would kill half of an experiment's animals. But Kevadon had no LD50. He had heard this stunning news from Grünenthal when he sat in the German firm's offices over two years earlier. And this would be the mantra for the detail men. In order for Merrell to edge out the other sedatives, Kevadon's advantage had to be clear. So Van Maanen directed the men to a statement in their binder: "Kevadon is so safe that it has been impossible to establish an LD-50 in animals." Except this wasn't entirely true. Flor Van Maanen's department had, in fact, managed to kill rats— lots of them.

Given Grünenthal's assurances that the drug had been tested thoroughly, Merrell's research division had bypassed normal toxicity studies using a range of doses. Instead, Van Maanen had gone straight to megadoses, feeding mice five thousand milligrams per kilogram (one hundred times the starting human tablet dose). The lack of a single fatality seemed strong confirmation of the drug's safety.

Recent experiments with lower dosages in lab rats, however, had produced disastrous results: In experiment 1257-40, "Acute Toxicity Study in Rats," more than *half* the rats given a mere five hundred to one thousand milligrams per kilogram died. In July, when Van Maanen's division tried again, it was worse: *All* the experimental animals died, most within a day.

Next, the research department decided to test thalidomide with a more advanced animal and gave it to a dog. Within two hours the dog was trembling and vomiting. For a few hours, the animal seemed better, but by morning, the dog was dead.

The results were confounding. It was impossible, Grünenthal had promised, for thalidomide to kill an experimental animal. The German paperwork related instances in which people safely downed more than fifty tablets at once. Yet in Van Maanen's lab, animals given thalidomide were dropping left and right.

Van Maanen hypothesized that the sucrose in Merrell's own rat and dog studies had boosted thalidomide's absorption. Thalidomide was insoluble—the powder did not dissolve in water—so they couldn't just make animals drink it. The sucrose was a carrier fluid to help administer the powder in a tube directly into the rats' stomachs or to inject it into their abdomens. So even though half the animals died—a result that should have established an LD50—Van Maanen deemed the experiment compromised. Even though all animal data was required with an FDA application, Merrell withheld the dead-rat and dead-dog results.

But Van Maneen knew that thalidomide held a few other surprises: Rat experiments in the biochemistry and pharmacology departments had revealed that once in the body, thalidomide changed structure. It became more polarized, more ionized. Such transitions weren't totally unprecedented, but Merrell's researchers didn't understand why the drug was transforming.

Other results, too, confused the Dutch scientist. An early experiment with a monkey (because monkeys were expensive, they only tested with one) left the monkey perky. The sedative, it seemed, did not sedate—or kill—man's closest experimental proxy. But untangling the drug's chemical mysteries was not Flor Van Maanen's job. The drug's fate was now in the hands of these salesmen.

Joseph Murray, the firm's FDA liaison, the man who would have to field questions from the government agency, listened quietly to Van Maanen explain the toxicity data. Flor's animal data—the selection presented—was solid. But animal data wasn't what worried Murray. It was the human data.

Raymond Pogge had been the first to sound the alarm eighteen months earlier: Despite Grünenthal's paperwork, the firm lacked "specific human safety data" for the FDA. Pogge then enlisted thirty-seven clinical investigators, including Ray Nulsen, whose forthcoming paper in the *American Journal of Obstetrics and Gynecology* was a key part of the Kevadon pitch. Unfortunately, Nulsen and others had skimped on patient reports. Murray had warned his bosses a year earlier of all the gaping holes in their human trial data. The few patients surveyed had taken the drug for under thirty days, and their doses ricocheted wildly—from fifty milligrams a day to eight hundred milligrams a day. One doctor had submitted data on nine patients after just two weeks.

Merrell's final FDA application referenced 3,441 case histories—but only about 850 came from Merrell's trials. The other 2,600 cited cases came from Grünenthal. But those, too, lacked patient detail. The FDA required physical exam reports—each patient's weight, blood pressure, sleep trends, age, sex, and symptoms—with subjects taking the drug at consistent doses for stretches of time. None of which Merrell had.

Murray's bosses had pushed the promotional side of thalidomide hard from day one, sidelining research. By April, even corner-cutting Raymond Pogge didn't think there was enough data to argue for thalidomide's safety. When Pogge quit, the Kevadon trials fell into the hands of Pogge's underling in the medical department, thirty-four-year-old Thomas Jones. Initially hired as a research associate, Jones was in his very first job in pharmaceuticals. When Jones stepped in for Pogge in May, he took over correspondence with Ayd, Lasagna, Nulsen, and other "investigators." But what Jones had finally given Murray for the official FDA application was still woefully short on human "data."

This, among other reasons, made announcing Kevadon's imminent FDA approval seem recklessly optimistic. A year earlier, a weak drug application might have sailed through. Dr. Jerome Epstein, an FDA medical reviewer, had for years orchestrated blind eyes and concessions for Merrell products. Bendectin, Pogge's three-ingredient morning sickness drug, had been green-lit within weeks. But in December of 1959, Epstein had resigned, leaving Merrell's application for triparanol—a cholesterol pill (MER/29)—in the lurch.

The new medical reviewer, Frank J. Talbot, seemed poised to deny the drug when he heard of doctors reporting hair loss and vision side effects. When Merrell's director of research issued a heated internal memo—headed "READ AND DESTROY"—warning that the FDA was "acting as God Almighty" and overstepping its power, Murray acted swiftly. Well practiced in coercion, within a day he wrested a private guarantee from Talbot that triparanol would be approved imminently.

On April 19, 1960, with official FDA clearance, Merrell flooded pharmacies. Marketed as a magic bullet, triparanol promised to lower cholesterol levels "irrespective of diet." The product stood to do gangbusters profits—in the arena of $500 million annually. Not only was triparanol sold to stores at a 200 percent markup, but it was also a long-term therapy—patients would refill endlessly. Merrell ran ads in pharmacist-oriented journals and set a thirty-three-cent retail price—drugstores would also enjoy a 200 percent gain.

To introduce triparanol to the public, Merrell spent lavishly and hired

William Douglas McAdams, Arthur Sackler's New York advertising agency. The triparanol campaign—a huge success—even included a creative pitch to *Redbook* profiling the new cholesterol drug in a story entitled "How to Keep Husbands Alive."

But the product had problems, and aggressive advertising couldn't stem the bad news. Cataracts, hair loss, and blindness complaints poured in. A young toxicologist, Beulah Jordan, had quit the year before over worrisome results from the company's own animal experiments.

The firm knew triparanol was living on borrowed time. "SHOW MORE ENTHUSIASM," an in-house newsletter urged detail men, "AND SEE IT REFLECTED IN YOUR BONUS CHECK!!!" If doctors complained to sales reps of triparanol's side effects? Blame another drug, "even if you know your drug can cause the side effect mentioned." With a potential $42 million a month in revenue, each day the drug was on the market could mean at least another $1 million for Merrell.

As the triparanol clock was running down, the firm needed a new profit maker. Enter thalidomide. They had secured enough raw material for 15 million tablets. The Kevadon brochures had been printed. Pills, stamped. Detail men now had the talking points. Everything, Murray knew, simply hinged on FDA approval.

So on Tuesday, October 25, he slipped away to call Ralph Smith at the FDA. Smith, Frances's boss, was a known ally of industry. In fact, Smith was the "agency superior" who had stormed Barbara Moulton's meeting a year earlier to fast-track a drug approval.

Murray asked Smith which medical reviewer had been assigned the thalidomide application, but Smith gave Murray a name he didn't recognize—Dr. Frances Kelsey.

Whoever she was, she was about to get the Murray treatment.

As a sleep-inducing agent, Kevadon is at least as potent as the most effective barbiturate, and so safe that it has never harmed a living thing (animal or man) regardless of dosage level.

—*William S. Merrell Company,*
Kevadon brochure, 1960

WILLIAM S. MERRELL CO.

INTERDEPARTMENT MEMO
NOVEMBER 17, 1960

To: All Kevadon representatives
From: Charles W. Gill
Subject: Cease Fire—You Made It
Via Air Mail—Special Delivery

At the Kevadon meeting our goal was set at 750 studies involving 15,000 patients. We thought it would take a month's full-time work to reach this goal. Either we underestimated the product or underestimated you—perhaps a little of both. At any rate, you have taken the program off so fast that you're already way over the goal on the number of patients and will probably have reached the goal on the number of studies by the time you get this letter.

Nine

By late November, Thomas Jones, Merrell's director of medical science, was feeling good about the Kevadon program. Since the Cincinnati conference, detail men had been crossing the country, strutting into hospitals with their Kevadon visual aids, recruiting top-level physicians. Hundreds of doctors had signed on as "clinical investigators." Sample bottles were mailed out by Merrell's shipping department, tracked by a secretary. So thoroughly had every step of the studies been farmed out that Jones didn't have to oversee any of it.

Instead, he got to work cajoling the handful of physicians Pogge had enlisted to make sure their publishable studies crossed the finish line. To that end, Jones flew to Los Angeles to meet with Sidney Cohen, who headed a UCLA alcoholism clinic and the Skid Row Volunteers of America Clinic. Cohen wanted $4,000 for a 150-patient study, more than other investigators had asked for. But Jones thought data on Kevadon's use in alcoholics would broaden the drug's market, so over a dinner at the Netherland Hilton, he talked Cohen down to $3,000.

Other psychiatrists, too, wanted in on the clinical trials, and Jones shelled out another $3,000 and $3,600 for vast Kevadon studies on emotional tension and neuroses.

By late November, Jones had finalized his inner circle of credentialed Kevadon investigators, and the detail men had set up an additional 762 trials. But the patient tally was robust. More than twenty-nine thousand Americans were now set to take the drug.

All was going smoothly for Jones until a strange report arrived from a detail man in Tennessee. An obstetrician at the Acuff Clinic in Knoxville was asking about Kevadon's effect on the fetus, and the query landed on Jones's desk.

Thomas Jones knew that the firm had zero animal data showing the drug's effect on the fetus, but Ray Nulsen in Cincinnati had been using Kevadon on pregnant patients for over a year, and his paper, soon to be published, asserted the drug was harmless if it crossed the placenta. Also, Dr. Edward Holroyd in California, head of obstetrics at Rio Hondo Memorial Hospital, had just written to tell Jones that he was treating fifty women with one-hundred-milligram doses. Holroyd even wanted to add another two hundred women to his study.

Jones must have felt confident in replying to E. B. Linton, the thirty-six-year-old Knoxville obstetrician who would turn out to be the only known trial doctor—out of more than a thousand—to raise the question:

It has not been established whether or not there is any transfer of Kevadon across the placental barrier. However, we feel that, even if transfer does occur, it would be completely safe.

Jones signed the letter and got back to work.

Sooner or later we will not be able to stop publication

of the side effects of Contergan.

— Dr. Gunther Michael,

Chemie Grünenthal memo, 1960

Ten

After only a year on the market, thalidomide sales in Germany had sky-rocketed. Selling ninety thousand packets of thalidomide a month in Germany alone, Grünenthal aimed higher. The firm ran another fifty ads in German medical journals and mailed 250,000 more brochures to doctors and pharmacists.

But in December 1958, a concerned Frankfurt doctor wrote to the firm: Contergan seemed to cause giddiness and balance disturbances in his elderly patients. The next year, 1959, brought more complaints: A pharmacist noted that patients on Contergan were losing warmth in their extremities. By July, another pharmacist, relating that his customers were suffering constipation and nerve damage, suggested Contergan might have "a negative effect on the circulation." Then came a scathing report from Pharmakolor AG, Grünenthal's Swiss licensee: Twenty doctors in Switzerland were reporting "severe side effects" from thalidomide, including trembling hands. "Once and never again. This is a terrible drug," declared a prestigious Basel doctor whose wife had tried a single tablet.

In October of 1959, Dr. Ralf Voss, a Düsseldorf-based nerve specialist, alerted Grünenthal that his sixty-three-year-old male patient using Contergan for over a year had developed polyneuritis. Peripheral or polyneuritis, a condition known to develop gradually, begins as numbness or prickling in the hands and feet, escalating to painful stabbing, burning, or tingling. Walking can become painful. Muscles atrophy and hands and feet grow wildly sensitive. People lose coordination and fall easily. The accumulated pain can be debilitating.

"Do you know anything about Contergan being the cause of damage to the peripheral nervous system?" Voss, worried, asked the firm.

Despite all the negative reports that year, and those dating back to the drug's first clinical trials, Grünenthal responded: "Happily we can tell you that such disadvantageous effects have not been brought to our notice."

A week after Voss's report, however, Grünenthal learned of two more nerve damage cases: A doctor using the drug for several months had suffered "sensory disturbances in his toes and fingers"—as had his sister-in-law. Grünenthal named "vitamin B deficiencies" as the likely culprit.

But by December, Voss had alerted Grünenthal to three more patients—all of whom used thalidomide for over a year—suffering peripheral neuritis.

"We have no idea how these cases of peripheral neuritis could have been caused by Contergan," Grünenthal assured Voss. "We shall pay appropriate attention to this matter in the course of further clinical studies."

When two additional doctors reported "severe circulatory disruptions in the lower extremities" in their patients, Grünenthal declared not only that "a causal connection with Contergan is unlikely" but also that the firm hadn't "heard or seen anything like it up to now."

Grünenthal kicked off the following year, 1960, with a promotional blitz: Sales reps promoted Contergan in about twenty thousand meetings with doctors, while a quarter million leaflets touted thalidomide as "harmless even over a long period of use." By March 1960, Contergan was Germany's most popular sleep aid, and it soon comprised half of Grünenthal's revenues.

But the bad accounts continued: A surgeon taking Contergan complained to Grünenthal of "paraesthesias and hypoaesthesias" in his hands and feet. Once again, the firm replied, "We have received no such reports to date."

By April 1960, neurologist Ralf Voss decided to take his warning public at a medical conference in Düsseldorf. He railed against thalidomide, detailing the extraordinarily painful symptoms of his three patients, at which point another doctor announced to the room that at least four of his own patients had *collapsed* after taking thalidomide.

The press had paid no heed to the April 30 meeting, but the medical community reeled at the suggestion that the wildly popular Contergan had serious side effects. A barrage of nerve damage reports soon hit Grünenthal. Boxes of the product were returned to pharmacies. By mid-May, Grünenthal had sent a memo to its sales teams acknowledging the "severity of side effects," yet the firm rebuffed demands by doctors and pharmacists to sell the drug by prescription only, which would shrink sales. "Everything," Grünenthal decided, "must be done to avoid this."

Instead, the company worked to generate positive spin. Heinrich Mückter—the man who had overseen the drug's creation—enlisted a doctor to study the drug's long-term effects in rats so that by July he could proclaim that even at extremely high doses "no pathological changes could be detected." Grünenthal asked Firma Paracélsia, its Portuguese licensee, for "a quick publication, perhaps in three months, with reports of fifteen to twenty successful cases who have tolerated the drug well." Then, despite the surging reports of thalidomide's neurotoxic effects, Grünenthal fast-tracked a study on children. At the University Clinic in Bonn, Dr. Konrad Lang—who had never before tested a drug—gave megadoses of thalidomide to forty minors, most with brain damage, without their parents' knowledge. Consuming ten to twenty times the adult dose, the children fared poorly: Two died (a three-month-old from heart failure and an older child from a congenital heart defect), one went temporarily blind, and another suffered circulatory collapse. Even though 10 percent of subjects suffered dramatically bad outcomes, Lang chose a glass-half-full approach and assured Grünenthal that "Contergan could be described as a rapidly-acting sedative particularly suited for use with children."

In addition to cultivating positive accounts, Grünenthal squelched negative news. Thus far, the reports of peripheral neuritis had gone straight to the firm's Stolberg office. But when Grünenthal learned in October 1960 that a Königstein neurologist was preparing to publish a paper on thalidomide-related nerve damage, company envoys tried to deter him. When the doctor stood his ground, the firm used a "friendly connection" with the editor of *Medizinische Welt* to stall publication. In the meantime, the same journal, to Grünenthal's delight, ran a paper praising Contergan's "atoxicity" and "lack of side effects after long use."

"We intend to fight for Contergan to the bitter end" was the message circulating within Grünenthal.

Only on November 2, 1960, a full year after Ralf Voss first wrote to Grünenthal of his patients' symptoms, did the firm update its labeling: "As with most drugs," the packaging now noted, "a more or less prolonged use of Contergan may evoke hyper-sensitivity reactions in certain predisposed patients. Immediately after withdrawal of the drug these allergic reactions will disappear."

But as 1960 drew to a close, Grünenthal's sales force grew uneasy. The package warning was murky. Prestigious clinics and doctors were questioning Contergan with "greater and greater intensity." The sales team pleaded for clear information. "We should be briefed above all very exactly," the Düsseldorf sales office advised management.

But the sales force didn't have to wait for Grünenthal's management to come clean. Because a few weeks later, a doctor in Britain would publish a letter in the *British Medical Journal* about thalidomide and peripheral neuritis. For the first time, Grünenthal's embellished safety claims were publicly challenged. And across the Atlantic, a medical reviewer at the FDA would read the *BMJ* letter and begin to doubt the drug's fundamental safety.

December 31, 1960

IS THALIDOMIDE TO BLAME?

SIR,—I feel that four cases which have occurred in my practice recently are worthy of mention, as they may correspond to the experience of other practitioners. They all presented in more or less the same way—each patient complaining of: (1) Marked paraesthesia affecting first the feet and subsequently the hands. (2) Coldness of the extremities and marked pallor of the toes and fingers on exposure to even moderately cold conditions. (3) Occasional slight ataxia. (4) Nocturnal cramp in the leg muscles. Clinical examination in each case has been essentially negative, and during this time I have not noticed similar cases in my practice.

It seemed to me to be significant that each patient had been receiving thalidomide ("distaval") in a dose of 100 mg. at night, the period during which the drug had been given varying from eighteen months to over two years. Thalidomide is generally regarded as being remarkably free of toxic effects, but in this instance the drug was stopped. Three of the patients have now received no thalidomide for two to three months, and there has been a marked improvement in their symptoms, but they are still present. The fourth patient stopped taking the drug two weeks ago, and it is therefore too early to assess the effect of withdrawal.

It would appear that these symptoms could possibly be a toxic effect of thalidomide.

Turriff, Aberdeenshire.   A. LESLIE FLORENCE.

Q: You also made no investigation to see whether the baby born [on January 5, 1961] to your patient, Betty Morgan, was a baby that might have been produced by medication you had given to Betty Morgan: did you?

DR. NULSEN: No.

Q: You just assumed that whatever medication she got from you couldn't have caused this?

DR. NULSEN: Yes.

— deposition of Ray O. Nulsen, 1976

Eleven

Frances rang in New Year's 1961 cozily at home. She and Ellis were teaching the girls to play bridge and making plans to find a larger house.

It was a needed break after a stressful end of the year: George, the family dog, had fallen sick and died. A blizzard blanketed the city, burying their station wagon in snow. And Frances's father, Colonel Oldham, the affectionate and funny man who called her "Baby" well into her adulthood, had passed away. Frances had flown to Vancouver for the funeral—her first commercial airplane trip ever—returning to Washington officially an orphan.

Frances's return to the FDA offices in January brought the pressures of work back: Joseph Murray of Merrell began hounding her with phone calls and mailings and arrived at her office with new data. When another project sidelined her attention—Frances had been enlisted in the FDA's fight to "suspend" sales of Eaton Laboratories' Altafur, a drug deemed ineffective—Murray grew irate. Frances had become unreachable, working nights, traveling to Boston and Chicago for hearings, increasingly run-down and sick. Murray accused her of causing delays and complained to her boss. Murray said he was under intense strain to move Kevadon along and the vice president of Merrell himself was considering getting on a plane to confront Frances.

But when Frances's schedule finally cleared, any plan she had to move forward on Kevadon halted. Mail from England, delayed due to a strike, finally arrived, and she picked up a *British Medical Journal* from December 1960. As was her custom, she read every page, including the end-page correspondence. There it was, a letter to the editor: "Is Thalidomide to Blame?"

A Scottish physician was suggesting that the new sedative had toxic effects on nerve endings. Four of his patients taking thalidomide had developed paresthesia of the hands and feet, leg cramps, coldness of the extremities,
ataxia—a painful array of symptoms called "peripheral neuritis."

The letter had been printed months earlier . . . but not a peep from
Merrell about these reported side effects. Frances was livid.

When Joseph Murray called to check in, Frances tested him: She
stayed quiet about what she'd read to see if he would mention it. To her
horror—nothing. After months of her asking for data on long-term effects
on humans! Frances then told him that according to the *BMJ*, Merrell's
wonder drug had neurotoxic side effects. Murray calmly admitted to having seen the letter, but only recently. The matter seemed of little concern
to him.

At that point, Frances ended the call and deemed Merrell's resubmit-
ted application incomplete. She demanded a laundry list of new paperwork: any data looking at the possible relationship between long-term
exposure to the drug and nerve damage; detailed data from Merrell's animal experiments; and the names of all trial doctors administering thalidomide to human patients for four months or longer.

By the end of February, she got her list: fifty-six physicians. These were
Raymond Pogge's first doctors, plus a few signed on by Jones.

But Murray made no mention of the seven-hundred-plus doctors enlisted by the company's detail men—doctors, at that moment, dispensing
the drug to more than twenty thousand Americans.

Murray's nonchalance about the peripheral neuritis news was a sham. A
week earlier, he had written urgently to Denis Burley at Distillers asking
for "any comments you may have on the peripheral neuritis report." Merrell management was so nervous about how this development would affect
their FDA application that the firm soon sent Joseph Murray and Thomas
Jones abroad to investigate.

On Monday, March 6, 1961, the duo arrived at the Distillers main office in London to meet with its top executives, including Kennedy. The
British firm, it turned out, had known about the peripheral neuritis problem long before Leslie Florence's letter in the *British Medical Journal*.

In fact, Florence had first alerted them to his concerns in February of

1959, ten months after the drug hit the market. As a general practitioner in Turriff, Scotland, Florence had been giving one-hundred-milligram doses of Distaval (thalidomide) to adult patients—plus himself and his wife— and fifty milligrams to his three-year-old son, whose eczema upset his sleep. But when Florence's legs grew dimpled and swollen, he wrote to Distillers: "I do not think it is in any way bound up in Distaval, but merely mention it in case any similar cases have occurred." Nonetheless, Florence wanted "a list of side effects—if any."

Denis Burley, medical adviser at Distillers, sent Florence an inventory of thalidomide's rare side effects: rash, dry mouth, constipation, and reports of nausea, vertigo, and vomiting at some one-hundred-milligram doses. But Burley made no mention of the numbness and dizziness reported in the early Grünenthal trials and claimed he was entirely "unable to ascribe" Florence's leg problems to Distaval.

The following year, Distillers received more reports linking peripheral neuritis to the drug, enough that by August of 1960, the company started quietly referencing the condition on the drug's packaging. By November, the firm notified Mückter at Grünenthal that "in the last year we have come to realise that long term thalidomide therapy (3 months or more) may give rise to peripheral neuritis."

But when Florence and his patients took a turn for the worse— Florence's legs ached with numbness, and his patients complained of agonizing tingling in their extremities—Florence decided to go public with his concerns. The *British Medical Journal* ran his letter about thalidomide on December 31, 1960.

Florence's letter opened a floodgate. Some *seventy* additional cases of peripheral neuritis had since been relayed to Distillers. Burley, in the meeting with the Merrell men, confessed that the number was rising daily.

Jones and Murray quickly sensed the peril to their FDA application and bombarded Distillers with questions: After how long did symptoms develop? At what dosages? Was there a treatment? And did anyone know *how* the drug damaged nerves?

The Distillers executives suggested Jones and Murray speak to the complaining doctors.

Leslie Florence was their first stop. Florence, a jovial, rosy-cheeked man who brought his dog to work, politely explained to the Merrell men the excruciating cramping and "pins and needles" his patients had felt. His sample group was small—four cases—but Florence also described his own painful symptoms. When he had stopped taking thalidomide, the cramping had ended, but the pins and needles—despite what Distillers was claiming—persisted.

Next, Jones and Murray visited an Edinburgh neurologist who related eight mild peripheral neuritis cases. Like Florence, Dr. J. A. Simpson hammered home a worrisome point: Withdrawing the drug did *not* stop the pins and needles. Another neurologist, at Middlesex Hospital in London, described twelve cases—some quite severe. One patient had lost significant muscle mass in the thigh. Again, stopping the drug had not ended the agonizing pain.

At the week's end, Jones and Murray returned to the Distillers office, where a doctor from Grünenthal, Hans-Werner von Schrader-Beielstein, and a pharmacologist from Distillers, George Somers, joined the discussion.

As Jones and Murray presented the findings of their interviews, Somers grew visibly agitated. He was, in fact, sitting on a secret: A year earlier, while he was testing liquid thalidomide, *all* his lab mice had died. Like Van Maanen at Merrell, Somers suspected that the sucrose carrier had dangerously enhanced the drug's absorption. Alarmed, he had told his bosses that Grünenthal's liquid thalidomide for children posed "a very real danger of deaths." But Distillers let its own liquid version continue to be used in human trials.

The peripheral neuritis complaints had weighed further on the already worried Somers. Nerve damage linked to thalidomide *tablets* meant the drug might be toxic even in solid form. He had told his bosses to go public with the news, but they countered that the dangers had "got out of perspective." The firm simply removed "non-toxic" and "atoxic" from its promotional materials.

As Jones and Murray presented their findings in the Distillers offices, Somers erupted: He confessed to the whole room that for a full year he had been sitting on data showing acute toxicity of liquid thalidomide. He handed over his paperwork.

Grünenthal's von Schrader-Beielstein jumped in to explain that his firm was already probing the matter. It was looking into whether Somers's mice might have been of an unusual strain. Grünenthal, he wished to make clear, had not suppressed results. In fact, the Merrell men could soon hear the whole story at Grünenthal headquarters: Murray and Jones were invited to Germany.

In January 1961, thalidomide sales in Germany had hit 1.6 million deutsche marks for the month alone. The drug had surpassed all other hypnotics, used daily by more than one million West Germans.

But the *British Medical Journal* letter struck an irreparable blow to Grünenthal. The peripheral neuritis risk was now public; the evasions were up. Word traveled fast, and the drug began falling out of favor. In January 1961, two Grünenthal executives trying to license thalidomide in East Germany were turned down because the country's health authorities knew of the nerve damage reports.

And in February 1961, Ralf Voss—the neurologist who had repeatedly complained to the firm of his patients' suffering—demanded the drug be placed on prescription. *None* of his fourteen patients had recovered.

A Bonn University clinic medical director soon after forbade use of thalidomide at his clinic and told Grünenthal to remove it from the market completely. The director of a nerve clinic accused the firm of making dangerously misleading claims.

Increasingly desperate, Grünenthal sales representatives tried to "foster confusion" when doctors asked about peripheral neuritis. One proposed combining thalidomide with decoy ingredients to blame for side effects. The firm even hired a private detective to dig up dirt on naysaying patients and doctors, smuggling a fake female patient into the offices of a neurologist planning a disparaging paper. But the only suggestive discovery made by Grünenthal's detective was the name Ralf Voss—along with other thalidomide critics—on a Bayer visitor log. This allowed Grünenthal to posit, briefly, that in an act of corporate sabotage, the rival firm had orchestrated the entire anti-Contergan campaign.

But after the number of nerve damage complaints reached four hundred, Grünenthal privately conceded that "for a large percentage of these cases, no other explanation remains than that Contergan is the trigger." To counter any impression that profit trumped safety, the firm announced it would voluntarily apply for a prescription requirement.

But in March of 1961, when the Merrell team arrived at Grünenthal's offices, the Germans downplayed the situation. Thomas Jones and Joseph Murray first met with Grünenthal's Dr. von Schrader-Beielstein and Dr. Günther Sievers in Hamburg. The Grünenthal men did not tell the Americans that the drug had been restricted to prescription—they would wait another three months to advise Merrell of this—and admitted to only forty-eight reports of peripheral neuritis. They emphasized that many doctors had used thalidomide on vast numbers of patients for a long time without "any complications apart from occasional allergy."

As proof, Sievers and von Schrader-Beielstein took the Merrell men on a local meet and greet: Dr. Michael Winzreid, a German psychiatrist who had used thalidomide on some one thousand patients, told Murray and Jones he didn't have a single peripheral neuritis case. Another psychiatrist in Düren said he had given almost four hundred patients long-term daily dosages of 100 to 300 milligrams—sometimes as high as 1,500 milligrams daily. Only three patients, he claimed, had mild adverse reactions— nothing verging on nerve damage.

Finally, Jones and Murray were introduced to a pair of detractors: Two doctors at the University of Cologne had nine patients with paresthesia and limb cramping. Some had muscle deterioration in their thighs and numbness in their hands and feet. On withdrawal of thalidomide, the cramping disappeared slowly, but the paresthesia lingered.

By the time Jones and Murray reached Grünenthal's Stolberg headquarters, the firm wasn't disputing the occurrence of peripheral neuritis. Instead, one of its executives, Dr. Gotthold-Erich Werner, fingered vitamin B_1 deficiencies as the culprit, not thalidomide.

Surprised, the Merrell men pressed for proof. When Werner admitted he had none, things got heated. Werner's claim appeared baseless. But eventually all the men in the room agreed that an investigation into vitamin B_1 metabolism in patients on thalidomide might prove fruitful.

The Merrell team returned to the United States, aware of at least 150 cases of peripheral neuritis linked to thalidomide in Great Britain and Germany. Murray would have to figure out how to present this sobering information to the FDA. Grünenthal, for its part, began to turn its attention to a new, more alarming problem that had arisen with thalidomide: complaints about deformed babies.

I agree with you that handling this subject in an

informal way is preferable to written reports.

—*Thomas Jones (William S. Merrell Company)*

to Denis Burley (Distillers),

April 28, 1961

Thalidomide and Peripheral Neuritis Report

Twelve

Barbara Moulton, Frances's closest confidante, was now a regular fixture at the Kelsey house. She stayed over to watch the girls when Frances and Ellis traveled for work; she helped Frances strategize before big FDA meetings. When Barbara started dating a newly divorced government economist—Eppes Wayles Browne, Jr.—she immediately brought him to dinner to meet the Kelsey clan.

But the highlights for Frances were the weekends spent at Moulton's farm. The sprawling West Virginia property, located near Charles Town, included an eleven-room stone house and 140 Holstein cows. Frances's daughters, Susan and Christine, were dazzled by the estate and by Moulton's brazen fondness for cigarettes and booze. They were amazed when their hostess slept unabashedly late on Saturday morning. Equally impressive was her Sunday-morning ritual—Moulton bolted out of bed and led the girls to milk the cows. Moulton, passionate about her herd, tracked milking patterns like baseball statistics.

Moulton reveled in making her own rules, but in the professional sphere, she had paid for this dearly. Almost a year since she testified before Congress, her search for government work was coming up dry.

Frances, aware of her friend's exile, had been practicing restraint in her FDA communications. Where Moulton was brash and outspoken, Frances exercised self-control. But when Joseph Murray returned from Germany, trying to blow off the whole peripheral neuritis issue, Frances erupted in anger.

On March 30, Murray strode into her office with a colleague, Thomas Jones. Murray put forth a strange theory: The reports of nerve damage might stem from vitamin deficiencies, not thalidomide. Their interviews

overseas, he claimed, had indicated that peripheral neuritis affected a minuscule number of people and resolved quickly if the drug was discontinued. Reports from their own American trial doctors, he added, suggested
near-negligible nerve problems.

Murray offered a meager amendment to the Kevadon package insert:
"Pins and needles of the fingers and toes, numbness and muscle cramps
have been reported in a small percent of patients receiving thalidomide
continuously for 3 to 6 months. Immediate withdrawal of the drug is recommended since this has resulted in prompt reversal of symptoms."

Frances pushed back. Why would a doctor give a patient thalidomide
when there were safer sedatives? And where was the information on the
drug's metabolism and absorption she had demanded months earlier? If
they kept giving her the runaround, she'd find the answers herself. In fact,
she was about to attend a pharmacology conference where she could dig
for information.

The threat rattled Murray, and the men headed straight to her supervisor, Ralph Smith. For seven whole months they had been waiting on their
application, waiting on Frances. They wanted help. Murray had known
Smith for years but couldn't get a read on him. Smith just peered at the
men through his clear-framed glasses and scribbled notes. Having been
publicly accused by Barbara Moulton of issuing dangerous "instructions
from above," Smith did not look eager to intervene.

Dejected, the Merrell team left. A lot had been riding on this FDA trip,
because back at Merrell's headquarters, the future of triparanol (MER/29)
was looking bleak. The cholesterol drug was amassing piles of awful reports. The president of Richardson-Merrell was predicting "damage suits."

If MER/29 was off the market, the company would start to sink. In the
two-plus years since Merrell had paid Grünenthal to license thalidomide,
buying the raw material, manufacturing pills, and enlisting its entire sales
force, Merrell had yet to earn a single cent from the drug. The firm was
getting "really angry" and was considering "drastic measures."

So Murray lobbied Frances harder. He set deadlines—decide in a
week, or else. . . . His language grew threatening. He said his company
was prepared to exert pressure and Merrell's vice president would visit
Commissioner Larrick to demand an official "yes or no." A "no," he made
clear, would be appealed at a hearing.

But the animal toxicity reports Frances had requested had yet to appear, and Murray hadn't come close to addressing her request for studies showing *how* thalidomide worked in the body.

Her patience wore thin. And then came a report from the Mayo Clinic saying that their cholesterol pill triparanol caused a litany of troubling side effects, which Merrell had blatantly hidden from the FDA.

Further convinced of Merrell's dishonesty, Frances drafted a warning to Murray about Kevadon: "Abandon any idea of obtaining clearance for this drug except on the basis of the submission of adequate information to demonstrate its safety." And if they refused additional studies? She would recommend a hearing to determine if the application should be once and for all formally refused. She issued another "incomplete" on the firm's most recent paperwork and then—this was risky—accused Murray of lying about peripheral neuritis: He had clearly failed to "make a frank disclosure" about the side effect.

Frances's letter incensed Merrell. Her statements were "libelous," Murray railed over the phone. The next day, he arrived with his colleague, Robert H. Woodward, demanding to speak to someone senior. The men sat with William Kessenich, medical director of the Bureau of Medicine, and relayed their frustrations. Kessenich arranged a group meeting the following day.

On May 11, Frances listened to an exasperated Murray as he blamed his silence about peripheral neuritis on a "failure of communication" between Merrell and its overseas affiliates. He begged the agency to at last "expedite" the Kevadon application.

But Frances was frosty. She still wanted case reports on peripheral neuritis patients, plus the animal data she'd requested months earlier. At that point, Frances leveled a totally new demand.

She'd been recalling her wartime work with Ellis on quinine in rabbits and its effects on a rabbit embryo. If Kevadon could induce neuropathy after just three or four months, what would happen during pregnancy, with a fetus exposed for up to nine months?

Frances demanded to see evidence that the drug was safe during pregnancy.

Part III

THE
FIGHT

Upper and lower extremities appear to be fins. . . .

Dr. Nulsen here.

—nurse's report on Baby Girl X,

born May 10, 1961, Cincinnati, Ohio,

4 lbs., 4 oz.

On April 5, 1961, Thomas David Diamond, first son of Mr. and Mrs. Thomas Dixon Diamond, was born at the Abington Memorial Hospital, in Abington, Pennsylvania, just outside of Philadelphia. Unfortunately, little David was born with severe birth malformations. Although each of the malformations that David had were previously reported individually in the medical literature, no one either at Abington Hospital or the Children's Hospital in Philadelphia, where the boy was treated, had seen or read in the medical literature of a single case where all of these malformations were manifested in one child.

—Arthur G. Raynes, Esq.,
attorney for Mr. and Mrs. Diamond

American Trial Lawyers Association Midwinter Meeting, 1969,
San Francisco, California

When I was born, the doctors handed my momma a piece of paper to institutionalize me and said, "Here, you sign this, we'll take care of her. You don't have to worry about it." And so she signed it, because that was what they did then. But my dad said he had to see me. He wanted to see me before they gave me up, and as soon as he saw me, he knew he couldn't send me away. So he brought me home. Both his family and my mom's family were really mad and disgusted with him. . . . But I don't think I would have survived an institution. . . . It's a miracle that I'm here.

—Dorothy Hunt-Honsinger,
born June 1961, Meadville, Pennsylvania

Thirteen

In a vast suburban Baltimore house, a stately gray-haired woman in her sixties sat at the head of a dining table and lifted a bell to signal to Mrs. Clark, her housekeeper, to clear the china and serve dessert.

It was a Sunday evening in January 1962.

Helen Taussig, a renowned cardiologist, loved entertaining at her Roland Park house, as well as at her summer home by Nantucket Sound. She had never married or had children, but as one of the first female full professors at Johns Hopkins University, she had amassed a flock of former medical students and fellows who felt to her like family. Anointing themselves her devoted "knights," they gathered regularly for Professor Taussig's "Round Table" conversations. The warmth of her sloping blue eyes and broad smile put patients and colleagues at ease.

That evening, her guest of honor was a young German physician named Alois Beuren, a foreign fellow at her Johns Hopkins clinic from the year before who had trained with her in pediatric cardiology. On his return to Germany, Ali had begun researching Williams syndrome, a rare illness characterized by "elfin faces," growth delays, mild mental retardation, and congenital heart defects.

But that night, Ali was eagerly telling his mentor about another matter, a bizarre epidemic that had recently terrified the German medical community. Across the elegant table, Ali spoke of an outbreak of birth defects in West Germany. A condition known as phocomelia—in which babies were born with flipper-like "seal limbs"—was turning up in staggering numbers across the country, despite previously being so rare that most doctors would never encounter a single case. What Ali thought might particularly interest Helen was that many of the babies suffered heart defects.

Through her rimless glasses, Helen studied Ali's lips and listened carefully—no easy feat, as she was almost entirely deaf. The chime of her own dinner bell often eluded her. Lipreading and a hearing aid guided her through most conversations, but she had also trained her hands to sense sound and was famous in the hospital for her ability to read a child's heart rhythms by touch alone. Helen's deafness stemmed from a childhood bout of whooping cough. But an early struggle with dyslexia had left her with preternatural powers of concentration, which she now trained on the young man at her table.

"What is more," Ali told her, "they think it is caused by a sleeping tablet."

When the dessert plates were cleared and the dinner ended, Helen Taussig retired for the night. But the next morning, the magnitude of Ali's news seized her—a drug entirely safe for the mother ravaged the unborn child. Children had been the focus of her entire career, and many times over she had risked her reputation trying to help them. Her mind raced. How widely was this drug used? What did this mean for the purported safety of other drugs? She decided she must go to Germany.

The youngest of four children in an exceptionally accomplished academic family, Helen Brooke Taussig was born on May 24, 1898, in Cambridge, Massachusetts. Her father, Frank Taussig, was the Henry Lee Professor of Economics at Harvard and co-founder of the Harvard School of Business Administration. Her mother, Edith, was one of the first women enrolled at Radcliffe College and had imbued her children with her love of botany and zoology. During summers on Cape Cod, Helen was urged to explore nature—hiking, gardening, and studying the beautiful intricacies of flowers. But when Helen was eleven, her mother died of tuberculosis, leaving the Taussig children under the purview of their father.

Helen was also struck with tuberculosis, which limited her to half days of school. On top of that, reading, spelling, and number recognition proved a labyrinth for young Helen. Getting through a single sentence was like running a mental gauntlet. No one in that day understood dyslexia, and Helen's teachers thought humiliation might be the cure, so they shamed her daily. Helen's father, fearing Helen might not complete grammar school, took time from his academic work to intensively tutor her.

His efforts, combined with Helen's determination to decode each word, letter by letter, cultivated her formidable focus. Not only did she complete grammar school, but she became an academic star, eventually following in her mother's footsteps and entering Radcliffe.

But college proved rocky for Helen. Her father remarried and moved to Washington to become a member of the Tariff Commission. Helen's grades plummeted, and she grew tired of being known in Cambridge circles as "Professor Taussig's daughter." Increasingly hungry for independence, she transferred to Berkeley for her final two college years. In 1921, her Phi Beta Kappa AB degree in hand, she celebrated with a trip to Yosemite in the thick of winter, an adventure she would brag about for years.

When Helen returned east, interested in pursuing medicine, she soon learned that her gender would bar her from the best opportunities. The dean of Harvard's new School of Public Health told Helen that while she could take classes, an actual degree was off limits. Eventually, she finagled special permission to take two courses at Harvard Medical School—bacteriology and histology (the study of tissues). Even then she was relegated to classroom corners and banished to a separate room to examine slides.

Fortunately, an astute mentor sensed Helen's intelligence and suggested she switch to Boston University's medical school. At BU, Helen still wasn't permitted to get a medical degree, but she could take a full course load—physiology, pharmacology, cardiology, and anatomy (Harvard forbade women from studying the *whole* body). Cardiology quickly enthralled her and she next applied to Johns Hopkins. In 1890, five feisty Baltimore women, all well educated and unmarried, four of them daughters of Hopkins trustees, had agreed to raise capital to build a medical school on the sole condition that it take women. In 1893, the first female medical students—three—had enrolled. In 1924, Helen Taussig joined a cadre of ten women (in an incoming class of seventy).

Her MD at last in hand, Helen then won a yearlong fellowship at the Johns Hopkins Heart Station, which she followed with an internship in pediatrics. An astute adviser, Dr. Edward Park, fearing the sexism Helen would face practicing medicine, suggested she pick a little-known—thus less competitive—subspecialty, congenital heart malformations.

Just as Frances Kelsey would thrive in the once-obscure domain of pharmacology, Helen flourished in her fringe field. Then the sounds of the world around her began to fade, and Helen realized she was going deaf. Doctors blamed a childhood whooping cough episode for damaging her inner ears, and by 1930, Helen could no longer follow a basic conversation or use the single device her whole career depended on: the stethoscope.

Desperate, she bought a locket-style hearing aid that hung like a necklace beneath her dress. When she lost the thread of a conversation, she had to whip the device out from her dress and wave it in front of the speaker's face. Vacillating between hollering and whispering, Helen soon taught herself lipreading. At lectures and seminars, she sat up front to carefully study the presenter's mouth.

But the fundamental diagnostic means of her specialty—listening to the heartbeat of a child—still eluded her. An amplified stethoscope helped moderately, but the speaker box loomed cumbersomely beside young patients. So Helen taught herself to "listen" with her hands. At home, she placed her fingertips on sofa cushions to feel the vibrations of radio music. She touched everything, focusing, concentrating, attuned to the slightest shift in movement and sound. Soon, with her palms alone placed on the chest of a child, she could not only measure a heartbeat but even detect a murmur or arrhythmia that other doctors, with mere stethoscopes, had missed. Helen, as no other doctor ever had, became known for the extraordinary keenness of her touch.

In 1930, thirty-year-old Helen Taussig was named the physician in charge of the cardiac clinic at Harriet Lane Home for Invalid Children. Mastering the new fluoroscope—a powerful X-ray-like device—she began to detect patterns in the hearts of "blue babies"—cyanotic children with blue lips and skin. Taussig posited that opening the ductus arteriosus with an artificial shunt might save the young children, and sought a heart surgeon willing to brave such an operation on an infant. Dr. Alfred Blalock, the new chair of the Department of Surgery at Johns Hopkins, agreed to try it. He enlisted his assistant Vivien Thomas—a Black wunderkind whose financial straits and race had kept him from medical school—and the duo commenced experiments with dogs. After two hundred canine practice rounds, in November 1943 they successfully performed the surgery on Eileen Saxon, a nine-pound one-year-old, and within months

Helen was recommending the procedure widely. On May 19, 1945, the team published "The Surgical Treatment of Malformations of the Heart" in *The Journal of the American Medical Association,* which drew cyanotic children from all over the world for the new "Blalock-Taussig operation" or "blue baby surgery."

In 1947, Helen published her groundbreaking opus, *Congenital Malformations of the Heart,* and soon became the first woman elected to the sixty-five-year-old Association of American Physicians. As more prizes followed, students from around the world flocked to work with her, always eager to discuss current medical research. So by the time Alois Beuren sat at her dining table that chilly winter night in 1962, he was excited to relay information about the phocomelia outbreak in Germany, and Helen was rapt.

So worrisome was the news that Helen began a frenzy of trip planning. She telephoned the Maryland Heart Association and the International Society of Cardiology Foundation and within forty-eight hours secured a $1,000 travel grant. She wrote to the German doctor Ali had named as the expert on the crisis—Widukind Lenz—and arranged to meet him in Germany. Ali, who soon returned to Germany, made introductions from overseas, and Ali's boss, a professor of pediatrics at the Children's Clinic in Göttingen, agreed to meet with Helen. She now had a unique opportunity to investigate, up close, the cause of a heart malformation, and to gather clinical evidence.

This would not be Helen's first trip to Germany. In October of 1960, she had attended a pediatric conference where she had unknowingly passed a small exhibit with X-rays and photographs of two infants with phocomelia—a condition defined as the "congenital absence of the upper arm and/or upper leg, the hands or feet or both being attached to the trunk by a short stump." The word was an amalgam of two Greek words: *phōkē* (seal) and *melos* (limb). For the doctors who had arranged the display, their cases had seemed a stunning find. Few physicians ever encountered phocomelia, and a sixteenth-century drawing by Goya in a medical encyclopedia usually served as the sole visual medical reference. The doctors had no idea that at the time of that conference, more than six hundred phocomelic babies had just been born in Germany. By the time Helen boarded her plane to investigate, the number had risen to several thousand.

It would be an understatement to say that my wife

and I were happy in the Spring of 1961.

—*Karl-Hermann Schulte-Hillen,*

Germany

Fourteen

Around midnight on April 24, 1961, when Linde Schulte-Hillen's contractions began, her husband brought her to the Hamburg hospital. Throughout the night, twenty-one-year-old Linde lay in a room with six other women separated by grayish-green plastic curtains. Clipped to her bed was a bell, which she had been instructed to ring if her pain intensified. It did not. Labor progressed slowly and Linde, calm, barely touched the bell, listening only to the moans of the surrounding women.

In the morning, her husband, Karl, a thirty-two-year-old law student in the last months of his studies, left the hospital to head back to the university. He promised Linde a quick return. It was exam time, and he had a crucial appointment. But by midday, while Karl was still gone, Linde's contractions had intensified. At 1:00 P.M., as a physician and midwife urged her along, Linde pushed a baby boy into the world.

His name was Jan.

At first, the birth seemed normal to Linde. She did not see Jan when he came out. The nurse simply instructed her to avoid touching the sterile cloth placed between her legs. Linde complied, lay back, and glimpsed her baby at a distance, being whisked from the room.

But as she lay there, exhausted, Linde sensed a bustling in the hallway. People were running to and fro. She could not fight her tired eyes drifting closed, but she soon woke to a nurse at her side.

"Is your husband . . . crippled by any chance?" the nurse asked.

"Is the baby not okay?" Linde gasped.

The nurse then explained: Linde's baby boy had short stumps instead of arms.

"Maybe they will grow?" a confused Linde asked.

"No," the nurse said coldly. "They will probably fall off."

The nurse's demeanor began to alarm Linde. As far as Linde knew, the problem was only with her baby's arms, but Linde sensed her son being given up for dead. She questioned the woman, only to learn that Jan had been set on the nursery floor, rather than in a crib. He had not even received the standard eye drops or shots.

It had been only fifteen years since the Nazi regime had targeted disabled people for sterilization and mass extermination. Almost a quarter million Germans with mental or physical disabilities, deemed burdens to society, had been involuntarily euthanized under Hitler's T4 plan. Linde, fearing her newborn son was being written off as "wasted life," demanded to see Jan. But the nurse refused and left the room, leaving Linde, alone, to stare at the blank wall, agonizing over her son's fate. What did life hold in store for such a child?

Meanwhile, Karl had returned to the hospital, unaware his son had already been born. He smoked in the waiting room until a doctor appeared. The chief of the hospital, in fact. Karl's throat went dry. He sensed something was amiss. For over a month, he had been fearing a problem with the birth. Six weeks earlier, he had gone to see his sister, Annette, in nearby Kiel, where she and her husband had just welcomed their second child. But the baby girl—inexplicably—had been born with shortened arms. Karl had kept the news quiet, so as not to worry Linde, but the strangeness of it—his sister's first child had been perfectly healthy—troubled him.

"You have a son," the doctor now told Karl in the hospital waiting room. But the words came awkwardly, and the man looked embarrassed.

"You can't mean that he hasn't any arms!" Karl erupted.

"How did you know?" the doctor asked.

Without answering, Karl stormed off to find Linde. Karl considered himself tough. He was certain he could handle what lay ahead. But his heart raced anxiously for his young wife, who, nearly a decade younger, knew little of suffering.

Karl found Linde alone in her bed, her face wrecked from crying.

"The boy is ours," Karl announced. "Our child." The arms didn't matter, he assured her.

But Linde turned to the wall. "I'm not even able to give you a normal child," she cried, then begged him to leave. Karl knew he could no longer keep the secret. He must absolve her of guilt.

"You are not alone," he confessed. "I have seen my sister's child . . . and it . . . is like ours."

Linde turned to him, shocked. What had happened to these babies?

Linde (short for Dietlind) Bergert was a slim seventeen-year-old with golden-blond hair and dark brown eyes when Karl Schulte-Hillen spotted her at a university dance. Tall and broad-shouldered, Karl had a rugged confidence that struck Linde as very manly. Her handsome suitor—the son of a lawyer—seemed to do everything with great deliberation, knowing what he wanted and going after it. Linde was what he wanted.

Karl had been raised by strict parents in Menden. The second of four children, he was a chubby boy, forced to jog to school alongside his father's car to get fit. At fourteen, Karl was drafted to serve on the Russian front in the deadly frost. During the day, Karl dug trenches, and at night, he slept in newspaper and hay, huddled with other soldiers to stave off the biting, subzero temperatures. When the war ended, a weathered teenage Karl hopped a transport back west and walked the last tiring miles to Germany.

Back home, Karl helped support his family through the bleak postwar years. He took up carpentry, grew cauliflower and potatoes, and hunted wild animals for food. Eventually, missing the life of the mind, Karl signed up for university night classes. After he got his baccalaureate, he met Linde at the dance and proposed quickly.

Since Linde was just beginning her university studies, the lovebirds lived frugally. Karl, who had decided to follow in his father's footsteps and pursue a law degree, juggled odd jobs to make rent. After the happy students had been engaged for three years and married for one, Linde became pregnant. But Jan's birth nine months later abruptly wrenched all joy from their lives.

Despondent after learning of his son's condition, Karl wandered the cobbled streets of Hamburg, fixating on people's hands and arms. He could not fathom what had happened. But he knew he must be strong—Linde was suffering the worst of it.

His sister, Annette, had given birth at home, spared the violent shock.

The baby had been quickly swaddled, out of Annette's sight, giving her husband time to lay roses on the bed before gently handing her their uncovered baby. "Things are not always the way one would wish," he'd calmly told her, promising to stand by the child.

Annette, already a mother and a decade older than Linde, remained calm. She had also grown up in the tough Schulte-Hillen household.

"It's our child," Annette said, without tears. "We must give her all our love and help."

But Linde had been alone for the birth, at the mercy of a heartless hospital staff. She was still suffering greatly, and Karl knew he had to help her navigate the emotional challenges ahead. For that, he needed to know what had happened.

When Karl heard that a third woman in the area had birthed a child with identical defects, he returned to the hospital. What had caused his son's deformities? he asked the chief doctor. Would he and Linde be able to have another child? A healthy child? No, said the professor, Jan's case had to be hereditary. Preposterous, thought Karl. Not only had this kind of defect never appeared in his family, but he knew from biology that he and Linde would have to share some rare genetic trait to pass it to their son. This would mean Annette and her husband also shared the trait—except their first child had been spared. And what of the other Hamburg woman? Three babies in a month? Karl pressed the doctor: Had he *ever* seen anything similar?

The doctor issued a firm denial and walked off.

Karl, frustrated, stood alone, until a nearby man beckoned him over. From his clothes, the man appeared to work in the hospital, but it was unclear if he was a doctor or technician. He did not offer his name.

"What did the boss say to you?" the man asked.

"That he'd never seen a baby like mine," Karl answered.

The man considered this, then said, "He isn't telling you the truth. . . . I have seen this before. Here." Then he rushed off, and Karl, stunned, went to find Linde.

The days since the birth had been grueling for Linde. She lay in the crowded hospital room, watching mothers cuddle their healthy newborns. It had taken three days for the hospital staff to let her see Jan—by which point she had grown afraid to look at him. When she finally did hold him, she felt gutted. As if her own arms had been cut off. She demanded the staff cut away the unnecessary sleeves on his swaddle jacket—she would pay for the jacket herself, the extra arm fabric a pointless taunt.

She had been begging Karl to take her home, but it was only on Jan's fifth day that they were released. Linde was relieved to be home, but Karl feared despair would soon overtake her. Conferring on how best to guide their families, Karl and his brother-in-law agreed: no shame, no guilt.

"This means telling everybody the whole truth," Karl explained to Linde, "without hiding anything whatever." If they showed the slightest shame, or any desire to hide the tragedy, the bad attitude would bring trouble, especially to Jan. They must "face things squarely," Karl declared.

Nagging at Karl's mind, however, was the fear that someday his son would grow up and ask: "What's the matter with me? What happened to me?" And while Karl could let go of shame and guilt, he would need an answer for his boy.

I would find it an exceptionally heavy setback if we give the impression that sales are more important to us than the responsibility which we carry as a pharmaceutical manufacturer. On the active side of our balance sheet, the firm's reputation is in my opinion at least as worthwhile as the Contergan sales in DM.

—Chemie Grünenthal internal memo,

May 10, 1961

Fifteen

Late in the evening of Thursday, May 4, 1961, thirty-three-year-old William McBride got a call at his home in Blakehurst, Australia, to attend a complicated birth. McBride, an ambitious workaholic, ran one of the largest obstetrical practices in Sydney, Australia. He was on call twenty-four hours a day, seven days a week. A tall man with intense blue eyes and a beak of a nose, his brown wavy hair was always side parted. He was wildly successful for his young age, and his confidence stirred envy in colleagues. But no one outside the Sydney medical community had ever heard of him. That was about to change.

Saying goodbye to his wife, Patricia, McBride got into his car and drove from his small suburban home into the city. In the darkness, he switched on the radio and heard the crackle of news: On the other side of the globe, John F. Kennedy had just completed his first one hundred days as president of the United States. It was late autumn in Australia and one of the coldest days in thirty years. When McBride arrived at Crown Street Women's Hospital—a four-story late-Victorian building, the largest maternity hospital in Sydney—he headed straight to the beige surgical room where the sterile instruments had been laid out. Dr. Paton, the thirtysomething-year-old anesthetist, grumbled about the chill.

On the operating table lay twenty-three-year-old Alice Wilson. The wife of a pharmacist, Alice was McBride's private patient. He had overseen her whole healthy pregnancy. She had entered the hospital uneventfully that day when her labor had started, but by nightfall an erratic fetal heartbeat—the pace would quicken, then slow—alarmed the duty nurse. A cesarean was ordered, and McBride was called.

McBride lost no time scrubbing in and commencing the operation, and the procedure went smoothly. But when the baby was finally lifted from its mother, McBride and his team stood in shock: The baby was missing both arms, and on each hand—hands that seemed to sprout directly from the shoulders—was an extra finger.

They scrambled to do the routine treatments: clearing the newborn's air passages, administering oxygen and vitamin K injections. When Dr. Paton slapped the newborn's feet, the sound of healthy cries filled the room, and relief settled in.

"It seems quite normal otherwise," remarked Paton, bewildered.

Since the mother was still fully sedated and he could postpone delivering the awful news, McBride returned home, tired and confused.

Snow fell thickly through the night, and McBride's drive to the hospital the next morning proved arduous: roads were closed, trees were toppled. But he was determined to check on Mrs. Wilson's baby. When he finally arrived at the hospital, the attending nurse reported that the baby had been vomiting. X-rays revealed a bowel blockage. Alarmed, McBride transferred the baby to the Royal Alexandra Hospital for Children for emergency surgery. During the operation, the surgeon noticed another dangerously underdeveloped bowel area blocking digestion. Within the week, the baby was dead.

McBride was rattled. In seven years of delivering babies, he had never seen internal or external damage as severe as what he'd seen in Baby Wilson. Then, three weeks later, on May 24, McBride was called to attend the labor of another private patient, Susan Wood. Once again, an erratic fetal heartbeat necessitated a cesarean. Upstairs, in the same operating theater, with the same attending nurses, McBride lifted up Susan Wood's newborn and saw that Baby Wood looked almost exactly like Baby Wilson. This baby, too, began vomiting. Within five days, that child had died as well.

Among the ward nurses, suspicion stirred. Since the start of the year, a surge of pregnant women had entered the hospital and miscarried, many of the fetuses displaying odd malformations. Even more troubling: All these women were Dr. McBride's patients. The nurses relayed this to the night supervisor of the labor ward, Sister Patricia Sparrow, who alerted

McBride to the "outbreak." But it wasn't until June 8, when McBride delivered another misshapen baby, to Shirley Tait, that the connection hit him with full force. When Baby Tait died after birth, the labor ward erupted in tumult. Three babies with wildly rare abnormalities born within weeks?

Meanwhile, John Newlinds, the Crown Street medical superintendent, had realized that the hospital's congenital malformation rate was running triple the national average. He and his wife, a pediatrics registrar, had already set up a large wall map, using colored pins to mark the addresses of the ill-fated mothers, trying to untangle the mystery. But the couple had kept their map secret because a cluster of pins around the Atomic Energy Commission's nuclear reactor south of the city might stir public panic.

On June 8, Baby Tait's birth suggested to Newlinds a more obvious link—William McBride.

"For God's sake, Bill," Newlinds demanded, chasing McBride down in the corridor that day, "what is going on?"

On September 16, 1960, a senior sales representative for the Distillers Company, Walter Hodgetts, had visited William McBride in his private practice. A tall, gruff man, Hodgetts could turn on the charm in a sales pitch. He had a stellar sales record, and on that September day, he was peddling a top-selling sleeping pill that had been on the British market for two years—Distaval.

Having recently heard of the drug from a colleague at Bankstown Hospital, McBride gave Hodgetts a quick "yes"—he would try out Distaval as a labor sedative.

When a pregnant woman arrived at Crown Street with hyperemesis gravidarum—severe vomiting that risked miscarriage—and sedation and IV fluids failed to help, McBride recalled Distaval. The obstetrician considered himself cautious when it came to dispensing medicine; his grandfather's first wife reportedly died on a hot summer day when she went to a Sydney pharmacist to buy citric acid for an elderflower cordial and was mistakenly given cyanic acid—akin to pure *cyanide*. McBride knew Distaval was marketed primarily as a sedative, but like many doctors of his day, he thought extreme morning sickness stemmed from anxiety, the angst over unexpected or unwanted pregnancies. Recalling Hodgetts's assurance of the drug's unparalleled safety, he ordered two Distaval pills from the hospital pharmacy and gave them to the sick woman. To his delight, her vomiting ceased. After that, McBride made Distaval his go-to remedy for nausea during pregnancy.

By May 9 of the following year, he was still so impressed with the drug that he wrote to the Distillers firm: McBride found Distaval "extremely efficient" in managing "morning sickness and hyperemesis gravidarum" and also an effective labor sedative. "I would be only too pleased to support any application to have this drug put on the National Health Service," he assured the firm.

On May 24, 1961, Distillers confirmed:

We are in receipt of your evaluation of "Distaval" and would like to take this opportunity to express our appreciation for your interest and co-operation.

—F. Strobl, Sales Manager

This letter lay on McBride's desk weeks later, after he had delivered the third malformed baby. As he sat in his office, sifting through patient medical cards, he wondered if the women might have suffered similar illnesses during pregnancy, or if they all lived near the Lucas Heights nuclear reactor. But he soon noted "nausea" as a common complaint and saw that, in each case, he'd administered Distaval.

Back at home, McBride locked himself away from his wife and children, probing the written material on Distaval. In his study, he thumbed page by page through the product's red-covered "Advisory Service Bulletin." According to the safety information, thalidomide had zero risk of acute toxicity—mice given massive doses had survived, and even human overdoses appeared safe. After swallowing twenty-one one-hundred-milligram tablets, a seventy-year-old British man had slept for twelve hours and felt only brief, lingering drowsiness. A two-year-old had fared fine after swallowing seven hundred milligrams. And long-term toxicity—tested in rats, guinea pigs, rabbits, and mice over thirty days—appeared nonexistent.

Nothing in the twenty-page bulletin bumped McBride except for a single line: "Thalidomide is derived from glutamic acid."

Another glutamic derivative, aminopterin, used to treat cancer, had been known for a decade to induce abortion in early pregnancy. McBride still had *The Year Book of Obstetrics and Gynaecology* with the first published report of that.

Scouring the Distillers brochure, McBride now realized nothing indicated that Distaval had actually been tested for safety during pregnancy. He then recalled a piece in the *British Medical Journal* earlier that year. Tearing through the piles of journals on his floor, he found the Leslie Florence letter about thalidomide and nerve damage. If thalidomide *was* harmful, what would happen if it crossed the placental barrier?

Penicillin and morphine were known to traverse the placenta—the former, protecting the fetus from infection; the latter, dangerously depressing fetal heart rate. If thalidomide bore any similarity to aminopterin as a glutamic acid derivative, then the drug might disrupt the embryo's ability to metabolize glutamine, an essential amino acid for cell growth. This was why aminopterin stopped tumor growth and fetal growth. Would thalidomide likewise disrupt development of the fetus?

That was it! McBride wrote furiously into the night, titling his paper "Thalidomide and Congenital Abnormalities." Simple animal experiments, he posited, would confirm if thalidomide crossed the placenta. Hours later, exhausted, he turned off his desk lamp.

The next morning, he set off to work in his car by 8:00 A.M., his handwritten manuscript beside him in his briefcase. His secretary could type it up for submission to *The Lancet*—a London-based journal with an international readership and a reputation for publishing quickly. Speed was of the essence.

At the hospital, McBride telephoned the Distillers office, where he reached Fred Strobl, the sales manager who had sent the grateful note weeks earlier. McBride shared his suspicion and told Strobl to report the news to the firm's headquarters in England. But to McBride's surprise, Strobl found his theory preposterous. The drug had been available in England and a host of other countries for years before it entered the Australian market—how would such a thing go unnoticed?

At lunch with John Newlinds, a frustrated McBride explained that he would have to launch his own animal experiments to prove the connection. But Newlinds didn't want to wait for animal experiments. He telephoned the hospital's chief pharmacist, Mrs. Sperling, and ordered Distaval removed from the pharmacy.

It was June 1961, and the Crown Street Women's Hospital was one of the first in the world to suspend thalidomide.

If you have one man in Australia and one man in Germany independently reaching the same conclusion, it is highly unlikely that they are both crazy.

—Widukind Lenz

Sixteen

It had been a grueling spring for the Schulte-Hillens. Intent on distracting Linde from her sorrow, Karl had urged her to return to her schoolwork, but it wasn't helping. Linde was dejected, lethargic. When she looked at baby Jan, she wept. Friends—uncomfortable at the idea of a handicapped child—had turned their backs. Neither Linde nor Karl could keep up with their studies, and Karl struggled to prepare an important brief for his final law exam. Stress threatened to overwhelm them.

But Karl had a mission: to find out what had harmed his son. His father, a notary in Menden, had asked doctor acquaintances about any similar births and now reported to Karl that around Menden there were a dozen cases like Jan's. One child was already two years old. Karl returned to the hospital and confronted the chief doctor, demanding an investigation. Surely the defects weren't genetic. But the man refused a probe, and Karl realized he would have to launch the inquiry himself. Karl's father contacted a Public Health Service doctor who promised to query area obstetricians. Then Karl and his brother-in-law began a thorough review of Annette's and Linde's activities during pregnancy: Had the mothers been exposed to polluted water? Or had they contracted toxoplasmosis from dogs or farm animals? But the various mothers in Menden, it turned out, did not share a water source, and when Karl had the family basset hound examined and Linde's blood checked, no toxoplasmosis turned up. Thinking that drugs could affect an embryo, Karl asked Linde and his sister what they had used—but his sister had taken only a traditional stomach remedy and Linde hadn't needed any medicine.

Soon the Public Health Service doctor gathering data went silent, so Karl took to calling anyone he knew with connections to medical specialists. He was determined to spare other children Jan's plight—if he could only figure out what had caused it. Finally, on the evening of June 18, Karl got a promising phone call.

"There is one man in Germany capable of throwing himself whole-heartedly into a case like yours," the friend, a medical student, told him. "He's a brilliant man—once he tackles a problem, he never leaves it until he has found the answer."

The doctor, Widukind Lenz, worked at the university children's clinic and specialized in genetics. The day before, a gynecologist at the university hospital had given Karl the same name. An appointment was made to meet Lenz the next day.

Karl's luck was improving: That very night, baby Jan smiled for the first time. The exhausted parents rejoiced to see the keen intelligence in their son's eyes. Certain Jan was mentally fit, the couple resolved to raise him like any other child. For the first time in months, Karl was hopeful as he entered the children's clinic the next morning.

Lenz, Karl had been told, was an obsessive scientist. He lived simply—wearing the same army coat for years, riding a bicycle instead of owning a car—and cared solely for his work. Unknown to Karl was the fact that the doctor he was meeting was the son of Fritz Lenz—a Nazi geneticist. The senior Lenz had for years promoted racial cleansing, recommending "sterilization of all the unfit and inferior"—including the disabled—before Hitler even rose to power. In fact, Fritz Lenz thought some 30 percent of the German population had no right to reproduce, deeming their sterilization the "central mission of all politics." His son, Widukind, however, rejected "race hygiene" and spent the war tending patients in a Luftwaffe factory. Widukind, who spoke five languages and wrote poetry, was kind, hardworking, and quietly intense.

As soon as Karl met the soft-spoken Lenz, he launched into the tale of his son and his niece. The wiry geneticist took copious notes and asked questions about Karl's family, but finally, as though exhausted, said: "We doctors are constantly listening to parents like you who are indignant when we explain to them that a certain deformity in their child is hereditary."

Karl's throat tightened—was Lenz writing him off? He tried to explain about the other children in the region, but Lenz interrupted—"Let's just stick to your own family, shall we?" He had seen none of the children in question, and everything Karl offered was hearsay.

A week later, Karl returned with Jan so that Lenz could examine him. Lenz said little as he studied the three fingers sprouting from the baby boy's shortened arms.

As weeks passed, Karl heard from other doctors in Germany—one in Frankfurt, one in Bavaria—who had delivered babies with similar malformations. A single hospital in Münster had apparently seen twenty children born without arms. With each update, Karl telephoned Lenz, but Lenz seemed uninterested.

Lenz, however, had taken Karl's concerns to heart. The night he had examined Jan, he returned to confer with his wife, Alma, a pediatrician. If there had been similar births in the area, genes were likely not at play— but if not genes, what? Lenz and his wife racked their brains to think what the mothers might have been exposed to. New pesticides on tropical fruits? Something poisonous lingering from wartime uranium experiments?

The next day, Lenz telephoned the gynecologist mentioned by Karl to confirm about ten cases in Menden, plus three babies with phocomelia in nearby Beckum, all born within the same week. He was advised of fifteen recent cases in Münster and traveled there to meet with Professor Wilhelm Kosenow, who told Lenz that in October 1960, at the annual pediatric meeting in Kassel, he had exhibited X-rays and photographs of two babies born with "seal limbs." Soon afterward, he had begun hearing of similar cases in the region. He had launched an inquiry and alerted the Ministry of Health office in Düsseldorf. Lenz phoned Karl to share the news. For the first time since they'd spoken, Lenz's alarm was palpable. "It's as if we were up against a medical epidemic," Lenz said.

Karl rushed to see him, eager to strategize next steps. But Lenz assured Karl he had submitted Karl's name to the Ministry of Health—they should hear something soon. Karl stiffened. Was Lenz simply turning matters over to a bureaucratic commission?

"You can't give up!" Karl implored. In the past few days, Karl had heard from a nurse in Hamburg that in one district alone she knew of seven cases like Jan's.

Karl's passion swayed Lenz. Something was harming pregnant women, and the scope of the epidemic could be staggering. But when had it started? And where? How many cases were there? And how would they locate them? Given Nazi-era attitudes toward people with disabilties, many children were likely being hidden in attics, without medical care.

In late summer, Lenz and Schulte-Hillen placed ads in newspapers, seeking out similar babies. People commonly brought sandwiches to work wrapped in newspaper so that on breaks they could eat and read the news. Posting anything in the paper quickly spread the word, and Lenz and Karl soon collected a list of names and addresses. Karl's father, too, continued to help. When meeting with clients at his law practice, the elder Schulte-Hillen would launch into the woeful tale of his two grandchildren with shortened arms, prodding clients to admit that they knew of a similar baby in their own village. The grandfather soon passed along ten additional names and addresses, and Lenz and Karl hit the road to find the children. Since Lenz, a decade older than Karl, had only a bicycle and did not know how to drive, the duo set out in Karl's old Volkswagen Beetle, zigzagging all over West Germany.

The two men could not have been more different: Schulte-Hillen, though a lawyer from a prominent family, sported a perpetual tan and muscular shoulders. His time digging trenches on the Russian front showed in his roughened hands and hulking movements. Karl's loud, jovial personality commanded attention.

Lenz, by contrast, was serene and professorial. Half-rim glasses fronted his delicately chiseled face. His hair was thinning. A pinched mouth and intense blue eyes hinted at a focused, somewhat obsessive mind, which often rendered him forgetful of practical matters. He exuded a calm stoicism. Pleasantries and jokes were not for Lenz.

As the duo navigated the countryside locating families, they had disturbing meetings. Some infants, hidden away, were brought forth only after Karl showed photographs of Jan, and Karl sensed that many mothers simply shunned their babies. Worried what a household racked by despair would do to these children, Karl resolved to explain to these families the source of this epidemic.

Lenz had begun hypothesizing that a virus or radiation or bad meat from butcher shops might have caused the deformities, but these lines of inquiry led nowhere. Only when Karl's brother-in-law returned from Sweden, where doctors told him of lab experiments in which pregnant animals absorbing certain chemical products had given birth to deformed infants, did Karl and Lenz propose administering a questionnaire to each mother: What did she eat? What products did she use? Was there anything she had begun to consume or use more than usual?

As Lenz and Karl continued their visits throughout the fall, Lenz read a research paper by a doctor in Kiel documenting an additional twenty-seven cases of phocomelia, positing that a new pharmaceutical might be to blame.

Lenz already knew of one mother of a phocomelic baby who had taken large quantities of a sedative called Contergan (thalidomide) before and during her pregnancy. She had begun to suffer neuropathy in her hands and feet, and when her baby was born in December of 1960 with mal-formed arms and legs, she immediately blamed the drug. Her husband, a doctor, had shared her concern with colleagues who had reportedly re-layed the matter to Chemie Grünenthal. Nothing had come of it.

Lenz now visited the family of another child born with truncated limbs. As Lenz explained his quest to find some kind of noxious agent that had caused the injuries in utero, the father announced:

"I think it is Contergan." His wife had taken large quantities of the sedative during pregnancy.

Lenz now saw that Contergan, wildly popular in Germany, appeared on several questionnaires.

"Come and see me," he told Karl over the phone. "I'm getting some-where at last."

In no time, the men were back in the Volkswagen, rushing to confer with the mothers again. Many women now admitted to using the sedative but had considered it too innocent to mention. Four mothers produced receipts and medical records.

Lenz—certain he had the culprit—telephoned doctors around Ham-burg to check their own cases. By November 15 he had fully confirmed that about half of the mothers they knew of had taken thalidomide. Lenz then tasked Karl with the difficult final step—to ask Linde and his own sister if either woman had taken the drug.

Karl reluctantly telephoned Annette. While she admitted that on vaca-tion the year before, a young woman at the hotel had given her a Contergan tablet, she insisted she hadn't taken a single pill since and that the incident had been before she was pregnant.

Karl asked the date of the vacation.

"The beginning of July," Annette answered.

Karl—doing the math—completely lost his temper. "You little idiot! You hadn't found out you were pregnant yet—but you were!"

With Linde, the conversation played out even more brutally. Linde adamantly denied taking any drugs during pregnancy, yet she and Karl knew all evidence pointed to thalidomide. If she hadn't taken the sedative linked to other cases, then what had happened to Jan?

Finally, Karl had a flash.

"Linde!" he said. "Remember the day your father died?"

When Linde's father had died the summer before, Linde and her sister Ute had gone to the train station, clad in black, to meet their younger brother and sister, who had been studying in London. But the English family hosting the siblings had failed to explain why they had been summoned to Germany, so the scene at the station was fraught. By evening, nerves were so frayed that Ute stepped out to the apothecary and returned with a tube of pills. Ute took two, as did her mother, her brother, Karl, and Linde.

Recalling that each Contergan tube contained twelve pills, Karl and Linde now scoured the house. If only ten had been handed out that night, the remainder might still be there. They soon found a container marked "Contergan."

Linde, a twenty-one-year-old student between exams, just one month pregnant, had taken the pills the night of August 10, 1960. And the drug had seemed so harmless, so totally unremarkable, that the entire family had forgotten.

Two small white pills, Karl thought, looking at the container, for my son's two arms.

If I were a doctor, I would not prescribe Contergan anymore. Gentlemen, I warn you, I will not repeat what has already been said before. I see great dangers.

—Heinrich Mückter,
Chemie Grünenthal,
July 1961

All of us have eaten a lot of Contergan.

—*German father of a baby with phocomelia,*
November 1961

Seventeen

In May of 1961, as both William McBride and Karl Schulte-Hillen were investigating what had caused the outbreak of birth defects, Grünenthal was contending with more bad news about the drug's first widely reported side effect: peripheral neuritis.

In quick succession, a trio of attacks hit the medical press. On May 6, Dr. Frenkel's paper, delayed for months, finally appeared in *Medizinische Welt*. Three days later, *Deutsche Medizinische Wochenschrift* ran papers by two different doctors about thalidomide-linked nerve damage. By month's end, 1,300 cases of thalidomide-induced peripheral neuritis had been relayed to Grünenthal, and Distillers was reporting an additional 75. Privately, the German firm feared the numbers were far higher—doctors seeing some improvement likely did not report the condition.

Morale plunged within the Grünenthal sales offices. In Hamburg, representatives found it "difficult psychologically to promote the product unreservedly" because "medical ethics obliged them to discuss side effects in detail." Salesmen no longer wanted their families touching the drug.

By July, Grünenthal's inner circle predicted lawsuits. The Gerling Group—their insurance firm—mapped out the firm's legal liability, and the situation looked abysmal. Not only was Grünenthal's animal testing paltry, but the drug should have carried a warning fourteen months earlier; after all, in May 1960, the firm had warned its own field offices about the possibility of nerve damage. In court, Grünenthal would undoubtedly be asked what actions it had taken after learning "the extent and severity of the side effects." Since the firm had failed to issue *any* printed warning, it would be subject to claims of "negligence." Grünenthal's lawyers told the company to settle rather than let any cases go to trial.

By that point, opinions within the firm about Contergan's future were splintering. Dr. Günter Nowel, tasked with managing the firm's application for prescription status with the Interior Ministry for West Germany, was incensed to learn that Ralf Voss had warned the firm about peripheral neuritis as far back as 1959. Nowel railed to his superiors that he had been "inadequately informed" and that the firm's reputation and his own were being undermined. Heinrich Mückter, the man who had grown wildly rich from the drug's sales, told colleagues, "If I were a doctor, I would not prescribe Contergan anymore. Gentlemen, I warn you . . . I see great dangers."

Others believed selling the drug by prescription, with a warning about peripheral neuritis, was a viable option. Packaging soon bore a red imprint: "Take only as directed by a doctor." But the German health authorities had been slow to enact Grünenthal's prescription recommendation, and the drug was still being sold over the counter throughout most of the country. Not until August 1, 1961, did three German states—North Rhine–Westphalia, Hessen, and Baden-Württemberg—finally place Contergan on prescription. The eight remaining German states failed to make a change even when Der Spiegel, two weeks later, ran the first mainstream press exposé of thalidomide-linked peripheral neuritis.

Under German law, however, the health authorities bore no responsibility for inaction. Full liability landed with Grünenthal. If its prescription recommendation had only been followed swiftly, the firm griped, "we would not now be faced with such a dangerous and uncomfortable situation so injurious to the reputation of our organization."

Meanwhile, Contergan victims were gathering strength. "There are dozens of us," said an angry letter to Grünenthal from one town, "and some are suffering from severe problems . . . living with these problems for weeks and months." They accused Grünenthal of trivializing the side effect as a fluke and insisted on a full recall. The number of sick people, they argued, was appallingly high: "Get rid of Contergan!" Doctors also advocated the drug's ban. "I am appalled that the product still can be, and is, prescribed," one physician wrote to the firm. How could the minuscule print mentioning peripheral neuritis properly alert doctors?

In fact, Grünenthal knew that a mere 5 percent of physicians had noticed the new written warning: "Medical practitioners are not at all informed," the firm's leadership admitted behind closed doors. Moreover, the new fine print falsely promised "symptoms would disappear without treatment if the substance was discontinued."

"This is just not true," objected the head of a neurology clinic.

Another doctor—suffering peripheral neuritis himself—was "downright horrified" by the firm's blatant misinformation. He had been in pain for almost two years.

Soon eighty-nine lawsuits were filed and Grünenthal was hit with its first reimbursement request from a health insurance fund; the fund sought to recoup treatment costs for its peripheral neuritis victims. Settling with a health fund, however, was a risky move for Grünenthal. Any settlement could "unleash an avalanche" of reimbursement claims, and Grünenthal predicted thousands more peripheral neuritis cases. The firm's private talks with doctors suggested that 10 percent of thalidomide's long-term users actually developed side effects. The drug had sold so astoundingly well and for so long that the expected caseload looked like it could crest ten thousand. Thus far, the company knew of 2,400 German victims— likely the tip of the iceberg.

Peripheral neuritis also undercut the medical community's confidence in the drug. The bloom was off the rose. As thalidomide failed to live up to its grand promise of atoxicity, new questions emerged. A Finnish doctor, connecting the same hypothetical dots Frances Kelsey had, queried Grünenthal about the drug's safety for a fetus: If thalidomide crossed the placenta, could it harm a child? The firm's answer: "Improbable."

And yet, over two years earlier, the firm had been alerted that the drug might induce birth defects. In April 1959, a doctor whose son was born with ear and eye defects told a Grünenthal salesman that he thought thalidomide exposure in utero had caused the damage. The doctor knew of two other babies born with defects whose mothers had taken the sedative while pregnant. Then, in June of 1959, animal evidence suggested the drug's danger to the fetus: A German researcher studying amphibians in Brazil warned Grünenthal that his thalidomide experiments on frogs showed "teratogenic effects"—the drug was inducing birth defects. The researcher sent Grünenthal photos of the harmed frogs, along with a report, requesting funds for further research. Grünenthal sent no reply.

November 1960 saw more grim news. A German pharmacist claimed a female customer who had taken Contergan while pregnant had given birth to a baby with liver damage. The company replied that, "based on all observations and findings, we can negate any causal connection."

By early 1961, the pregnancy question came with greater frequency. In March, a doctor from National Drug Company, a Richardson-Merrell subsidiary in Philadelphia, asked Dr. von Schrader-Beielstein if the drug endangered the fetus. Grünenthal admitted that it had no "empirical knowledge" on the matter and that animal experiments "might be useful," but the German firm did not conduct such experiments, despite the drug's wide use in treating morning sickness.

But Grünenthal's in-house animal experiments should have alerted the firm: Three rats given thalidomide (to study peripheral neuritis) turned out to be pregnant, and their litters suffered: Two had notably small litter sizes and the third birthed a single stillborn. The firm, it seems, ignored this data.

"Everything is done to keep this apple of our eye secure," Grünenthal leadership reminded employees.

In September 1961, just as Karl and Lenz were locating victims throughout the countryside, another significant report made its way to the firm. A doctor who had delivered a malformed baby in March had just learned of other children in the area born similarly. The families all suspected Contergan. Again, the firm stayed silent. Soon after, a Grünenthal doctor reportedly quit when Mückter's research department refused to investigate.

Behind the scenes, Grünenthal's upper ranks appeared rattled. If there is a smoking gun in this saga, a moment when Grünenthal and Merrell began to consider the possibility that the drug caused birth defects, it is likely September of 1961. A team from Stolberg flew to the United States to meet with Richardson-Merrell from September 10 through 16, a uniquely long visit between the two firms. While no known documents detail what was discussed, it seems pregnancy made the agenda. On the second day of the Grünenthal visit, Thomas Jones wrote to three obstetricians conducting large Kevadon trials: He asked for more data concerning possible side effects. "The question has been raised as to whether Kevadon exerts any deleterious effect upon the infant," Jones explained to the doctors. Specifically, he asked about "fetal abnormalities."

By this time, Dr. Nulsen in Cincinnati—Raymond Pogge's golf buddy and the official author of the firm's paper on Kevadon use in pregnancy—had delivered at least two babies with truncated limbs. In a proper clinical trial, these births would have been reported to Merrell, and presumably to Grünenthal during its Cincinnati visit. Grünenthal was there, after all, to discuss "experiences and problems related to Kevadon."

Weeks after the Grünenthal envoys returned home, animal data from an independent researcher once again cast suspicion on thalidomide: Fritz Kemper at Münster University, dosing chickens with thalidomide to study the peripheral neuritis link, was shocked to see the drug caused much broader damage. His chicks lost weight and their feathers darkened. Autopsies revealed yellowed bones, scarred and blackened livers, and shrunken gonads. He advised Grünenthal of his results and posited that the drug might alter sexual function by blocking folic acid absorption. Since chickens served as a better proxy for humans than most experimental animals, Kemper guessed that Grünenthal's limited animal experiments had missed the drug's full effects. To that end, Kemper planned his next experiment—to study thalidomide's effect on the fetus using chicken eggs. In essence, an independent researcher now took it upon himself to conduct the animal research that Grünenthal had neglected for years.

Grünenthal registered no public alarm at Kemper's news, yet around the same time—in October 1961—a chemistry graduate trainee visiting Grünenthal's Stolberg headquarters noticed Contergan bottles labeled "NOT FOR PREGNANT WOMEN."

That caution, however, never left the building. No such alert would accompany thalidomide in any of the forty-six countries where the drug was sold. Grünenthal would say nothing publicly about the danger the drug posed to the fetus until two doctors on opposite sides of the globe sounded the alarm.

Q: In September of 1961, were you ever informed by anyone at the William S. Merrell Company that the Food and Drug Administration through Dr. Kelsey, had asked for more data on the particular question of whether thalidomide was safe during pregnancy? . . . As a result of that meeting were you asked to develop any particular animal studies regarding this particular problem of safety for use in pregnant women?

A: Not to my recollection . . .

—*Florus Van Maanen deposition, 1971*

The pharmacologic properties of drugs should be

studied in vitro and in vivo in the fetus.

—American Academy of Pediatrics,

"Committee on Fetus and Newborn:

Effect of Drugs upon the Fetus and the Infant,"

October 1, 1961

I was born in Melbourne, Australia. My father was a doctor. The drug house promoted it as a sleep aid to doctors because the idea was doctors could get a two-hour nap and wake up refreshed. My father actually used it and it worked well. So my mother was having problems in her pregnancy. Given that my father had used it and it was a drug that had no side effects for him, and the drug representative had assured him that things were safe, my father had no anxieties when he prescribed thalidomide for my mother.

—Jeff Green,

born September 1961

Eighteen

Resolute and repentant, William McBride devoted the Australian winter of 1961 to determining how thalidomide harmed babies.

Enlisting the hospital's supply of rabbits, mice, and guinea pigs—animals normally used for hormonal testing—he set up experiments in a chilly shed in the parking lot. On June 14, a little over a week after he told the hospital superintendent, John Newlinds, that he suspected thalidomide, McBride began feeding seventy-five milligrams of the drug to newly pregnant rabbits and mice.

Knowing his results would take weeks, McBride resumed his obstetrical work, hearing nothing more from Distillers. But word of his warning may have been traveling up the firm's chain of command. One week after McBride's phone call, at a company dinner at a hotel in Adelaide, the head of Distillers Australia purportedly cautioned everyone to curb their expectations for sales: "We've had a report from a doctor in Sydney last week about Distaval abnormalities in the fetus," Distillers salesman John Bishop recalls company head Bill Poole announcing to the table. Bishop was particularly rattled by the warning that night because he'd been giving his wife the drug for months, and she was eight months pregnant.

Most of the company's rank-and-file detail men, however, got no warning. In early July, when Walter Hodgetts, the salesman who had talked McBride into trying out Distaval, ran into McBride on the street, he was aghast when the obstetrician told him about the harmed newborns. He wrote up McBride's account, noting that McBride's probe showed that Distaval use was the only link between mothers.

What happened next is up for debate.

According to Hodgetts, he handed his report to Fred Strobl at the Distillers office—the same man who had presumably taken McBride's call weeks earlier. Hodgetts and Strobl both assert that they then marched into the office of Bill Poole, who had just warned his inner circle at dinner about McBride's news. In Hodgetts's telling, Poole called senior executive and Distillers board member Ernie Gross to relay the news. Poole, however, would later deny this phone call took place and would claim, under oath, that Hodgetts did not tell him anything about McBride's concerns at the time. (John Bishop, however, would never forget Poole's dinner-table warning about the drug. The following month, his daughter was born with severely malformed hands and arms.)

In fact, no one in Distillers' upper ranks would ever cop to personally getting the news, though many would acknowledge it was "discussed." Assistant sales manager Hubert "Woody" Woodhouse recalls that in June and July of 1961, he, Strobl, and Poole routinely drank whiskey together after the office closed, debating the financial implications of McBride's theory. And someone at Distillers' headquarters in London was apparently shaken enough to send Walter Hodgetts back to Crown Street hospital to inspect the birth records. Hodgetts charmed the formidable record keeper, Mary Brown, into sharing the relevant documents. But when he relayed the detailed information on the multiple disfigured babies to his superiors, no action to restrict the drug was taken. Two years later, angry with how his Distillers superiors had proceeded, Hodgetts would storm the German embassy in Australia to denounce the firm.

Meanwhile, McBride worried his theory was fraying. His mice, the first animal subjects to give birth, hadn't produced a single deformed offspring. Soon the rabbits, too, produced normal babies. McBride was confounded and mortified. So convinced had he been that his rodent experiments would prove thalidomide's teratogenic effects that with colleagues he'd let slip the words "Nobel Prize." His peers thought him deluded. McBride, after all, was an obstetrician, not a toxicologist or pathologist. What's more, pregnant patients who had taken Distaval months earlier were now delivering perfectly healthy newborns in Crown Street hospital. A professor of pharmacology at Sydney University, Roland Thorp, whose department had worked with thalidomide, told McBride that his hypothesis was dubious. In mid-July, McBride suffered another blow when *The Lancet* rejected his paper. How could they not want to publish a warning of incontrovertible magnitude! McBride was devastated. Worry set in on September 4, when a fourth phocomelic baby was born at the hospital to a mother who had taken Distaval. McBride was at his wit's end until he spotted an editorial in the September 30 *Lancet*:

IATROGENIC DISEASES OF THE NEWBORN

That one person's meat may be another person's poison can be especially trying when the two individuals are connected by a placental circulation; thus the drugs taken by the pregnant woman may enter and upset her fetus. Moreover, drugs prescribed in doses relatively safe for older children and adults may harm the newborn even when given in proportionate amounts. . . . All the drugs prescribed by all concerned with each patient should be carefully recorded and their possible role in the etiology of unexpected disorders in the infant should be carefully examined.

McBride felt a rush of vindication; the letter seemed a nod to his rejected paper. The problem: Neither the word "Distaval" nor the word "thalidomide" appeared in the text—so no one had been warned of the specific danger. Meanwhile, the October 1961 Distillers brochure touted: "It is with absolute safety that 'Distaval' can be administered to pregnant or breastfeeding women without any adverse effects on the mother or child."

But in November, the tides shifted. Six months after the strange births began at Crown Street, a former schoolmate of McBride's came to visit. A graduate in pharmacy studies from Sydney University, I. Goldberg happened to work for Distillers, and McBride immediately fumed to his old friend about the drug firm's indifference to his suspicions. Goldberg was floored—what suspicions? As McBride explained the birth deformities, Goldberg went pale. He'd heard nothing of this link. Goldberg left to dispatch someone from Distillers to take McBride's statement. Assistant sales manager Woody Woodhouse (one of the four men in the Sydney office already aware of McBride's theory) arrived at Crown Street, where McBride announced he was ready to send warnings to various international medical journals. Woodhouse pleaded with him to hold off until Distillers had a chance to take the drug off the market. McBride, not looking to punish the firm, complied.

On November 29, 1961, McBride received a letter from Denis Burley of Distillers UK:

> We are most concerned over the evidence you have presented to us and completely agree that pharmacological work should be carried out to see whether any further evidence can be obtained. However, on Monday we received another report from an overseas source also making a similar suggestion to yours, on much the same evidence, and we therefore felt that we had no alternative but to withdraw Distaval from the market immediately pending further investigations.

The overseas source was Chemie Grünenthal, and the suggestion of the drug's teratogenic properties had come from the quiet Hamburg pediatrician Widukind Lenz.

We've asked these [Grünenthal] gentlemen to withdraw their drug and they've replied that they are unable to do so for financial reasons.

— Ministry of Health,
Düsseldorf, Germany,
November 24, 1961

Nineteen

Lenz was exhausted.

On November 15, 1961, he at last had telephoned Chemie Grünenthal to let the company know that Contergan was linked to the mass of phocomelic births. Lenz spoke to Heinrich Mückter—who, unbeknownst to him, had overseen the drug's creation—and relayed his research, insisting the product be immediately recalled.

But Mückter acted blasé. Declaring it the very first he'd heard of any association between thalidomide and birth defects, he ended the call saying he would send someone in a few days to discuss the matter further. After six months of painstaking investigation, Lenz was outraged. This drug was all over Germany. This was an epidemic. Each day lost could mean five more abnormal babies! Hanging up, Lenz immediately wrote up his warning and mailed it to Grünenthal:

> In view of the incalculable human, psychological, legal, and financial consequences of this problem, it is, in my own opinion, indefensible to wait for a strict scientific proof of the harmfulness or harmlessness, as the case may be, of Contergan. I consider it necessary to withdraw the medicament from sale immediately until its harmlessness as a teratogenic agent in man is conclusively proved.

Agitated, Lenz revisited the mothers with phocomelic babies who had *not* noted taking Contergan and scoured their medicine cabinets. He demanded the names of their doctors so he could review prescriptions. In no time, he had determined that, like Linde, these women had used the drug but forgotten. He now had fourteen detailed, incriminating case histories.

Then Mückter telephoned Lenz, his tone entirely changed. He apologized for being caught off guard by the previous call and asked if a Grünenthal representative could visit Lenz that Monday. Lenz agreed, but within hours the delay worried him: What guarantee did he have that the meeting would get Grünenthal to pull thalidomide from the market? Lenz thus made a bold decision. That Saturday, he was set to take part in a conference in Düsseldorf for the Pediatricians Association of North Rhine–Westphalia, where Drs. Wilhelm Kosenow and Rudolf Pfeiffer— who had presented on the two phocomelic infants in Kassel the previous year—were going to discuss the country's phocomelia outbreak. Except Lenz was the sole member of the German medical community who knew the cause.

"I'm going to speak to them about the drug," Lenz told Karl.

Lenz took the train to Düsseldorf, conferring with a professor of pediatrics who was himself the grandfather of a child born with phocomelia. At the conference, Lenz sat quietly through Kosenow and Pfeiffer's presentation until the question-and-answer session, at which point he dramatically announced, "As a man and a citizen, I can no longer accept the responsibility of keeping to myself the observations I am about to make." Lenz explained to the room that his research indicated "a certain substance" was causing the outbreak. "Each month's delay in sorting this out," he warned, "means the birth of perhaps fifty to one hundred horribly mutilated children." Lenz called for the substance's immediate withdrawal, though out of caution he did not, at first, name the drug. Yet as the meeting ended and horror-struck doctors chatted anxiously, one desperate man approached Lenz: Was the substance Contergan? His wife had taken that drug, and they now had a child with phocomelia. Lenz confided to the man and five trusted colleagues that yes, the offender was thalidomide.

On Monday, as Lenz sat in his clinic awaiting the Grünenthal representative, he was surprised when three men arrived: Dr. von Schrader-Beielstein; Dr. Günther Michael, head of clinical research; and the company's legal adviser, Dr. Hilmar von Veltheim. Sensing trouble, Lenz asked the men to wait, racing up and down the halls to enlist an independent observer. But no one would bite. Returning alone, Lenz suggested to the Grünenthal team that they postpone their discussion to the afternoon, when they could join his meeting with the Hamburg health authorities. The Grünenthal men agreed.

Lenz had meticulously prepared a detailed presentation of his fourteen case studies, but when the Ministry of Health meeting began at 2:30 P.M., the Grünenthal men attacked. As Lenz struggled to discuss his data, the executives interrupted repeatedly. A ministry official condemned the disruptions, but the Grünenthal men were far from done: They threatened legal action against Lenz for his "unjustified attack" on their firm, claiming his rumors and unvetted data amounted to "the murder of a drug by rumour." The health authorities, however, sided with Lenz, and as the four-hour meeting drew to a close, they asked the drug firm representatives to withdraw thalidomide. Grünenthal refused.

The next day, Lenz arrived at his clinic to find von Schrader-Beielstein and von Veltheim waiting for him. They demanded photocopies of his research and asked for a meeting that Friday at the Ministry of Health in Düsseldorf, the jurisdiction presiding over Aachen, where Grünenthal was headquartered.

Karl Schulte-Hillen, who was threatening to go to the press if the health authorities didn't act soon, asked to attend, so the two men set out together for the conference in Karl's Volkswagen. But Karl's arrival rattled the Grünenthal team. Upon hearing Karl was a lawyer, von Schrader-Beielstein insisted he leave. When the ministry urged Karl to comply, Karl stormed out, and an official chased him down the hall to explain that the drug firm was hinting at legal retaliation and they all needed to be careful.

Lenz, alone, then presented his evidence, which so worried the ministry officials that they, too, asked Grünenthal to take thalidomide off the market.

On the lunch break, the Grünenthal team telephoned their headquarters in Stolberg, and when the meeting reconvened, they asked Lenz to step out of the room. They privately told the ministry they had been authorized to put a "not to be taken by pregnant women" label on Contergan and to issue notices to pharmacists and doctors. But the ministry wanted the drug withdrawn entirely.

Enraged, von Schrader-Beielstein blasted Lenz. Lenz stormed back in to defend himself, and the sight of the usually taciturn pediatrician stirred

to outrage seemed to embolden the ministry. The officials leveled an ulti-
matum at Grünenthal: Withdraw the drug, or the ministry would ban it. At
that, von Veltheim, the Grünenthal lawyer, threatened legal action, and
his team exited into the night. The meeting had lasted all day.

On Saturday, von Veltheim and von Schrader-Beielstein rushed to
Grünenthal's headquarters in Stolberg for an emergency summit. After
relaying the events at the ministry, they advised Heinrich Mückter and
other executives that withdrawal of the drug seemed necessary. Mückter
then shared his own news. He had received a letter the day before from
Distillers UK:

> We have had a rather disturbing report from a consultant obstetri-
> cian of deformities in children which could be associated with the
> taking of thalidomide by mothers in early pregnancy for morning
> sickness. . . . The mothers of these infants had all been given Dis-
> taval in early pregnancy in a dose of 100mg night and morning. . . .
> The administration of Distaval seems to be the only common factor
> in these cases.

Confusion and anger swept the room. A doctor in Australia *shared*
Lenz's theory? Why had Mückter said nothing of this letter while
von Schrader-Beielstein and von Veltheim were protesting Lenz's claims
at the Ministry of Health? Von Schrader-Beielstein, a father himself, pro-
cessed this development. As the newly arrived doctor in the firm in 1956,
he had been the one to seek out safety testing of the drug for pregnancy.
The overall sentiment in the summit was that Grünenthal must withdraw
the drug. But Mückter disagreed. The drug would remain on sale. And
when protest erupted, he announced that responsibility for the choice
would fall on him alone. Mückter's sole concession was to send warnings
to doctors and pharmacists about Lenz's reports.

Even without Mückter's concession, Lenz's warning was about to
sweep Germany. One of the doctors at the Düsseldorf conference had
slipped word to a journalist, and on Sunday, November 26, all of West
Germany awoke to an article in the *Welt am Sonntag* newspaper headed
"Malformations from Tablets—Alarming Suspicion of Physician's Glob-
ally Distributed Drug."

Within hours, the Grünenthal executives reconvened. This time, Mückter acted fast, telegramming the West German Ministry of Health:

WE ARE TAKING CONTERGAN OUT OF CIRCULATION IMMEDIATELY UNTIL SCIENTIFIC QUESTIONS HAVE BEEN ANSWERED.

The Ministry of Health issued public warnings—radio and television announcements and notices in newspapers—saying thalidomide was linked to birth defects. And by Monday, November 27, almost every publication in Germany carried news of the drug's dangers. Grünenthal also began to alert doctors, pharmacies, wholesalers, and licensees, but the firm's warnings were half-hearted: "Because press reports have undermined the basis of scientific discussion," they wrote, and due to "the continuous pressure of Dr. Lenz," they were compelled to act. The drug's withdrawal, they implied, was a conciliation to unproven accusations.

But the die was cast. It was almost seven months to the day since Jan Schulte-Hillen had been born and Karl and Linde had vowed to find out what had harmed him. Karl had at last scored a victory against the drug firm. By November 29, all forms of thalidomide were officially banned from the German market.

December 6, 1961

Mrs. Elinor Kamath
Paul-Clemensstrasse 2
Bonn, Germany

Dear Elinor:

There seems to be something crazy about Dr. Lenz's report on
Contregan [*sic*]. Don't know what it is and how it grew. The fact
is that this same drug is being used in Britain under the name
Distaval and our correspondent there says there are no signs
of any teratogenic effects therefrom — just the peripheral
neuropathy.

Before you get too deeply imbedded in this story, do as I
suggested in my letter yesterday — wait a couple of weeks until
the thing settles down, and then let me know briefly how
matters stand. Then I will let you know if we want another
story.

Best regards.

Cordially,
Max Sien
Managing Editor
Medical Tribune

Twenty

Elinor Kamath was relaxing in her Bonn apartment, the windows frosted with a late-autumn chill, partaking in her favorite Sunday-morning ritual. It was November 1961. Her husband had just returned from the local *Pressehaus* with a thick pile of the French and German newspapers, and together the couple—both foreign correspondents in Germany—held their steaming coffees and flipped through the Sunday editions. Kamath, forty-seven, placed the small tabloid-format paper *Welt am Sonntag* (World on Sunday) in her lap. She dove in from back to front, her custom, but froze when she spotted an article on the bottom of the back page. A drug called Contergan, the article reported, had caused a spike in birth defects across Germany.

The month before, Kamath had been working at her desk one morning when her housekeeper, Frau Becker, arrived, agitated. At that point, Kamath and her husband, Mahdav, a correspondent for *The Times of India*, had been living in Bonn for two years, and Becker was a thrice-weekly feature in their lives. Though Becker spoke no English, Kamath had become fluent in German, and the worry in her housekeeper's face seemingly warranted a chat. Kamath suggested they take their coffees together in the kitchen. Soon, a fraught story came pouring out of the normally cheerful Becker: Her sister-in-law had just given birth, and the baby had no arms or legs. Kamath, who covered medical news and considered herself well versed in health matters, had to mask her shock.

A few days later, Frau Becker brought even stranger news: *Three* babies had been born without limbs, in a matter of weeks, in the same Bad Godesberg town hospital. Kamath's investigative alarm triggered, she reached out to a high-level doctor she knew at the hospital. But he issued a fast denial: The story of other babies was a conciliatory line fed to a distraught mother. Kamath let the matter go.

But now—this article! In the Sunday paper! Kamath *had* been onto something. A German sedative was maiming unborn babies. She immediately sensed the scope of the story and scrambled for sources. She dialed her English-speaking gynecologist to see if he'd been at the meeting of pediatricians, referenced in the article, where Lenz had denounced the drug.

"Have you seen the report in *Die Welt am Sonntag?*" she asked her doctor. "Were you at the Düsseldorf meeting?"

His answer stunned Kamath.

"I don't know who let that damned story out," he snapped. His swift denial was enough to tell her she was onto something colossal. She threw herself into research, first calling Widukind Lenz. Lenz explained how he had gone house to house in West Germany for months, surveying mothers of phocomelic babies, and had found one common link: thalidomide. Lenz now knew that the crucial window for exposure was between thirty-four and forty-nine days after the last menstrual period, with even a single pill being enough to harm a fetus.

Kamath compiled a report for the *Medical Tribune*, the international publication she wrote for part-time. An article there could reach physicians worldwide. She contacted Max Sien, her editor in New York, laying out the story and sending along her notes and the *Welt am Sonntag* clipping. But Sien wrote back to say the story seemed far-fetched. He wanted her to back off and give it time. Kamath was outraged. If this drug was being sold in other countries, it was a ticking time bomb.

Resolved to get the story out, Kamath clambered to collect her own evidence, visiting the Interior Ministry in Bonn and the Land Ministry in Düsseldorf and consulting professors at the University of Bonn. Well connected in the expat journalist community, Kamath urged foreign correspondents to get information about thalidomide from their respective countries, but they blew her off. Sydney Gruson, a *New York Times* correspondent—and future executive vice president of the paper—spurned the story. And the correspondent for Denmark's leading daily said he covered only stories of great political consequence. Kamath was crushed. No one grasped the urgency except a Swedish correspondent Kamath contacted—a woman—who knew thalidomide was sold in Sweden and told Kamath she would start digging.

On Wednesday, November 29, a worried Kamath played her final card. Antony Terry, a *Sunday Times* (London) correspondent, was a regular dinner guest in her home. Terry had deemed the thalidomide news trivial, but Kamath threatened to end all dinner invitations if he ignored the story. On December 3, 1961, Terry filed a piece for *The Sunday Times*, the first article to appear in England noting the drug's dangers.

Next, Kamath alerted government outposts. At the U.S. embassy, Kamath met with scientific attaché Dr. Ludwig Audrieth and his deputy Dr. Herman Chinn, with whom she had a good rapport. She handed the two envoys carbon copies of her data, and agreed to let Chinn use her research in a State Department report. Hoping to find an angle to interest the American press, she had been trying to determine if thalidomide had been used on U.S. military bases in Germany. But the medical military liaison in Heidelberg assured her that since the drug lacked FDA approval, it wasn't distributed on base, though the German wives of American military personnel could have purchased it in civilian shops.

This reminded Kamath of a recent gathering at the home of the Canadian ambassador. The joke of the party had been that the majority of the wives—seven or eight—were home that night because they were all in their eighth month of pregnancy, the result of a frisky embassy ski weekend early in the year.

Kamath now telephoned the embassy switchboard and asked an operator she knew if any of the babies had been born. The operator knew of two—both healthy. But she patched Kamath through to the assistant commercial secretary, and when Elinor explained the epidemic, he raced over to borrow her files. Thalidomide had been on the Canadian market for eleven months and the envoy wanted copies for Ottawa. The embassy immediately reached out to Grünenthal in Stolberg for more information.

On Christmas Day, December 25, almost a month after the news hit the German press, the *Medical Tribune* finally carried a small story—without Kamath's byline—on the potential dangers of thalidomide.

At that point, Kamath accompanied her husband to India, on home leave. At a medical conference there, she tried to spread news of the drug's risks, and she planned an eventual deeper dive into the story. But when she returned to the United States to visit family in January of 1962, a letter from her *Medical Tribune* editor advised her that he found the thalido-mide story only of "academic interest." The paper would publish no more for the time being about the drug's suspected dangers.

My name is Sabine Becker. I was born in Berlin in January 1962. I was my mother's first child, but I have been told nothing about the day of my birth. It's a big mystery. When I've asked, I've been told it was das Schicksal—*destiny.*

My arms were missing.

I was one of the last thalidomide babies born in Germany. If they had taken it off the market sooner, I would not be this way.

—Sabine Becker,

born January 1962

Twenty-one

Back in the United States, long before news of thalidomide's link to birth defects made headlines in Germany, peripheral neuritis was becoming a problem for Merrell.

Throughout 1961, news of the thalidomide side effect circulated so publicly from overseas that Merrell's own clinical investigators were growing worried. In July, Norman Orentreich of New York City, a high-end dermatologist who would go on to create the Clinique skin care line, wrote to Thomas Jones about seven international articles on the risk of nerve damage from thalidomide's "twin" sisters—Contergan and Distaval. Orentreich wanted to know: Had Jones seen all this news? Worse— Merrell's own trial doctors were witnessing the problematic side effect. Ralph L. Byron, Jr., of California wrote to Merrell that all four of his patients on Kevadon suffered "numbness, tingling, and a rather marked tremor." Byron deemed the symptoms "so distressing that we have not used it further." Sidney Cohen, chief of the psychosomatic section of the Veterans Administration Center in Los Angeles, was preparing a report on "Thalidomide Neuropathy," which Thomas Jones asked him to delay.

Merrell had to persuade the FDA this was all irrelevant. To that end, Jones invited his most impressive trial doctors to a daylong conference at the Washington agency, in order to sing the drug's praises. Frank Ayd, a Baltimore psychiatrist, had seen peripheral neuritis in several patients, but Jones thought the incidence low enough and considered Ayd prestigious enough that Jones simply asked him to downplay the issue with the agency. Sidney Cohen, who had used Kevadon on more than 150 alcoholics, was urged to tell the FDA that his sole peripheral neuritis case had been quickly cured by pyridoxine.

On September 7, 1961, almost a year to the day after the Kevadon application hit her desk, more than a dozen men filed into Frances Kelsey's spartan office. Thomas Jones and Joseph Murray of Merrell led the delegation, which included eight physicians from around the country, as well as Dr. Florus Van Maanen of Merrell. They were all there to champion Kevadon.

The doctors settled into the windowless room: Frank Ayd, G. Gordon McHardy, Basil Roebuck, Martin Towler, Sidney Cohen, Sol Levy, Hassan Azima, and Louis Lasagna—almost all were psychiatrists, and all were running vast Kevadon trials. In fifteen-minute rotations, they stood before Frances to tout Kevadon's sleep-inducing abilities and to argue its safety over other hypnotics.

Frances was skeptical as she sat through the choreographed presentations. No physician present offered scientific proof of the drug's safety, and Frances's recent queries within the medical community had turned up detractors. A doctor at the National Institute of Neurological Diseases and Blindness had cautioned her that in a drug recommended for chronic use, any neurotoxicity was serious. Frances's question about the drug's safety in pregnancy had still gone unanswered, and there wasn't a single obstetrician at the meeting. When asked, no doctor could speak to the drug's effect on the fetus. Murray's only response to her May query about pregnancy had been to let her know that the Nulsen paper was finally in print—as though that settled matters.

But Nulsen's so-called research had needled her from day one. Merrell's application claimed that Nulsen found pregnant women on Kevadon could wake and return to sleep easily, but Frances still hadn't seen any Nulsen patient reports. More worrisome, Nulsen's paper—"Trial of Thalidomide in Insomnia Associated with the Third Trimester"—suffered a glaring omission: any research on the early stages of pregnancy. A week after the presentations in her office, Frances issued another "incomplete."

Furious, Murray telephoned to say the firm had now been jumping through hoops for a year. Christmas—just around the corner—was peak sedative season. Having already missed Christmas of 1960, his bosses didn't want to lose another holiday. Murray asked Frances to give him the exact wording she wanted on the product label. He'd write it down, rush to the printer, then run over to her for a quick "OK." Frances reminded him that all labeling had to be formally submitted. She advised him that any label caution against use in pregnancy. But Murray was anxious about a "warning" that implied risk.

When he sent Frances a pile of data indicating what he thought was "the safety of thalidomide usage during pregnancy," Frances once again noted that Merrell still had no data on *early* pregnancy. How could they possibly say it was safe? If their trial doctors had given the drug to women in the first or second trimester, where were the reports? And if Merrell truly had nothing to prove the drug was safe in early pregnancy, why did it refuse to issue a caution?

My mom became pregnant in September of 1961. My parents' wedding anniversary was September 12, so I think I was an "anniversary baby."

I was born with two shortened arms with grossly abnormal hands, no thumbs, and both feet were clubbed and bent in. My left leg was unable to completely straighten out.

I was baptized and christened multiple times—twice in the hospital, by both a nurse and a hospital chaplain, and finally by the family priest in our church. No one thought I would make it.

Years later, I found my baby book. A nice book my mother must have bought, or been given, themed for a girl. My mother had written in my birth weight, birth date, and the time of birth. . . . She had also written in the name of the attending doctor. . . . It was Dr. Ray O. Nulsen. . . . She was a patient of Dr. Nulsen in Cincinnati.

The rest of the baby book was empty. She was too busy taking care of me.

—Gwen Riechmann,
born May 1962,
Cincinnati, Ohio

Dear Tom,

I trust that you returned safely to Cincinnati and that in the meantime you had good news regarding Kevadon. I must say, and this is off the record, that I have never seen anyone searching for as many negative things as the officials did at that meeting. . . .

As for my expenses, my round trip jet plane fare was $337.92. In addition I had quite expensive limousine services and spent, in round figures, (for limousine, insurance and incidentals) another $35, so that my expenses altogether would be $372.92. This naturally does not include the honorarium of $300. . . .

Sincerely yours,
Sol Levy, M.D.

—*Sol Levy, MD, Kevadon investigator,*

to Thomas Jones, Merrell,

September 12, 1961

I was born at the University Hospital in Columbus, Ohio. My father was going for his architectural degree. My father's parents came from Greece to Ellis Island and were not well off financially. My mother often accepted free trial drugs from her doctor to help with her morning sickness. I was born with deformities. My right leg was deformed and later had to be amputated. My left arm was smaller and shorter with only three webbed fingers, flipper-like.

—Gus Economides,

born November 1961

Twenty-two

Throughout the fall of 1961, Merrell was fighting on two fronts. While it muscled for Kevadon's approval, triparanol was sinking fast. A woman using the cholesterol drug for eight months had lost half her hair. The Mayo Clinic reported that the MER/29 patients suffering scalp and skin changes now had cataracts. As competing firms spread the bad news among doctors, customers began returning the Merrell product.

Another new FDA reviewer—John Nestor—proved a nightmare for the Cincinnati firm. After stonewalling Merrell's new MER/29 label, saying it would give doctors a "false sense of security," Nestor stormed a meeting between Merrell's big guns—President Frank N. Getman and Vice President Robert Woodward—and the FDA's William Kessenich, demanding that Merrell withdraw MER/29 from the market once and for all.

Merrell refused but knew it had to minimize risk. To that end, the firm started quietly taking the drug out of circulation, avoiding the word "recall." Detail men were told of a "major promotional revision," and doctors were advised the drug was out of stock. No alarms were to be sounded.

With Senator Kefauver's hearings under way, Merrell's leadership knew that any bad publicity could become "an example before a congressional committee of the necessity for more stringent laws and regulations." And even though a voluntary withdrawal might offer Merrell a leg up with the FDA for future drug applications, it would halt MER/29 sales overseas, whereas if the FDA *forced* MER/29 off the market, Merrell could keep selling the drug internationally, with warnings. Plus, if the firm withdrew the drug—thus acknowledging its dangers—liability claims would ensue. So Merrell braced for an "all-out fight" in the event of any "action by Government" and tried to rally the whole company. Merrell's president cited

Dr. William Hollander in a company-wide morale-boosting memo: Hollander, a trial doctor for MER/29 and Kevadon on a $2,400 retainer, declared that a recall of the cholesterol pill would "pose a threat to research progress in the United States and to the welfare of the people."

With MER/29 sales slowing, Merrell's fight for Kevadon's FDA approval took on greater urgency. Though more than sixteen thousand Americans were using the sedative, no one was paying for it. During its expensive, yearlong promotional campaign, millions of tablets had been dispensed for free. If the FDA didn't budge soon, the firm's finances looked grim.

In her new colleague, John Nestor, Frances had found a kindred spirit. Nestor was a fiery character who would make headlines later in life as the "Wheeled Avenger of the Beltway" and the "Left-Lane Bandit"; at age seventy-two, on a crusade to deter speeders, Nestor began setting off daily in the left lane of the Washington, D.C., beltway with his Chevy Malibu's cruise control set at the fifty-five-mile-per-hour speed limit.

One of ten children, Nestor had grown up in Franklin, New Jersey, where his father, the personnel manager of a zinc mine, taught him about the inequities of the world. After graduating from Georgetown's medical school, Nestor studied pediatrics at Johns Hopkins under renowned cardiologist Helen Taussig, who had helped develop "blue baby" surgery. Nestor then ran a private pediatrics practice in D.C. until a mishap with a prescription drug changed his life.

While on a trip to Florida, Nestor had used a sample of a new antibiotic to treat his sore throat. Even though he had read the insert, he suffered a second-degree burn from a phototoxic reaction to the sun. Enraged that a few hours of sunbathing on a hotter day might have killed him, Nestor called the FDA. What was wrong with the agency's safeguards that an antibiotic could trigger a potentially lethal reaction? But his rant was ignored. Only when Senator Kefauver's hearings mentioned the FDA's struggle to recruit doctors did Nestor grasp his destiny.

Nestor knew the FDA's salaries were paltry, but the relentless sales hype from pharmaceutical detail men so irked him that he was itching to wage war against the industry. Besides, the diaper rashes and runny noses of pediatrics had grown boring. Nestor was a man who liked a fight. Weeks after arriving at the agency, Nestor took over the dubious MER/29 application. Despite the mass of complaints detailing the drug's dangers, Merrell refused to withdraw it. More egregious: Merrell ran ads in seven major medical magazines touting the drug's safety, without citing the reports of hair loss, skin thickening, and blindness.

Frances hosted the forty-nine-year-old bachelor for dinner many times to decry Merrell's aggressive ploys. Most recently: Merrell president Frank Getman had arrived at Nestor's office with general counsel for Richardson-Merrell, Bradshaw Mintener—the former assistant secretary of health, education, and welfare (HEW)—and managed to convince deputy FDA commissioner John Harvey that the agency lacked the legal standing to recall triparanol. Compelling Merrell to issue a warning might mark the extent of the FDA's powers.

For Frances, this news would have been sobering. If the FDA couldn't force Merrell to withdraw an obviously harmful drug, it was urgent that she keep Kevadon off the market. Where other pharmaceutical firms would concede errors—she had just successfully pressured Wallace & Tiernan to recall their tranquilizer Dornwal after she was tipped off at an NIH meeting that the drug could cause bone marrow disease—Merrell looked disturbingly determined to keep selling MER/29.

But on the Monday after Thanksgiving, Frances got a stunning phone call from Joseph Murray. After fourteen months of veiled threats and heated meetings, Murray was reaching out to relay bizarre news: Thalidomide had been recalled in Germany because of a suspected link to birth defects. He hoped the suspicions would prove circumstantial, and to that end Merrell intended to keep its FDA application under consideration. For half a year, Frances had been asking about pregnancy safety. Just weeks earlier, she had called Merrell's affiliate, National Drug Company, inquiring about the drug's possible "hazard to the fetus." Given that the drug had been used widely for morning sickness overseas, the implications of the news were awful.

That night, Frances shared the grim update with Barbara Moulton, who had come to dinner with her new fiancé, Eppes Wayles Browne, Jr.—one of Kefauver's chief economists, whom Barbara had met when testifying. Despite the subcommittee's relentless exposure of drug industry malfeasance—price-fixing, false advertising—the press had wearied of the hearings. Public sentiment around pharmaceutical regulation now lay somewhere between ignorance and ambivalence. Kefauver's dream—to pass a robust drug law protecting the American people—had stalled. His committee needed a news story to spotlight the issue. Wayles Browne sat in Frances's house, listening intently.

Meanwhile, Merrell, under pressure from the FDA, wrote to the thirty-seven doctors named in its New Drug Application to share the news from overseas. But in an act of stunning negligence, it did not contact the one thousand additional doctors enlisted by its detail men. Distillers had pulled the drug from circulation in the UK in late November, writing to Grünenthal that "the reports are of such a serious nature that we had no alternative." But American doctors, many of whom saw pregnant women, continued giving free, unmarked thalidomide pills to tens of thousands of patients.

My friends call me JoJo. My parents were from the Philippines, and my dad was doing his doctorate degree at Cornell in entomology. When my mom was pregnant with me, she had morning sickness, so she went to see her doctor and he gave her medicine. . . . My parents were surprised to find a baby with short arms, no elbows, and three fingers on each hand.

—Jose Martynov Galvez Calora,
born January 1962,
Ithaca, New York

I was born in Oklahoma City. . . . Both arms were missing at the shoulders, and I had two short leg stumps above the knee. . . .

Soon after I was born, the doctor put my mom in a hospital room with another woman whose baby was stillborn. . . . They wanted my mom to get used to the idea that I was going to be gone, in an institution. They told my mom I would be significantly "retarded."

I am now a lawyer.

—Jan Taylor Garrett,
born February 1962

My mother was sedated—that's how it was done then—so I was delivered when she was asleep. They brought me to her and showed her how to nurse me and I was all wrapped up. They never told her anything was wrong with me, and they didn't unwrap me. . . . My dad eventually had to tell her. . . . He left the hospital, called her on the phone in her hospital room, and said, "She's crippled."

—*Carolyn Farmer Sampson,*
born March 1962,
Morristown, New Jersey

Twenty-three

On a crisp April day, Frances and her colleague John Nestor sped north forty miles to Baltimore to meet with Helen Taussig. Hours earlier, Nestor had received a stunning bulletin: His medical school mentor, just back from a trip overseas, had called the FDA to report that a drug in Germany was causing an epidemic of birth defects.

Since late December, when Merrell had relayed the information that thalidomide had been linked to birth defects in Germany, Frances had heard nothing more about the matter. The key report from the U.S. deputy scientific attaché in Bonn, Herman Chinn—three pages aggregating journalist Elinor Kamath's research—had reached the U.S. State Department in early January and found its way to the FDA and HEW (the Department of Health, Education and Welfare). But it never reached Frances, so she still knew nothing of Widukind Lenz's findings and assumed no concrete data yet existed to substantiate the connection.

On March 5, a whole three months after Germany recalled thalidomide, Merrell finally requested to withdraw its Kevadon application. Almost simultaneously, the firm pulled the drug from the Canadian market. Nonetheless, Merrell and its affiliate, National Drug Company, had claimed skepticism "that these birth defects can accurately be attributed to the action of 'Contergan' (thalidomide)." As proof, they noted: "There have been no reports of these bizarre defects [in the United States]." Merrell's letters to its clinical investigators described the decision as one of "prudence."

Behind the scenes, however, the Canadian Food and Drug Directorate had advised Joseph Murray of Merrell that numerous Canadian doctors had demanded a thalidomide recall. Murray had flown to Germany to discuss the matter with Grünenthal's von Schrader-Beielstein, but by the time the men connected, the vice president of Merrell had decided to pull the drug from the Canadian market: "This step was taken as a consequence of our thorough review of all data available to us from abroad and was considered necessary as a precaution to the future use of the drug until the unresolved question of its association with congenital malformation is answered." Merrell hoped that at some point down the road the drug could be re-introduced, but for the time being, Merrell's vice president told Grünenthal, "This totally unexpected development calls for certain modifications in our contractual agreement."

Around this same time, March 1962, Thomas Jones of Merrell learned that four abnormal babies had been born to patients of Ray O. Nulsen.

For Frances, the call from the illustrious Helen Taussig was the first concrete news about thalidomide in a month.

As the tall, gray-haired cardiologist beckoned Frances and John Nestor inside her home, she told them of hundreds of deformed babies throughout Germany and England. Taussig shared photographs and X-rays of the injured infants, and Frances reeled. For almost a year, she'd worried about what might happen if Kevadon crossed the placenta. But these effects—missing limbs—were worse than anything she'd imagined. Some babies had no arms or legs and couldn't even turn over. In all her years in medicine, she'd never seen any birth defect this severe.

Particularly haunting, Taussig pointed out, was the fact that *seven* injured babies had been born to Grünenthal employees—two babies without ears, and five with malformed arms and legs. A striking number, too, were the children of doctors. In her whole career, Taussig noted, she had encountered only two cases of babies with congenitally absent limbs. Yet some German pediatricians were now caring for upward of fifty such children. Taussig, who had called the FDA merely to report the news from overseas, was shocked to learn that the product was under consideration by the FDA.

Frances, Nestor, and Taussig could now assemble the troubling narrative: Grünenthal, Distillers, and Merrell were calling the data inconclusive. Yet Grünenthal had swiftly managed to prove by experiment that the drug did, indeed, traverse the placenta of an experimental animal, and Taussig wanted this information public. Widukind Lenz had been smeared, with Grünenthal circulating news of his Nazi father. A Canadian reporter had even been told that Lenz decided to vilify thalidomide because of psychic "visions." Lenz thought Grünenthal was orchestrating a cover-up. Taussig herself felt that the firm had "behaved disgracefully"— gunning for profits, refusing to admit the drug's risk. She was mystified that the German medical community seemed to oppose an in-depth probe.

She had instead undertaken her own probe: She determined that between 1954 and 1959, eight West German pediatric clinics had observed zero cases of phocomelia. In 1959, however, there were 12. In 1960, 83. In 1961, the clinics saw 302. In order to establish a control group, Taussig had visited a U.S. Army base, where an army doctor confirmed that not a single incident of phocomelia had been reported, there or on any other American base in Germany in either 1960 or 1961.

Then in mid-March, Taussig had seen tangible laboratory evidence. While at a meeting at the Children's Hospital in Leeds, Taussig and a colleague had received a call from George Somers, the guilt-ridden pharmacologist for Distillers, asking them to come over immediately. At his lab on the outskirts of Liverpool, Somers dramatically whisked a cloth from a dish to reveal a newborn rabbit with limb deformities. He'd given the mother thalidomide. Taussig ordered X-rays.

Returning to the United States, Taussig resolved to publicize the drug's dangers. Other than Elinor Kamath's small piece in the *Medical Tribune*, the only American media attention so far given the issue was a short article in a February edition of *Time* magazine—"Sleeping Pill Nightmare"—the result of three months of needling by an American father whose daughter, living in Germany, had a phocomelic baby. The *Time* article noted the drug's wide overseas use but said it had been distributed in the United States only "under heavy restrictions." Two days later, Taussig delivered a public warning at a special session of the American College of Physicians in Philadelphia. But her description of the overseas outbreak aroused scant interest. The next day, at a news conference in Philadelphia, she strengthened her message. It was "the most ghastly thing you have ever seen," she told reporters. She urged new laws to ensure all drugs were tested on pregnant animals before going to market. *The New York Times*, reporting on both speeches, assured readers that "because officials were suspicious of it," the drug had not been approved by the FDA.

But Frances knew the drug had been used in clinical trials, and Taussig's reports worried her. She immediately asked Merrell and National Drug Company if all the doctors who'd been given thalidomide samples had been warned, and she demanded a complete list of their names.

In the meantime, that April, the MER/29 debacle was casting serious doubt on Merrell's integrity. Nestor had gotten wind that a former Merrell toxicologist was accusing the firm of doctoring data. The story was wild: A monkey harmed by MER/29 in Merrell's lab experiments had disappeared from company premises before the requisite autopsy. Yet the same monkey was described in data for the FDA as being alive and well. The toxicologist had been asked by her lab superiors to fudge data. Make it appear that the experiments had run longer, she had been told, and omit bad results.

When Nestor finally stormed Merrell's Cincinnati offices with a certificate of inspection, the two-day investigation turned up troves of falsified data for MER/29—plus a compromising company memo from Merrell's president headed "READ AND DESTROY." Cornered, Merrell at last agreed to pull MER/29 from pharmacies. But the firm advised doctors this was merely "out of an abundance of caution . . . until all possible controversy is put to rest." The company, in fact, reaffirmed that MER/29 was safe when used as recommended.

But the FDA finally submitted its MER/29 findings to the Justice Department. Within months, Merrell was under criminal investigation by a grand jury and three congressional committees. The FDA New Drug Division circulated an internal memo cautioning its staff that any information submitted by Merrell required "thorough verification."

Meanwhile, when two weeks had passed without a sign of Merrell's Kevadon clinical investigator list, Frances alerted her bosses. The FDA sent field officers to Merrell headquarters, who for three days prowled the Cincinnati office, asking about the Kevadon program. But the names of the trial doctors were still nowhere to be found.

Joseph Murray tried to placate Frances, insisting that the company had duly warned its doctors. In December, within days of learning the news from Germany, he had purportedly alerted American "investigators then active with Kevadon" to the initial information and told the doctors not to give it to pregnant women or women who might become pregnant. Then on March 20, after Merrell formally withdrew its FDA application, those same doctors—"as well as others who had received the drug"—were asked to end their studies and return supplies. As proof, Murray gave Frances copies of the letters, but it would later emerge that in February, Merrell had followed up with investigators to insist there was still "no positive proof of a causal relationship between the use of thalidomide during pregnancy and malformations." Plus, Merrell had advised doctors, pregnant rats given thalidomide had not shown a single malformation.

On the day Frances received Murray's timeline of its warning letters, the list of clinical investigators at last arrived. It now made sense why it had taken so long to compile. As Frances read page after page, name after name, tallying all the locations and specialists, her unease mounted. More than 1,200 doctors had been dispensing thalidomide throughout the United States. And more than 240 of them specialized in obstetrics and gynecology.

These drug fellows pay for a lobby that makes the steel boys look like popcorn venders. In the end, they mounted against Estes the most intense attack that I've seen in a quarter century in Washington.

—Paul Rand Dixon,

U.S. Senate Antitrust and Monopoly Subcommittee

Twenty-four

On April 12, 1961, Kefauver rose in the Senate and at last submitted drug bill S. 1552. While the presidency might never be his, he had won his third Senate term, and a piece of major drug legislation, the first since 1938, seemed dazzlingly within his reach.

The bill aimed to lower prices and increase safety. After three years of an exclusive patent, drug firms had to permit license of their products. To ensure quality, the FDA would authorize drug manufacturers and inspect plants. HEW would eliminate indecipherable generic names. And any promotional materials with a trade name now had to show the generic name with equal prominence.

To improve safety, ads would have to disclose side effects and efficacy. Package inserts, with warnings and contraindications, would go to doctors, not just pharmacists. And HEW would publish an annual list of worrisome drugs. In addition, Barbara Moulton's proposals from a few years earlier had finally been codified: The sixty-day automatic approval for drugs was eliminated, and manufacturers would now have to prove each drug was both safe and effective.

The legislative hearings began in July 1961 and were set to last through February—a lengthy concession to Republican committee members trying to give the drug industry time to mount a defense. But the hearings were basically a rehash of Kefauver's investigative probe of 1960—exposés of drug industry malfeasance—with a few memorable new characters.

Early 1962 brought the enigmatic Sacklers to the stage. The three brothers—Mortimer, Arthur, and Raymond—had forged a highly integrated pharmaceutical operation that could develop drugs and then publish favorable research papers in their own medical journals. Arthur, head of Douglas McAdams, appeared before the subcommittee in January of 1962 to defend his firm's misleading ads for MER/29. "I would prefer to have thin hair to thick coronaries," Sackler snipped. At which point a Kefauver aide pointed out that since MER/29's efficacy had never been established, there was no assurance that MER/29 would protect Arthur's coronaries.

The press tracked the hearings closely, and mail from around the country championed Kefauver. Eleanor Roosevelt, following the proceedings, decried the industry's "price-fixing and monopolistic practices." It had been two decades since she had toured the FDA's "Chamber of Horrors," and she was aghast—all these years later—to learn that "hidden and serious dangers in drugs are not revealed in advertising or information supplied even to doctors." If drugs were sold before proper clinical trials were completed, patients had become "unwitting guinea pigs."

The White House, however, had mostly shunned Kefauver's efforts. The Tennessee senator had been President Kennedy's two-time rival in the national Democratic primaries, and relations between the two men were chilly. But on January 11, 1962, Kennedy appeared to do an about-face and champion Kafauver's work: In his State of the Union address, the president promised to "recommend improvements in the food and drug laws . . . to protect our consumers from the careless and the unscrupulous."

Confident that his twenty-six exhausting months of hearings and 12,885 pages of documented testimony had firmly established his case, on the morning of February 7, 1962, Kefauver adjourned the session. The drug hearings were over.

At that point, President Kennedy alerted the chair of the Judiciary Committee, the first hurdle for the new bill, that it was his "sincere wish that it [S. 1552] be enacted during the current session of the Congress." But even with the president's support, Kefauver and his team knew a long battle loomed to push the bill through Congress. They would have to "stir people up."

On April 12, a properly stirring story landed at their feet. John Blair's secretary—a young woman from Tennessee named Jo Anne Youngblood—raced into the office waving a New York Times article: "Deformed Babies Traced to a Drug." A Dr. Helen Taussig, it turned out, had just given a speech in Philadelphia to warn about an overseas epidemic of birth defects.

"This compound could have passed our present drug laws," Taussig had told reporters. "We must strengthen our food and drug regulation."

Kefauver, excited, dispatched Lucille Wendt—a bacteriologist, patent expert, and lawyer on his staff—to dig up everything she could on thalidomide.

WM. S. MERRELL COMPANY

DIVISION OF RICHARDSON-MERRELL INC.

PHARMACEUTICAL MANUFACTURERS SINCE 1828

CINCINNATI, OHIO

May 1, 1962

Dr. H. W. v. Schrader-Beielstein
Chemie Grunenthal GmbH
Stolberg, Rheinland
Germany

Dear Doctor von Schrader:

I have been reviewing the files on thalidomide and one discrepancy has caught my attention. You advised us in early December of 1961 that the first reports you had heard on the Dusseldorf conference were encouraging and that the consensus of the experts was that a warning letter would have been adequate instead of withdrawing the drug from the market. However, when we received the actual report some weeks later, our translation indicates the experts felt it was proper to remove the drug. Since there is no explanation for this discrepancy in my file, I would be very interested in any comments you may care to make.

With best wishes,

Sincerely yours,
F. Jos. Murray

I am the size of a two-year-old without my wooden legs. I was born missing a lot of bones. I have two fingers on my left arm, and just a thumb on my right. The doctors wouldn't let my mom see me right away. They tried to convince her that because I was misformed on the outside, I was misformed on the inside. They wanted her to give me up. But she insisted on seeing me.

My mom told me, and I believe my mom, that this was an act of God. That God wanted me to be this way. She said she only took aspirin. I don't think my mom would lie to me.

— Peggy Martz Smith,
born May 1962,
Fort Thomas, Kentucky

The evidence is overwhelming that thalidomide causes a specific and absolutely ghastly malformation. . . . It certainly is only by the "grace of God" that our country has escaped.

—Helen Taussig,
April 3, 1962

Twenty-five

Since she'd returned from Europe, Helen Taussig had been trying to measure the aftermath of thalidomide. In addition to pressing hospitals in Germany for updated phocomelia data—malformed babies were still born there weekly—she contacted medical authorities worldwide and soon had reports from Australia, New Zealand, and Japan. Canadian cases, she learned, reached into the hundreds, even though the drug had been sold there by prescription. But Merrell had championed the safety of the drug, and doctors had shared samples freely. A Canadian doctor with a phocomelic son admitted that he had given some to his pregnant wife.

As Taussig helped Canadian families navigate choices on amputation, prosthetics, and rehabilitation—she had become the authority on phocomelia—she braced for more cases from that country. Reports indicated that even after the March recall, some 10 to 15 percent of Canadian pharmacists refused to relinquish the drug. It was, they reasoned, still safe for men.

But Taussig hit a wall in her attempts to get data from the United States. She had learned of a phocomelic baby born at an American base in Nuremberg, Germany, but there were simply no reports of phocomelic births on American soil remotely traced to thalidomide. (For the time being, Merrell made no mention that they had learned in January and February of four deformed babies born to patients of Ray O. Nulsen.)

Further, Merrell skirted any inquiry that might establish a clear connection between thalidomide and birth deformities. The overseas cases, the firm told Taussig, so varied in environment and parentage, were posing "difficult limitations on analysis." It was "no simple matter," Murray complained, "to obtain detailed and significant histories on each human case." Murray, in fact, asked Taussig's help in determining "the appropriate way in which to approach this problem."

Taussig thought, at the very least, the drug might have left a trail of damage near the firm's headquarters, in Cincinnati. After all, so many of the first German cases had been linked to Grünenthal employees. But when Taussig queried Children's Hospital in Cincinnati, she was assured that the drug hadn't been administered anywhere in the city.

The source of this misinformation was Dr. Josef Warkany, president of the Teratology Society of America. In a bizarre irony, the very first American organization dedicated to the study of congenital birth defects had been founded in Cincinnati in 1960, a mere mile or so from Merrell's headquarters, just as Merrell was submitting its FDA application for Kevadon. The Society was the brainchild of Austrian-born Warkany, who in 1940 became the first person ever to show that environmental factors could cause birth defects. Warkany should have been *the* scientist to jump in and untangle thalidomide's ravages. Thousands of tablets had been given to pregnant women throughout his own city, where he gave lectures on teratology, and where Flor Van Maanen of Merrell attended his seminars. Yet someone had told Warkany that thalidomide hadn't been used in Cincinnati. Further, something Warkany had heard about the overseas phocomelia epidemic convinced him that thalidomide couldn't be responsible.

Undeterred, Taussig decided to run her own animal experiments. She wrote to Merrell requesting bulk thalidomide, and Joseph Murray provided her with five hundred grams. She was determined to produce laboratory evidence of malformations in rabbits and end the denials.

Taussig doggedly shared her findings at medical conferences up and down the East Coast. But while doctors reeled at the story, the press ignored her. After the *New York Times* coverage of her Philadelphia speech, the media had gone silent, and she couldn't bait medical journals. The American Medical Association refused her paper on the epidemic because *Time* had briefly covered the matter. Outraged, Taussig focused on the lay press, but her pitches to general magazines were also spurned. *Redbook* turned down her story to avoid unduly scaring expectant mothers.

Finally, on May 14 *The New England Journal of Medicine* agreed to publish her research. "We can no longer afford to get stuffy because an eager lay press picks up some information of importance," the editor conceded. After that, *Scientific American* snapped to attention and asked her for her material.

But Taussig's greatest chance to sound the alarm came in late May of 1962 when Congressman Emanuel Celler of New York invited her before his House antitrust subcommittee. Celler was in the process of introducing a measure in the House as a companion to Kefauver's Senate bill, and Taussig would speak to H.R. 6245, the Drug Industry Antitrust Act.

As in the Senate, industry pushback on the measure had been vigorous. The American Institute of Chemists depicted the bill as an attack on the Thomas Edisons of the day, whose "inventive spirit" would be tragically fettered should private pharmaceutical research laboratories be saddled with restrictions. The yeas and nays for the bill had come from predictable sources, a reprise of positions on Kefauver's bill. The announcement that Dr. Helen Taussig was on the schedule to testify riled the measure's opponents.

"Dr. Taussig may be a brilliant physiologist, but she is not a pharmacologist, and she has no right to testify about drugs," declared the AMA's Morris Fishbein, angered that an individual doctor was "campaigning" for the bill.

Nonetheless, the stately Taussig stepped into Celler's hearing room on Thursday, May 24—her sixty-fourth birthday. Frances sat in the audience to offer support.

After reading prepared remarks, narrating her travels to Germany and England, describing the work of Widukind Lenz and George Somers and the 3,500 babies so far harmed by the drug, Helen got to the photographs.

As she prepared to project her slides, she realized many people seated around the vast gallery wouldn't be able to see. She urged people to adjust their seats, and a congressman from New Jersey invited onlookers to move forward. Worried that her automatic projector might run too quickly for people to take in the pictures, she offered to run the slideshow twice.

When at last her images flashed on, Taussig narrated: "There is a baby and you will notice the little flippers of arms up here, one malformed leg. . . . Another baby, two arms, no hands . . . Another one here with the legs very seriously malformed . . . Another one, a bright lad, and look at the arms."

She'd been strategic in her choice of pictures: These were not, by far, the most gutting injuries she'd witnessed. Instead, she had chosen bright and lively children with truncated arms or missing legs. She wanted the committee to grasp that these children had "normal mentalities"—meaning they would, in time, understand their limitations. This, Taussig believed, was the heartbreak.

"There is nothing you see in the pictures," Taussig somberly told the crowd, "that is as terrible as seeing the children." The committee appeared duly stunned, and Helen continued, articulating her support for Celler's bill.

"A drug cannot be assumed to be safe for infants and children because it is safe for adults," she declared. The FDA must require that drugs be tested specifically for effects on the fetus. And any warnings about contraindications for pregnancy and children should be in massive type—as large and prominent as the brand name.

She endorsed the provision for an annual government list of problematic drugs and, like Moulton, argued that a drug's "efficacy" must be a factor in its approval.

As for thalidomide, Taussig said that had the sedative been invented in the United States, it would likely have ended up on the market given the lax drug laws. Then she gave a nod to Frances, seated in the gallery, noting that the drug was stopped from going on sale only by the great work of "one person in the FDA" who'd been "afraid that it might have some harmful effects on pregnancy."

But what harm would the next strange molecule bring? And when? What if it was harder to detect? "We ought to do what we humanly can to prevent future catastrophes," Taussig warned.

Taussig's hour-long testimony seemed to rouse Celler's committee, but it failed to reach the press. The drug hearings had dragged on so long that no one from the media had shown up to hear the Johns Hopkins cardiologist. There was neither a radio mention nor a newspaper clipping to memorialize the event, and John Nestor, livid that his former medical school mentor had been ignored, put in a frustrated call to Kefauver's team: Their whole drug bill might hinge on this one story—thalidomide—getting national attention. He urged them to get the word out.

But Kefauver knew this. In fact, his team had tried to talk Celler out of inviting Taussig to testify because it was too far from either bill reaching a final vote. If they could all wait a little longer, they would, at the right moment, leak the story Eppes Wayles Browne had heard: Merrell had hounded a medical reviewer and mother of two for almost two years in an attempt to force her to approve a dangerous drug. Between Kennedy's support and Frances's story, the fate of Kefauver's bill looked bright.

*When I was born, my arm looked like a chicken
wing. . . . They transferred me to the university hospital. I know from looking at hospital records that
they said that I was a girl when I was born, and then
when they transferred me, they said I was a boy. Un-
descended testicles. The doctors right off the bat told
my parents there wasn't anything that caused it, it
was just God's will.*

—*Darren Griggs,*
born June 1962,
Columbia, Missouri

It is chilling to think that under the current laws,

several companies could have suspected the terato-

genic effects of this drug and quietly developed their

marketing plans without disclosing the hazard.

—*Frances Kelsey, 1962*

Twenty-six

On Monday morning, June 11, Kefauver arrived at the Senate in great spirits. In his hand was a letter from the patent commissioner, enthusiastically supporting his bill's patent provision. Kefauver had recently tussled with fellow committee members over his requirement that patents on mixtures or modifications of existing drugs show "greater therapeutic effect." Others on the committee preferred "substantial" to "greater," but Kefauver was having none of it. He now had an official letter from the patent office to support "greater," and he was certain he had the votes to get S. 1552 reported out of committee that day.

But as he entered the Judiciary Committee hearing room, he was struck by the vast number of senators gathered. And when the meeting started and he showed his letter, they voted down his wording.

Worse, the minority leader, Illinois Republican senator Everett Dirksen, dubbed "the Wizard of Ooze" for his flamboyant speeches, distributed mimeographed copies of an entirely *new* set of amendments. Including a watered-down patent provision. These revisions—basically a new bill that went light on the drug industry—would be renamed the Eastland-Dirksen bill.

Kefauver, confounded, soon unraveled the backstory. Days earlier, the White House had decided that rather than champion Kefauver's drug bill, it would take credit for its own. Thus, Jim Eastland of Mississippi, chair of the Senate Judiciary Committee, was deputized to do *whatever* was needed to get a bill reported onto the floor for a vote. For Eastland, this meant icing out Kefauver.

In what would later be called "the secret meeting," Eastland's staff director, two representatives from HEW, two Republican lawyers, and two representatives from the Pharmaceutical Manufacturers Association all met with the blessing of Myer Feldman, Kennedy's right-hand man. The daylong June 8 gathering began with drug industry men presenting *their* ideal amendments, which by early evening the whole group had somewhat informally agreed to. Nothing was set in stone.

But by the following Monday morning, the PMA had typed up the handshake agreements to present to the Judiciary Committee as a new bill, ostensibly blessed by HEW.

Kefauver was irate. One of the HEW representatives, Jerome Sonosky, so shocked and embarrassed to see his Friday-afternoon scribblings in official amendment form, had to admit to Kefauver that he'd attended the meeting at the behest of the White House. Only . . . the White House had yet to see the new bill. Sonosky said that his boss, Wilbur Cohen, HEW's assistant secretary for legislation, had reviewed it all Friday evening, but Cohen denied it.

It was legislative hot potato. No one would admit to sanctioning the PMA's version, and no one wanted Kefauver's ire. Kefauver called HEW and the White House. In twenty-three years in Congress, he ranted, no administration had ever "emasculated a bill without letting its sponsor and chairman know."

A sacred line had been crossed.

Colleagues rallied to Kefauver's cause. Senator John Carroll of Colorado managed to filibuster until noon to stall a vote, and then objected to the continuation of the meeting to shut down the matter for the day.

Meanwhile, Kefauver, brooding in his office, told his team: "I'm going to the floor to have this out." Aides wanted him to cool off, but Kefauver headed to the Capitol.

Just after the buzzer rang to signify a quorum call, Kefauver announced he intended to speak. Word traveled fast. Myer Feldman at the White House immediately put in a call to Kefauver, and Kefauver stepped out of the chamber to take it.

"I haven't been so shoddily treated in twenty-three years in Congress," Kefauver told Feldman and hung up. When he returned to the chamber, the secretary to the majority urged him to stop. But Kefauver refused.

"Today a severe blow to the public interest was delivered in the Senate Judiciary Committee," Kefauver told the room. "Most of the drug manufacturing industry and its acolytes have been punching away for some time at S. 1552. . . . Today they swung a 'haymaker' and just about knocked this bill right out of the ring. I refuse to believe that my colleagues in the U.S. Senate will let this sorely needed legislation go down 'for the count.'"

Kefauver presented a copy of Kennedy's letter to Senator Eastland from April, supporting the original bill. "In this letter the president not only strongly endorses S. 1552 as amended, but also requested certain additions and minor changes, which by request I was prepared to offer."

Kefauver could not *believe*—he asserted this several times—that the new bill had the president's support. He had the patent commissioner's support for the language in his patent provision, and a letter to prove it. That was supposed to end the controversy over particulars. "Much to my amazement, at a meeting of the Judiciary this morning, I discovered that there had been a secret meeting."

The story of the hush-hush summit riveted the room. Virtually every piece of Kefauver's bill had been watered down to become "a mere shadow of the one approved by the Antitrust and Monopoly Committee" months earlier. Kefauver would later say that the only upside of the Eastland-Dirksen bill was that it didn't repeal the Food, Drug, and Cosmetic Act of 1938.

Essentially daring the president to acknowledge backpedaling, Kefauver then issued a challenge: "I want the people to know what has been happening. . . . I think the people are now entitled to know . . . what the administration's present position is." Then he sat down. A dead silence followed. No one had ever seen a senator defy the president, the leader of his own party, or even the chairman of the Judiciary Committee. Eastland, the "king of kings" who oversaw the passage of nearly half of all Senate bills, was inordinately powerful.

But Eastland calmly lit a cigar and accepted responsibility for the bill. He was sure the White House would back him. Then Dirksen—de facto cosponsor of the bill—closed the session with an odd tribute to Kefauver:

> He is as single purposed as an Apache Indian. He is as gracious as a Victorian lady. There is a rare diligence about him, and a rare consistency also. . . . His patience is certainly equal to that of Job. I think he makes Job look a little like an amateur.

At Kefauver's chambers that afternoon, a *Washington Post* financial reporter named Bernard Nossiter stopped by to see John Blair, Kefauver's economist, and offer condolences on the doomed bill.

"Don't be too sure," Blair replied.

Despite Kennedy's sabotage, Kefauver's thalidomide dossier was now complete. He knew the full story of FDA medical reviewer Frances Kelsey and her fight to block the German drug, and Kefauver's team was ready to pull this rabbit from their hat.

"If it hadn't been for Dr. Kelsey," Blair told the *Post* reporter, "thalidomide would have been selling here for the past year and we'd now have a medical disaster of major proportions on our hands."

Nossiter headed back to the newsroom and passed the tip to his editor.

I am desperately worried that because we have not had phocomelia in this country our doctors are going to oppose stricter legislation. If we had thousands of cases here they would all be up in arms and we would have no difficulty at all in getting legislation through. As it is, it may be a long hard fight.

—Helen Taussig,

June 19, 1962

Twenty-seven

Morton Mintz was a man of strong opinions.

The father of four and ex–navy officer had been working as a reporter at *The Washington Post* for four years and was known within the newsroom for his fervor. He loathed injustice, and he was a self-starter with a habit of going after big targets—no institution was too powerful to scare him off.

In 1959 and 1960 he'd written a five-part series on the health hazards of auto exhaust, taking to task behemoths like General Motors and Ford. In 1961 he began a yearlong probe into the Maryland savings and loan scandal that would result in multiple high-level government indictments. Mintz made enemies easily and proudly. He loved telling stories of the moguls who hated him. Famed Watergate reporter Bob Woodward, later in life, would single out Mintz as a beacon of bravery in a newsroom known for bravery. Mintz had a particular zeal for writing about congressional oversight—hearings in which the government dug into its own dirt—and he covered inquiries around the Capitol that most reporters blew off. He was one of the few journalists in town who routinely showed up for subcommittee probes of all sorts, riveted by every piece of Beltway minutia.

Mintz, the child of Lithuanian immigrants, had felt the pull of journalism early. When he arrived at the University of Michigan, he immediately began writing for *The Michigan Daily*, soon rising to editorial director, and became a campus correspondent for *The Detroit News*. He graduated in 1943 and served on a tank landing ship for the invasions of Normandy and Okinawa. He returned to the States in June 1946, fell hard for a friend of his sister's, Anita, whom he married within months, and then landed a job at the *St. Louis Star-Times*.

Mort was assigned basic cub reporter items for the paper: police blotter bits, obituaries, and caption writing. His pay was only ninety dollars a week, but when he switched from the *Star-Times* to the *St. Louis Globe-Democrat* in 1951, his salary and assignments improved. Soon after, he and Anita had their first child, Margaret. In November 1951, their second daughter, Elizabeth, was born with severe Down syndrome. This upturned the couple's life. Her care in a private facility cost one hundred dollars per month, amounting to 13 percent of Mort's gross pay. At age seven, her access to that care would end. Subsequent private care would run twice as much. But the state institutions for special-needs children were known as some of the worst in the nation.

Frustrated by their predicament, and realizing other families faced similar plights, in June 1954, Mintz pleaded his case before the mental health committee of the state senate. For nearly an hour, he mapped out his personal situation and shared research showing the better standards of care in other states. He offered suggestions for how new legislation could improve care in Missouri.

The speech bore the hallmark of Mintz's later work—exhaustive research bolstering a strong moral message. "This little girl of ours is an innocent human being," Mintz implored. "She has feelings. She can be hurt or helped, she is capable of being made happy or being made miserable, just as you and I, and she is our flesh and blood." She deserved, he said, "the opportunity to learn, to give and receive affection, to be as happy as a person so afflicted may be." The state care was so abysmal that should he and Anita have to leave Elizabeth there, "we should be weighed down emotionally with feelings of guilt, fear, and cruelty.

"I must tell you honestly and bluntly that I am appalled and baffled," he told the committee. "I am beset by disgust and indignation with the inertia, the apathy, the indifference, the ignorance that beset this state when it comes to providing adequate care for the mentally retarded. . . . Does it not haunt the conscience of our leaders . . . ? Does not the situation fire our leaders with zeal and determination to correct it?"

But the speech did not elicit the hoped-for change. And Mintz grew obsessed.

By 1955 his crusade to help Elizabeth morphed into an in-depth *Globe-Democrat* series on "mental retardation." He probed its effect on families and exposed government apathy, noting the glaring lack of research into causes or cures. His groundbreaking reporting on the formerly closeted matter earned praise from the chief psychiatrist at the National Institutes of Health, plus an award from the Missouri Association for Retarded Children: Mintz's journalism, they said, sought to bring the "basic rights of humane justice" to those considered "the least amongst us."

But as the clock ran out on Elizabeth's private care, Missouri made no improvements in the "backwardness and neglect" of its public institutions. With another child, Roberta, to factor into their finances, the couple decided to uproot themselves and move to Washington, D.C., where public care was better. Mort landed a job at *The Washington Post*.

The *Post* was not yet the Pulitzer Prize machine of the 1970s, when the Pentagon Papers and Watergate exposés would bring the paper national fame. But executive editor James Russell Wiggins had been shifting the paper toward original reporting; to that end, he had been growing the paper's staff to avoid relying on news services. Mintz, hired in 1958, was part of that initiative.

His 1959 series on air pollution had pitted him against the giants of the automobile industry. In 1960, he had drummed up attention for the Twenty-third Amendment, which would allow District of Columbia residents to vote in national elections. From October 1961 to June 1962, he had probed a Maryland banking scandal that resulted in the indictment of two congressmen and the speaker of the Maryland House of Delegates.

Mintz's byline was starting to carry some weight, but he was far from a superstar. And as a general-assignment reporter without a specialty, he sweated hard for each story: Every investigation required that he master a whole new field. In his mind this was an asset. He could build a rapport with the reader and communicate clearly because he, too, was coming to the story fresh.

He and Anita now lived in a two-story house in Cleveland Park with a nice backyard and a view of Tregaron—a sprawling thirteen-acre estate. Mintz could sometimes sneak in a game of tennis on the nearby courts. Daniel, their fourth child, had been born in 1961, and Elizabeth was living in a wonderful public care home. Mintz worked late during the week on deadlines, but Sundays were reserved for family dinner.

Sometime in early July of 1962, Mort's editor, Seymour "Sy" Fishbein, called him over in the newsroom. Fishbein laid out the story relayed from the Kefauver offices and suggested Mintz speak with the FDA reviewer.

Mintz was surprised. The FDA wasn't his beat. But Fishbein had decided the paper's medical reporter wasn't right for the piece and had been stalling until the man left for vacation. Fishbein wanted Mintz on this story. Mintz had the right capacity for outrage. And upon hearing the basics, Mintz was enraged. It didn't hurt that his mother had had a severe reaction to a Merrell cholesterol drug, triparanol—MER/29.

So, on July 11, Mintz went over to the FDA offices to interview Frances Kelsey about thalidomide. And the first thing he did—before he got to his questions—was explain about his daughter Elizabeth.

WEARS NO MAKEUP—HATES HOUSEWORK

DR. KELSEY WOULD PREFER TO
RETAIN ANONYMITY

*The practically unknown woman doctor who saved untold
American mothers and babies through her lone, stubborn
fight against a new drug has become a national celebrity
overnight. . . .*

WASHINGTON—DR. Frances Oldham Kelsey—a no-nonsense
woman with straight, severely cut gray hair, no makeup, stout
shoes, and a shyly quiet voice—is America's new sweetheart.

—The Boston Globe, *Sunday, August 5, 1962*

When will our real Mommy be back?

—*Susan Kelsey,*

diary entry, August 1962

Twenty-eight

On a hot, muggy Sunday in July 1962, Frances awoke to see her photograph on the front page of *The Washington Post*, beneath the headline "Heroine at FDA Keeps Bad Drug Off Market." It had happened at lightning speed. The Thursday before, a spritely blue-eyed reporter had come to her bare FDA office, asking about her every interaction with Merrell for the past two years.

Now the whole country was talking about Frances's battle to stop thalidomide. She had saved the United States from a dangerous drug. Frances couldn't quite wrap her mind around it.

The day the article came out was chaos. The phone rang off the hook—magazines, newspapers, and radio stations all wanted to speak with the tenacious lady doctor. The *New York World-Telegram & Sun* newspaper sent over a photographer to capture Frances's domestic side. He snapped pictures of her passing phonograph records to Susan and Christine in the living room, or posed with Ellis, standing over the girls as they sat side by side at the piano. They all found it absurd. When had the family *ever* hovered like that around the piano? The girls wore matching short-sleeved white blouses and headbands, while Frances sported a simple dark housedress. In the pictures, she looks warm, motherly, and attentive—as though she hadn't worked grueling hours in a windowless office for the past two years. No hint that she left the girls at home for days at a stretch to attend conferences. The choreography of making Frances look like a normal mom, a woman the public could identify with, had the family in stitches.

In the afternoon, she and Ellis slipped away to a backyard barbecue. Albert Sjoerdsma, a former pharmacology colleague from the University of Chicago, was hosting friends at his new home in Bethesda. Susan and Christine stayed home to mind the telephone, which kept ringing.

Frances and Ellis stood on the screened porch drinking Manhattans with the other adults while children played softball in the blazing-hot yard. Ellis was his boisterous self, but Frances was quiet, absorbing the absurdity of everything that had transpired. Suddenly Mrs. Sjoerdsma ushered Frances into her study. Christine and Susan back home relayed a call from NBC Radio, and Frances had to give a live interview. In another room, the guests and children gathered around the transistor radio to listen.

When Frances finally emerged from the study, a seven-year-old girl excitedly declared, "History is being made in our house today."

Frances was sure the hubbub would die down quickly. Over the next few days, however, the attention intensified. As the *Washington Post* article was reprinted in papers across the country, letters of congratulation and gratitude arrived at the house from nearly every state. (At the end of his article, Mintz had printed her address, as was normal in that day.) Susan and Christine checked the mailbox daily, gathering dozens of notes at a time. Some, like Santa Claus mail, were merely addressed to "Dr. Kelsey, Washington, D.C."

More letters arrived at her FDA office. Doctors, nurses, housewives, lawyers, and investment managers wanted to celebrate her "courage in fighting off these monstrous forces." Fans cheered her "true, honest, integrity and moral, as well as objective character." Frances seemed a remedy against the current "corruption of public figures." A woman from Ohio found it "heartwarming to know that there are dedicated individuals who adhere to their principles in spite of pressures that are brought upon them." Frances was crystallizing in the minds of Americans as a patriot fighting to "protect the citizens of this great country."

"IF our civilization survives," one woman wrote, "it will be because of people like you who have integrity and a sense of the value of human life." Frances seemed a fortification against the "big, selfish interests [that] prize the 'ALMIGHTY DOLLAR' above everything" that many saw overtaking the country.

Most interesting, however, was a mother from Brooklyn who mentioned Senator Kefauver's scorn for the weakened drug bill that had just come out of the Senate. The woman urged Frances to "show Congress how important a strict law in this field would be."

In fact, Kefauver had already enlisted Frances. On July 16, the day after the publication of the *Washington Post* article, the Tennessee senator invited Frances and her family to Capitol Hill that upcoming Wednesday. Mintz's article hadn't quite stirred Congress to action as Kefauver had hoped. Deputy FDA commissioner Winton Rankin said that while the American public owed Frances a "vote of thanks," the current law was clearly sufficient because it had let her block the drug. In effect, the thalidomide story was now being used to stop Kefauver's bill.

But Kefauver knew there was more to the thalidomide story than Mintz had covered. No feel-good victory was at play. Kefauver planned to get hold of Merrell's FDA paperwork and examine all its false claims. And if he could nudge Frances further into the public eye and show the full drama of her fight with Merrell, he could prove the need for a stronger bill.

On July 18, five weeks after his fiery Senate speech, Kefauver calmly stood before Congress and, with Frances and her family watching from the gallery, called upon Kennedy to award her a national medal for Distinguished Federal Civilian Service.

His original S. 1552, he reminded colleagues, would have stopped a disaster such as thalidomide. And that tipped it: The next day, Kefauver's original bill was finally released by the committee—a huge step forward.

But Morton Mintz's *Washington Post* story had another outcome: Mothers and fathers and nurses and pharmacists began calling the FDA, asking if any pills had circulated within the United States. Because no one in the American press yet knew that the drug had been used across the United States by more than 1,200 doctors, the public had no idea it was at risk.

Part IV

THE
COST

Twenty-nine

On July 23, *The Arizona Republic* ran a shocking front-page story, "PILL MAY COST WOMAN HER BABY," reporting on an unidentified pregnant Phoenix woman who, having read in the paper about Frances, realized she had taken thalidomide.

The woman's husband, a teacher, had procured the pills in London while leading an overseas school trip. After his wife—already a mother of four—ran out of the tranquilizers she was taking for "nerves," she borrowed her husband's stash, using upward of thirty pills in a month. The woman called her doctor, who cabled the London drugstore and confirmed she'd been taking pure thalidomide.

Since this was the first word of any American woman having access to thalidomide, the doctor scrambled for information, calling Frances at the FDA. Frances referred him to Taussig, and within days, he sent a Western Union telefax to Helen in Baltimore:

HAVE PATIENT TWO AND A HALF MONTHS PREGNANT HAVE ESTABLISHED DEFINITELY THAT SHE HAS BEEN SUBJECTED TO THALIDOMIDE PATIENT OBTAINED DRUG WHILE IN EUROPE

Taussig leveled with him: Given the quantity and timing of the thalidomide use, the odds of a healthy baby were grim. "Therapeutic" abortion would be justified.

The doctor, himself a father of four, counseled his patient that if she hoped for another child, "I would strongly recommend you terminate this pregnancy and start again next month under better odds." To drive home the danger of going through with the birth, he showed her a picture from a medical journal of five swaddled infants with only heads and torsos. The woman decided to terminate, and the doctor arranged with the hospital's three-person medical board for a procedure later that week. In the meantime, still shocked that this overseas toxin had wound up in her home—the woman deemed it her civic duty to warn others. She spoke with *The Arizona Republic*'s medical editor on the condition of anonymity, and the resulting published story sparked national interest: an *American* mother harmed by the notorious German drug.

Moreover, her plans for an abortion drew scrutiny. This was a decade before *Roe v. Wade*, and, except to save a woman's life, abortion was illegal—a back-alley or overseas endeavor. Over the next two days, the press descended on Phoenix. When the county attorney, a Catholic father of nine, threatened to prosecute the hospital, the hospital canceled the procedure and sued the state and county to force a judgment; the hospital wanted to know, in advance, if the abortion would be protected by law. Its legal filing, however, required release of the woman's identity.

On July 26, the story exploded even more sensationally: *The Arizona Republic*, in "Mother TV Star Here," revealed that the mystery woman was charismatic TV personality Sherri Chessen Finkbine, host of the Arizona edition of the nationally syndicated *Romper Room*. On the live morning nursery school show, the petite "Miss Sherri" led the Pledge of Allegiance before serving children milk and cookies with a "God is great" prayer.

Her wholesome image clashed so dramatically with the public's concept of abortion—the lawless choice of wayward women—that her decision to go through with the procedure sparked a heated national debate. Editorial writers nationwide weighed in to applaud or scold Finkbine, while nascent feminists began to advocate for reproductive rights. A Gallup survey of Americans coast to coast showed that 52 percent of those polled supported Sherri's choice, 32 percent disagreed, and 16 percent claimed to have no opinion.

But with the Finkbine house engulfed by media, any hope of having the procedure on American soil vanished. No U.S. hospital would risk the attention, so Sherri and her husband flew to Sweden, where the law protected her choice. On August 18, as Vatican Radio declared that "a crime" was being committed in Sweden, the fetus emerged, as predicted, with only one arm and no legs. It was not a baby, the Swedish doctor told Sherri, but an "abnormal growth."

Returning to Phoenix, the Finkbines faced further drama. Anonymous letters threatened to cut the arms and legs off their children, and FBI agents were assigned to a protection detail. Shunned by friends, colleagues, and even the doctor who had originally advised the procedure, Sherri lost her *Romper Room* job. For the rest of her life, she would be remembered as the woman who in 1962 dared to assert her right to an abortion.

Nonetheless, Sherri had accomplished her civic goal—the mother of four had alerted women across the country that thalidomide could be in their homes.

Most U.S. government officials had never heard of thalidomide until Helen Taussig testified before Celler's House subcommittee in May 1962. In the aftermath of her appearance, Merrell, in its first public comment on the matter, assured Congress that timely warnings had been sent to all of their clinical investigators and that thalidomide's link to birth defects was "still mere speculation."

In her FDA office, however, Frances was dubious and had begun tallying the Kevadon investigators in each state. Based on the scale of the trials alone—more than 1,200—how could Merrell's trials *not* have resulted in any birth deformities?

While the FDA leadership publicly accepted Merrell's stance, Frances began digging. She telephoned a former professor from her medical school days: Dr. Edith Potter, an authority on fetal pathology, worked at Chicago's Lying-In Hospital, where Frances's own daughters had been born. With at least eighty-one doctors in Illinois dispensing the drug, Frances suspected some injuries. Potter explained that the hospital kept no official registrar for birth malformations, but she knew of two cases of limb abnormalities that past March. One involved the baby's feet; the other involved both arms but wasn't "typical phocomelia." Neither mother, however, recalled taking any drugs. Potter promised to advise Frances of any developments.

News of six cases of phocomelia at Cincinnati General Hospital alarmed her. A Kevadon investigator there working in anesthesiology had apparently advised Merrell of these abnormal births in July, yet he maintained that "no women of childbearing years" had received the drug. Given the high number and proximity to Merrell's headquarters, Frances urged an inquiry.

As rumors spread within the government of the scope of Merrell's trials, health commissioners across the country began asking if the drug had been dispensed in *their* states, and the FDA began confidentially sharing numbers—77 trials in New York, 110 in Ohio, 72 in California, etc.—but regional health commissions were assured Merrell's trials had caused no cases of phocomelia.

After Mintz's *Washington Post* piece on Frances, however, the public, too, wondered about stray pills, and the Finkbine story galvanized the press. *The Arizona Journal* called the FDA: Was the agency checking on Merrell's trial doctors? The *New York World-Telegram & Sun*, tipped off by the New York City Department of Health, published a story about "federal red tape" hampering efforts to find the doctors who got thalidomide. The Ohio Department of Health—stunned by the number of trial doctors in the state—wanted names. Eventually, an Indiana FDA official broke ranks and gave his regional health agency the Kevadon investigator names. News that the names were out triggered more requests.

Commissioner Larrick—who had done astoundingly little since learning about the scope of the Kevadon trials—finally asked Merrell if all doses of the drug had been rounded up. Given that Merrell was under criminal investigation for falsifying MER/29 data and had fought tooth and nail to keep the product in circulation after its toxic side effects were known, Larrick's request appears oddly delicate: He was following up merely "because of inquiries which had been made of us as to whether or not some of the drug might still be available" and because "we found ourselves unable to answer this question with finality."

Merrell quickly redoubled its defense. A company press release affirmed that thalidomide was "never sold in the United States" and that phocomelia was only "circumstantially linked" to the drug. The FDA did nothing to clarify for the public that "sold" did not mean distributed. The agency officially backed Merrell, as did the media. The *Cincinnati En-*

quirer's nearly word-for-word summary of Merrell's press release assured readers that their hometown firm was handling matters responsibly.

But the firm's behavior grew clumsier by the day. Five days after Merrell's executive vice president met with Larrick to assure him that Vick Chemical, Merrell's affiliate, had *never* distributed thalidomide, he called Larrick back to clarify that Vick had, in fact, run human "trials." Other cracks in the firm's narrative emerged. Yes, after the news from Grünenthal in December, Merrell had sent warnings to physicians "actively investigating" Kevadon. But the firm didn't specify how many doctors they'd alerted. And why had Merrell waited until March to notify *all* investigators to return or destroy pills? More perplexing, Merrell had left it entirely up to trial doctors to decide how or *if* they would alert patients.

Both Frances and Helen Taussig grew increasingly disturbed as they began to hear of children born with phocomelia during the period of thalidomide's clinical trials. Taussig had just examined a Connecticut three-year-old with the signature thalidomide limb damage and heard of two more babies in Cincinnati. She was trying to hunt down the doctors who had tended the mothers, but these cases, she was repeatedly told, couldn't possibly be related to the drug. Yet Taussig sensed that doctors were entirely unwilling to imagine that a pill they had handed out had caused such harm.

Frances, likewise, realized the foolishness of waiting for Merrell to report birth deformities. She decided, instead, to get hold of birth reports for the relevant period and work backward. Even though Chicago didn't keep a registry, New York—where at least fifty-six doctors had given out the drug—did. Frances asked the New York City health commissioner for help and received a report of more than five thousand birth malformations in New York City alone. But she was confused by the dates involved. This mass of harmed babies had been born in 1958, a year *before* Merrell's trials started.

The FDA, however, had recently learned that three years before Merrell's trials, another drug firm—Smith, Kline & French—had also tested thalidomide. Under a 1956 licensing agreement with Grünenthal, SKF had shipped the sedative to more than sixty physicians. After a year of human testing, SKF dropped the drug and canceled the contract. No one seemed to know if those earlier pills were still lying around. And no one knew if those first investigators had grasped that samples marked "SKF #5627" were thalidomide. To worsen matters, SKF told Commissioner Larrick that one of its trial doctors might be linked to a birth malformation in 1957. The case, the firm explained, would take time to track down.

It was emerging that well more than one thousand doctors around the country had been giving out thalidomide since 1956. The toxic drug had permeated the whole United States for over five years. But this remained a well-guarded secret in the summer of 1962, known only by Richardson-Merrell, SKF, and select government agencies. Until someone—a frustrated FDA insider?—tipped off United Press International and the story that Merrell had 1,200 "trial" doctors dispensing Kevadon finally broke.

Reporters coast to coast then began hounding regional FDA offices. In Philadelphia, nearly one hundred newspaper, radio, and television inquiries hit the district office over three days. *The Louisville Times* demanded information from the FDA about Kentucky's forty Kevadon investigators.

In Ohio, home to a stunning 110 trial doctors, the media pounced. Were these private-practice physicians or hospital doctors? *The Columbus Dispatch* asked. A Youngstown radio reporter demanded names, and *Cincinnati Enquirer* reporters telephoned the FDA district director at home late one night for confirmation that "doses of thalidomide had been given in this area." The Ohio Department of Health, under "a great deal of pressure" from the press, begged the FDA for an assurance that the agency was handling the situation.

But the agency wasn't. All the FDA knew at this point were the names of the Kevadon trial doctors. How many pills or patients were involved still remained a mystery. And the agency's public assurances that no abnormal births had been reported was wildly misleading. Yes, no injuries had been "reported"—via Merrell—but the agency had yet to contact a single trial doctor. They hadn't even begun to look.

The FDA had found itself in uncharted territory. Since 1938, when the law began requiring animal and human tests prior to product approval, no unapproved drug had sparked a safety crisis. Drug trials were typically small and uneventful. The agency's challenges routinely stemmed from products already on sale that later proved problematic or ineffective. If the manufacturer refused a voluntary recall, hearings could remove a drug from circulation. But the vast premarket thalidomide trials had caught the FDA off guard. Legally speaking, the agency was on terra incognita. As a result, it was letting Merrell call all the shots.

For weeks, the FDA had been assuring the media that Merrell's trials had done no harm. But when the New York City health commissioner held a press conference to announce the death of a "deformed" infant likely linked to German Contergan, he held up Merrell's blue and white Kevadon tablets—to warn women. The press, in turn, made note of Merrell's widespread Kevadon trials—alerting the public that the drug had been given out in thirty-nine states, plus the District of Columbia.

Merrell quickly recast its story. News of the 1,200 trial doctors undermined the firm's we-never-sold-it defense. Instead, Merrell sent the FDA a dispatch touting its vast thalidomide recall and implementation of all necessary actions "at the appropriate time with highest sense of responsibility." Yet it was only the day after this statement to the FDA that Merrell actually followed up with its thousand-plus trial doctors. Thomas Jones had waited until the end of July—over a half year since hearing of the drug's dangers—to finally send out letters asking the Kevadon investigators to confirm they actually had no more thalidomide on hand.

The letters he'd mailed, months earlier, had not, in fact, shown the "highest sense of responsibility." His cursory March notes asking doctors to cease trials and return pills had also insisted that "no causal relationship" between thalidomide and birth defects had been proved. Jones didn't telephone investigators. He didn't task detail men to relay the warning. And he neglected the most obvious and crucial step: to alert *obstetricians* running trials. Jones was so blasé about the matter that he told three Kevadon investigators that he was still very interested in their studies and that they could keep dispensing the drug.

Scores of investigators would later claim either that they had never received Jones's March letter or that, given its lack of urgency, they had shrugged it off. Merrell's "intensive effort to recall and follow up" was pure fabrication.

But well into the summer, the FDA remained entirely in the dark about the firm's deception. As a result, the agency made no effort to assess how much thalidomide remained at large.

It was only when a congressional committee summoned Larrick and

Frances to testify publicly on the matter that Larrick took concrete action. The day before Larrick and Frances walked into the Senate, the FDA tasked inspectors nationwide with an emergency assignment. By close of business on Wednesday, August 1, an agent had to visit every American Kevadon investigator and ask: How much thalidomide had the doctor received and when? Had patients been told to get rid of the drug? Had the drug been given to pregnant women?

"In view of the great public interest in this situation," field officers were told, "this assignment is one of the most important we have had in a long time." After three whole months of sitting quietly on the names of hundreds of Kevadon doctors, FDA inspectors had twenty-four hours to find them.

DRUG MAN DOUBTS DANGER
FROM THALIDOMIDE IN U.S.

JULY 29, 1962

CINCINNATI (AP) Wide-spread fears of defective babies being born as a result of the clinical testing of thalidomide are probably exaggerated, a spokesman for the William S. Merrell Co. says.

There are people whose opinions have a right to some weight, who would say that the problem here has been exaggerated.

—*FDA commissioner George Larrick,*

August 1, 1962

Thirty

On a warm August morning, Frances entered the New Senate Office Building in a white collared blouse and a striped blazer, a gold pheasant brooch fastened to her lapel, a gift from Ellis. Her short hair combed back from her face, she surveyed the room. Throngs of TV crews, spectators, reporters, and photographers all trained their attention on her—the star witness.

This was not a hearing on Kefauver's drug bill but a subcommittee meeting on government operations helmed by Minnesota Democrat Hubert Humphrey. The senators were ostensibly probing the inner workings of the FDA, but everyone knew that the day's real topic was thalidomide—and that what was said there could make or break Kefauver's drug bill, S. 1552.

Frances's presence in the room was already a Kefauver victory. A week before, Kefauver had again proposed a White House award for Frances and slipped the press his letter to Kennedy. He knew that keeping Frances—and thalidomide—in the spotlight was his best hope for passing his bill.

As the hearing came to order that morning, South Dakota's Senator Karl Mundt, a Republican ally of corporate interests, surprised the room by fawning over Frances. Kefauver's aides had preemptively wooed him with news that not only had the Kelsey family lived in South Dakota for eight years, but they still voted there. Mundt now extolled his celebrity constituent—a dedicated doctor who symbolized the nation's best values. South Dakotans, he told the crowd, were proud of the Kelsey family. Frances's lapel pin was, in fact, the ring-necked pheasant—the official bird of South Dakota.

Senator Humphrey then took command of the meeting. Only by "the skin of its teeth" had the country escaped a thalidomide tragedy, he said. Adding that it was urgent that the government sort out how it communicated about emergency public safety matters, he handed the floor to Commissioner Larrick.

Though Frances had been invited as the media magnet, Larrick was still the voice of the FDA. After thirty-nine years at the agency, he sat at the table beside Frances, his clear-framed glasses resting on his hollow cheeks. Above his trademark bow tie, his neck was jowly, and his combed gray hair was thinning. He'd recently taken several medical leaves, and his failing health was public knowledge. The contrast between him and Frances was dramatic. He lacked her youth, her vivacity, her education. He had begun his career at a small agency that assessed simple products by sight, touch, or taste. Over four decades, science had vastly advanced pharmaceuticals, and regulation now required sharp scientific appraisal. Though Barbara Moulton's attack on Larrick had been unsuccessful, it had exposed his paltry credentials.

Larrick began with prepared remarks aimed at assuring the committee that Merrell had behaved responsibly. He offered an overall timeline: A few days after the news from Germany, Merrell had contacted doctors who had received the drug over the previous twelve months. The firm directed them not to give it to premenopausal women. "Later"—Larrick did not specify the time lapse—"the drug was recalled or its destruction was requested by the firm."

As for the FDA, Larrick boasted, "We are now checking every doctor who received supplies of thalidomide to be sure the firm's requests were heeded"—though he failed to mention that this investigation had commenced just twenty-four hours earlier. At any rate, no one, he assured the committee, had been harmed by Merrell's clinical trials. The few U.S. incidents of phocomelia, he claimed, stemmed from German pills.

In support of this notion that German pills had caused the few American cases, Senator Humphrey read aloud a telegram from an army major in his home state of Minnesota:

In 1959 my wife was prescribed thalidomide while we were stationed in Germany. My 2½ year old daughter was born with multiple abnormalities, complete absence of legs, partial formation of arms. Urge strong legislative action to preclude any tragedies of this nature in the future.

But Larrick was not there to champion legislative change. He felt the FDA's review process was, overall, a success. He boasted that the FDA now had a computer to gather data and that forty-four hospitals had been enlisted in an adverse-reaction reporting system (though Humphrey burst his bubble by noting that there were more than six thousand hospitals nationwide). Larrick's remarks were meant to calm, not stir, the public. And when he ceded the microphone to Frances, he praised her for preventing "the commercial distribution of thalidomide," as though she had proved the agency's efficacy.

As Frances began her remarks, flashbulbs erupted. Since the front-page *Washington Post* story, she'd been on radio and television dozens of times, yet still the public craved more. She walked the committee through the arrival of the New Drug Application for Kevadon and her discovery of the *British Medical Journal* letter on peripheral neuritis. She relayed Merrell's claim that its overseas partners had failed to advise it of the drug's neurological side effect, but Senator Jacob Javits of New York wasn't convinced. More than any other senator on the committee, Javits doubted Merrell. Wouldn't the drug firm's licensing agreement with Grünenthal, he said, have compelled an exchange of such information?

Further incensing Javits were the "clinical trials." Fifty-six physicians in New York had dispensed thalidomide to patients, but the state health department couldn't get straight answers from the FDA about who the doctors were, how much thalidomide they'd given out, and whether the patients knew what drug they'd taken. With Larrick in his sights, Javits demanded to know: Were doctors in the United States allowed to hand out experimental drugs without a patient's knowledge?

Yes, Larrick affirmed, this was completely legal.

Humphrey asked how many doctors in the country had been detailed with thalidomide. Larrick bristled at the word "detail"—in-person promotion applied only to drugs on sale. But he acknowledged that more than 1,200 doctors had received thalidomide. The law, he explained, allowed "unlimited" clinical trials.

"This is a loophole in the law, through which you could drive a South Dakota wagonload of hay," an astonished Senator Mundt declared.

As the testimony moved to Merrell's actions once it heard the birth defect news from Germany, Javits supplied what Larrick had omitted: Merrell had, in fact, waited until March to ask doctors to return or destroy thalidomide. A whopping four-month delay. Javits asked Frances to explain this lag, and she deferred to Larrick. But all the commissioner said was: "I think the firm proceeded with reasonable diligence." In reality, the FDA hadn't known until April that Merrell's return-or-destroy letter had taken so ridiculously long.

Then Javits asked if the FDA had considered commencing its own recall.

"We rarely have to order withdrawals," Larrick answered evasively.

Javits was stumped: The drug had been fully pulled from German shelves in November 1961, yet neither Merrell nor the FDA had done anything to remove the drug from circulation in the United States until March of 1962. And in March, the drug firm had made only the barest effort—a subdued warning letter sent quietly to doctors.

Javits then asked: Did the FDA even have the power to recall thalidomide?

"I think we do, yes," said Larrick, but since Merrell had acted with "reasonable diligence," the agency hadn't needed to.

Larrick then went the extra mile to defend Merrell, noting that the drug's pregnancy risk had not been "conclusively proved" in December. Larrick made no mention of the dispatch from Herman Chinn, U.S. deputy scientific attaché in Bonn, Germany, a report the FDA had been sitting on since January that detailed Widukind Lenz's research—the exact same research that had convinced German health authorities to fully recall the drug.

Larrick—shadowed by accusations of professional ineptness—seemed terrified to admit to the congressional committee how little his agency knew about Merrell's actions, how little the FDA had done. Before the Morton Mintz article spotlighting Frances, Larrick had likely assumed the thalidomide episode would fade into obscurity. Now that it was garnering more attention than any other drug during his tenure, he was scrambling to appear on top of things. Perhaps this is why he proceeded to tell the committee an egregious lie. Larrick announced that the Kevadon trial doctors had "obeyed" Merrell's recall orders. Since the FDA investigation had essentially begun that morning while everyone sat in the committee room, nobody at the agency had any idea if Merrell's doctors had or hadn't returned or destroyed pills.

Javits wasn't buying it. He asked Frances: Did *she* think Merrell acted with "due diligence"?

"My understanding was," Frances answered, "when the drug was still in the investigational stage that . . . our authority did not extend there." Javits had asked about Merrell, but Frances, out of nowhere, condemned the law: *Our authority did not extend there.* In direct contradiction of Larrick, she said the FDA lacked the legal power to recall a drug in the clinical trial phase.

Frances brought none of Taussig's dramatic visuals or Moulton's fervor to Capitol Hill, but she was clearly advocating for a new drug bill. As though she'd come that day to make this one assertion, minutes later she restated her claim: The FDA did not have "the clear-cut authority to stop investigational drugs."

If this was her strategy, it worked. Javits, for the rest of the hearing, couched his proposals in "Had you the authority . . ." And soon everyone in the room agreed the FDA lacked important legal muscle. By way of explanation, Larrick himself eventually read aloud the portion of the current law exempting experimental drugs from FDA oversight (section 505). If the drug was sent to "an expert qualified by scientific training and experience to investigate the safety of such drug," it escaped oversight. But Frances pointed out that the term "expert" was being widely abused. Inexperienced investigators were running drug trials, she said, submitting amateurish testimonials, not proper studies. A serious problem that needed fixing.

With this, Javits named the elephant in the room—S. 1552, Kefauver's bill. Javits asked Larrick how the proposed amendments might better drug approvals. But Larrick refused to weigh in. Opinions on legislation were "political"—not for the commissioner of food and drugs. But Humphrey pushed back: Would the new bill help the FDA get better information about drugs and improve communication on scientific information?

"Yes," Larrick reluctantly conceded.

His point made, Senator Humphrey closed the session, thanking Dr. Kelsey—the "fine South Dakotan"—for her help. And then he officially seconded Kefauver's motion that the president award her a medal.

President Kennedy, for his part, had spent the morning first with the U.S. ambassador to Cambodia and then in a meeting on nuclear disarmament. After heated discussions on the Nuclear Test Ban Treaty, the president emerged to find that Humphrey's committee had thrust thalidomide back into the news. Frances's Senate appearance had riled the press, and reporters now wanted answers about the FDA probe on thalidomide. By late afternoon, Kennedy knew he had to publicly weigh in.

At a press conference, standing before several hundred reporters, Kennedy issued what would be remembered as a warning for women to check their medicine cabinets. But it began as a plea for a new drug bill. American consumers, Kennedy said, deserved better protection. He thanked Frances—an emblem of the country's strength—for preventing the commercial distribution of thalidomide but noted "the drug was given to many patients on an investigational basis." To avoid future catastrophes, he proposed a 25 percent increase in FDA staff, the largest single hike in agency history, as well as legislative safeguards. In particular, Kennedy wanted a bill that would allow the swift recall of any dangerous new drug. Thus, approximately five hours after Frances told the Senate that the FDA lacked the legal standing to recall thalidomide, Kennedy moved to grant the agency that power.

As the president transitioned to a discussion of the test-ban treaty, a reporter circled back to thalidomide: Was there anything the government could do about the drug *without* a new law? Kennedy said that nearly two hundred FDA inspectors were on the case and that all doctors, hospitals, and nurses had been alerted. Nonetheless, it was "most important" that American women check their medicine cabinets.

For six months the U.S. government had known that the drug, distributed nationwide, was linked to serious birth defects. For six months it had done nothing in response to the report of its own overseas attachés. Yet on that August day, Commissioner Larrick and President Kennedy put forth a story of robust FDA action. Which was false. All doctors, hospitals, and nurses had not been alerted. And while Kennedy's medicine-cabinet warning would crystallize as a key moment in the thalidomide saga, it was an off-the-cuff answer. Warning the public of the drug's wide availability had never been the government's plan.

MERRELL WINS CLEARANCE
IN THALIDOMIDE INQUIRY

AUGUST 2, 1962

WASHINGTON The William S. Merrell Co., Cincinnati chemical firm was given a clean bill of health here today for its activities
in handling of the drug thalidomide.

It was determined that many doctors gave the drug to other doctors who were not investigators and those doctors in turn gave other doctors the drug and thus the distribution pattern became very, very large and difficult to follow up.

—*James Nakada, director,*
FDA Kevadon recall,
1982

Thirty-one

Hours after Kennedy issued his televised warning, FDA field offices began reporting their findings to headquarters.

They were dire.

Hundreds of Merrell's investigators had failed to sign official statements explaining how or on whom they would conduct thalidomide studies. The drug had circulated widely, without tracking, and the sparse records kept had been lost or destroyed. The few doctors who had submitted patient reports to Merrell had not kept duplicates. Almost no doctor could readily tell the FDA which patients, exactly, had taken the toxic drug.

In Raleigh, North Carolina, where Kevadon had been stocked at a hospital pharmacy for use by multiple doctors, the pharmacist had no record of how many tablets the hospital had received or where they had gone. At a New Orleans hospital, even though the pharmacy had stocked the drug for over a year, no doctor would admit to using it.

Frances's claim of sloppy "experts" was proving frighteningly accurate.

Meanwhile, across the country, August vacations slowed the inquest. In the Buffalo area, half of the listed investigators were out of town. And in Chicago, seven doctors were traveling and unreachable.

Chicago—where eighty-eight doctors had been running trials—exemplified the full ineptness of Merrell's "recall." Inspectors collected more than 100 tablets from two doctors with thalidomide on hand—*after* a Chicago Board of Health recall had already rounded up 3,076 tablets from area doctors.

In some cases, doctors had gotten the drug from colleagues who had failed to relay the warning letter. And not all doctors parted easily with the sedative. The Philadelphia Eagles' team physician, who had been giving Kevadon to the football players, insisted that despite the pregnancy side effects, the drug was a *great* sleep aid for men. Other doctors had apparently hoarded supplies for personal use. Baltimore inspectors found two doctors, not on Merrell's investigator list, sitting on thalidomide stashes. One had been taking it himself; the other had given it to his wife.

FDA inspectors were also increasingly balking at the scope of their mission. In Seattle, an obstetrician told them he had given several hundred pills to pregnant women at a charity outpatient clinic and destroyed the records. The women had all delivered normal babies, he claimed, but he had not contacted them since Merrell's March letter. The inspectors determined that "charity out-patients" — poor women — "would be impossible to locate," and they closed the file. In other locations, unwieldly hospital archives deterred inspectors from more than "a cursory examination" of patient charts. When inspectors in the Baltimore area learned of a baby "born without arms and legs" to a registered nurse, they dropped their query when no paper trail linked her to an official Kevadon investigator.

The most stunning discovery was an obstetrician in North Carolina — a Merrell trial doctor — who admitted to FDA agents that during his Kevadon trial, one of his six subjects had delivered a stillborn child with webbed feet and a three-chambered heart. Even there, inspectors were reticent. When the doctor refused to share his patient's name, the FDA agent agreed that "under the circumstances the name did not seem important." As a result, the woman was not informed that the drug might have harmed her baby.

In the end, FDA representatives made contact with 1,073 of the 1,231 doctors to whom Merrell had officially shipped the drug. Sixty-seven of them still had thalidomide on hand. HEW relayed this information to the press but stayed mute on the scores of additional doctors found dispensing the drug and the mass of pills collected. The nurse's armless baby and the stillborn with webbed feet were not mentioned publicly.

In fact, through early August, the FDA still contended that no babies had been harmed by Kevadon. The few U.S. cases of phocomelia, they repeatedly assured the press, stemmed from German pills.

And yet, in Cincinnati, FDA inspectors and the local press heard rumors of *several* phocomelic births. On August 5, the *Cincinnati Enquirer* reported on the cases, adding that "none have been traced to any mothers who had any contact with the drug." An unnamed local obstetrician said that, yes, he had tested the drug, but not in early pregnancy. And he claimed that no birth malformations were seen. The article described Merrell as "absolved of blame" by the recent Senate hearing.

The unnamed doctor was, of course, Ray Nulsen, and he was parroting exactly what he'd told FDA inspectors days earlier in his office: He'd only given the drug to eighty-one women in the third trimester, to no ill effect. But the *Cincinnati Enquirer* article stirred trouble for Nulsen.

After reading the *Enquirer* piece, a middle-aged woman and her twenty-two-year-old daughter-in-law stormed into Merrell's headquarters holding three blue pills—thalidomide. The younger woman had taken the pills throughout her pregnancy, and her baby girl, born with four misshapen limbs, had died at eleven months. Both women were patients of Dr. Nulsen.

Faced with this news, Nulsen acknowledged the women as patients but denied giving the drug to the young mother. Merrell at first claimed to believe him, telling the FDA it suspected "ulterior motives" on the part of the "aggressive" mother-in-law: Maybe *she* had gotten the drug from Nulsen and passed it along? (In fact, Merrell's Thomas Jones already knew at this point that Nulsen had witnessed at least four birth deformities while testing the drug.) The FDA sent a team back to Nulsen's office, but the obstetrician was vacationing and refused to cut short his trip for a second interview.

In the interim, the FDA agents visited the two accusing women. They found the mother-in-law very credible, and the baby's mother showed them the small beige envelope in which Nulsen had given her the drug. Once a month, she had picked up an envelope with about sixty pills, labeled merely: "One or two tablets at bedtime for sleeping." She also gave the FDA a pill to test. But when the FDA representatives asked to borrow records of her baby girl, the mother refused to part—even briefly—with her few precious photographs. Her husband would copy the birth and death certificates and medical records, but she was adamant that her daughter not be discussed in the news.

Midinterview, they were interrupted by the arrival of two high-ranking

Merrell executives. At first, the mother-in-law orchestrated a secretive shuffling between rooms to keep the Merrell team from spotting her government guests. But eventually, the FDA men made a brazen exit— astonishing the Merrell executives. The encounter was awkward, but the two sides were not wildly at odds. They had all come to the conclusion that Nulsen was lying. The FDA had a letter from Nulsen—dated mere days after the woman had given birth—stating that he had seen no babies harmed in his Kevadon study. And Merrell had located records showing that Nulsen had received thalidomide tablets in the thousands and had unequivocally "used the drug in all stages of pregnancy"—news it soon shared with the FDA. Merrell said it was now hearing of other abnormal births linked to its go-to local obstetrician, and seemed eager to wash its hands of him.

By the time FDA officials returned to Nulsen, their suspicions ran high. Nulsen hastily read aloud from a patient chart that looked heavily doctored: dates noted the wrong years, in different kinds of ink. Somebody, it seemed, had clumsily tried to remove any indication he'd given the pregnant woman thalidomide. But one detail gave him away: The woman's chart noted that in her first trimester she'd been given APC (aspirin/phenacetin/caffeine). Raymond Pogge had concocted MRD-640, an APC pill turbocharged with thalidomide, and Nulsen, the FDA knew, had used it on hundreds of women. The FDA had this evidence, as well as a letter in the drug application noting that he'd given thalidomide to between 500 and 750 patients for insomnia and anxiety: hundreds more than the 81 third-trimester patients he had admitted to in his first FDA interview.

But Nulsen was adamant about this case—he had not given the mother the drug. And none of his nurses or assistants, he said, would have dispensed it without his say-so. His office was busy, though, verging on chaotic. And he commented that pregnant women could do "strange things"—like swap medicine or even take pills for an unwanted pregnancy. So it was not impossible that the drug had, in fact, originated with him. When the inspectors asked if Nulsen had ever delivered another infant with phocomelia, his denial was, the FDA noted, "very emphatic."

The next day, *The Cincinnati Post & Times-Star* reported on the dead baby girl: "Cincinnati Baby's Death Is Linked to Thalidomide." In response, Commissioner Larrick, while still praising Merrell for being "extremely frank" in sharing information with the FDA, finally had to acknowledge publicly that 207 pregnant women across the country had been given the drug. Nulsen was not named, but Larrick acknowledged that the majority of those women — 121 — lived in Cincinnati.

The Cincinnati media snapped to action. One reporter, tipped off that a local doctor couldn't account for eight hundred tablets, demanded details from the FDA's Cincinnati office. But the FDA clammed up. Helen Taussig's hunch that Merrell's home turf would turn up a trail of Kevadon damage was proving eerily correct. But the Cincinnati medical community, rather than bring these cases to light, closed ranks.

The day before the mother-in-law and daughter-in-law had shown up at Merrell with their blue pills, another woman had given birth to an infant with bilateral phocomelia at Cincinnati's Jewish Hospital. As Ann Morris lay in bed, in shock, the delivering doctor asked her if she had gone to Canada and bought thalidomide. No one mentioned Kevadon or the Merrell Company. No one mentioned the local obstetrician running vast, informal trials. Or the additional Kevadon trial doctor based at that very hospital. Or the rumored missing pills. Ann's obstetrician was not an official Kevadon investigator, so the FDA would not have spoken to him, even though the FDA already knew that Merrell's trial doctors had passed the drug around freely. Between practices. Within hospitals. No one — not the Merrell Company or the physicians who'd received the original shipments — knew where the drug had ended up, and most of the women who'd received it had no idea what it was. The FDA's entire investigation had dangerously hinged on the honor system — "when a physician stated that he had contacted his patients or was going to contact his patients," the agency wrote at the time, "this fact was accepted."

Ann and her husband, Doug, put their baby, Carolyn Jean, in foster care, as advised, expecting she would soon die. They returned to their apartment, heartbroken. All Ann knew about thalidomide came from her recent issue of *Life* magazine sitting at home, showing page after page of armless infants from Europe. "What a terrible thing that happened in Germany," Ann thought. It would be decades before she suspected the same drug had maimed her daughter.

August 9, 1962

TRUMAN FELT

PUBLIC RELATIONS COUNSEL

1131 NATIONAL PRESS BUILDING

WASHINGTON 4. D.C.

Director
Division of Public Information
Food and Drug Administration
Fourth St. & Independence Ave. SW.
Washington, D.C.

Dear Sir:

I have been retained by the William S. Merrell Co. of Cincinnati
to help keep them abreast of Washington developments in drug
regulation and would be pleased to be placed on your mailing list
for all FDA releases.

My address is shown above.

Thank you for your cooperation.

Very truly yours,
Truman Felt

Thirty-two

On August 7, 1962, Frances crossed the White House lawn to stand inches from President Kennedy. It felt like a fairy tale. It was a little overwhelming. He laid a gold medal around her neck as photographers and film crews captured the event: America's heroine, at last getting the President's Award for Distinguished Federal Civilian Service. Though known for eschewing "fuss and feathers," Frances wore a blue dress, a matching blue hat, and a pair of midheels for the occasion. The public was thrilled to see their plain-Jane sweetheart dolled up. But *The New York Times* reminded readers: "She does not use cosmetics, and hence wore no lipstick."

Among her eleven guests in the Rose Garden that day were Ellis and her daughters, E. M. K. Geiling, John Nestor, and Barbara Moulton. As attendees milled cheerfully amid the magnolia trees, political tensions simmered. Washington insiders recalled Moulton's agency exposé and takedown of Commissioner Larrick, and her presence at the ceremony—combined with Larrick's absence—sent a clear message.

But the day's greater political intrigue came from the sullen presence of Senator Kefauver. Because Kennedy had not taken kindly to Kefauver's incessant pressure to honor Frances, her award was officially deemed the idea of Anthony Celebrezze, the new HEW secretary. Only at the last moment was Kefauver even invited to the event. Throughout the afternoon, Kefauver was sidelined in press photographs, lurking at the fringes of the jubilant crowd. As Celebrezze ceremoniously presented Frances to the president, Kefauver watched in frustrated silence.

Kefauver and Kennedy were more at odds than ever: Now that the public had been stirred by the thalidomide news, the White House wanted to assume full credit for any new drug bill. With the help of HEW and the

FDA, on Sunday, August 5, while in Hyannis Port, Kennedy had released the text of what was now being called the "President's Amendments." It wasn't lost on the Senate Judiciary Committee that the new bill looked a lot like Kefauver's original tough-on-industry version, which they had previously decimated. Nevertheless, the committee chair, Jim Eastland, endorsed JFK's rebranded amendments, and Hubert Humphrey declared to the Senate that the president had taken the initiative on drug legislation.

A follow-up closed-door Judiciary Committee session to which Frances, Larrick, and HEW's legal team were invited completely shut out Kefauver. But Frances plugged his agenda. She had grown deft at using her scientific expertise and moral weight to argue legislative points. Just as Geiling had done in 1938, she now mapped out the key components for a new law: She told the committee to restore Kefauver's initial amendment that would end the automatic approval of drug applications within sixty days. And she pressed to eliminate all hearings and red tape involved in a drug recall. In the case of imminent danger, a recall should be easy. The committee agreed and the meeting was adjourned.

Within weeks, the committee unanimously voted to release the *fourth* version of S. 1552—the closest thing to Kefauver's bill since he first introduced it. A floor vote would now be possible. When reporters sought his response, Kefauver conjured surprising graciousness. "This is a very good drug bill. . . . I think it will give a great deal of added protection to the American people."

As the Senate at last deliberated in its vast, marble, two-storied chamber, Kefauver and Humphrey both stood and offered an amendment from their desks—unanimously accepted—requiring that prescription medicines be tested on animals before human use. But Senator Javits went further. Javits proposed requiring physicians to obtain patient consent to administer an unapproved drug.

Many in the room bristled, including Kefauver, who feared the powerful AMA would torpedo any bill that undermined physician rights. But a HEW representative then rushed in with a press release showing the updated findings of the FDA thalidomide recall.

"Tablets of thalidomide, unidentified by name, and which may be mistaken for other drugs, still are at large in family medicine cabinets," the report stated. In fact, 2.5 million tablets, they said, had been distributed nationwide, with almost twenty thousand Americans given the experimental drug. The document then made its way to Eastland, who studied the sobering information and declared to the chamber, "That does it, gentlemen." Twenty copies of the release circulated throughout the gallery, and Javits's amendment, modified to protect the "interest of patients," passed unanimously.

Kefauver made one last push, before the final vote, to lower drug prices. Cost concerns, after all, had kicked off his drug inquiry. But the amendment was tabled.

Thalidomide had vaulted the drug bill to the top of everyone's agenda — but safety was now the matter of the day. No one was fretting over profit margins. At seven that evening, the bill passed unanimously.

"The Senator from Tennessee has waged a long and lonely fight for an adequate drug bill," Senator Paul Douglas declared to the chamber. "Because of the many terrible tragedies which have occurred in European countries from the use of the drug thalidomide and the cases which have occurred in this country, it has been proved that the Senator has been right all this time. . . . Can we learn from this lesson; or can mankind educate itself only by disaster and tragedy?"

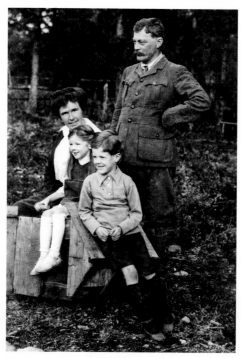

Frances Oldham with her parents and older brother
near their family home on Vancouver Island, circa 1919
Courtesy of the Family of Frances Oldham Kelsey

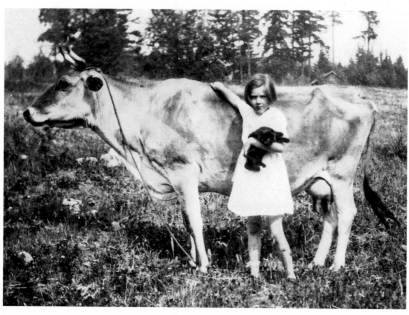

Frances, age seven
Courtesy of the Family of Frances Oldham Kelsey

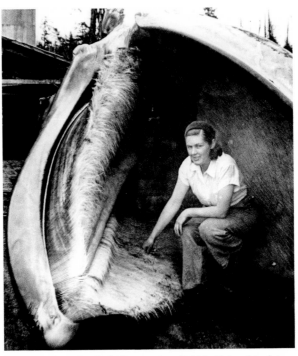

Frances, Kunghit Island whaling station, British Columbia, late 1930s
Courtesy of the Family of Frances Oldham Kelsey

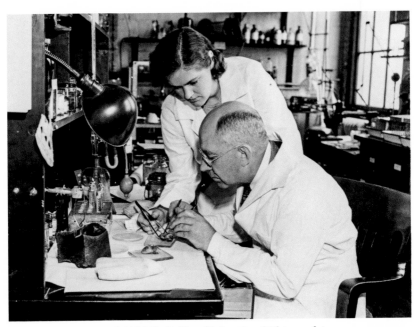

Frances with E.M.K. Geiling, University of Chicago, late 1930s
Courtesy of FDA

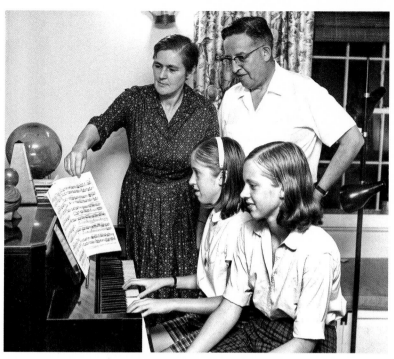

Frances with husband Ellis and daughters
Christine and Susan in a July 1962 press photo
AP photo / William J. Smith

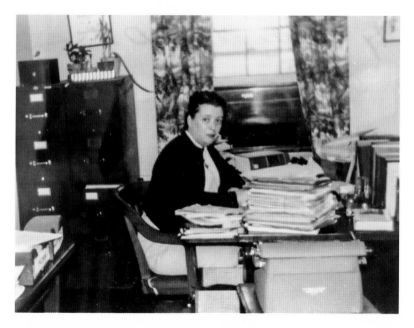

Barbara Moulton Browne in Washington, D.C., 1960s
Courtesy of the Family of Barbara Moulton Browne

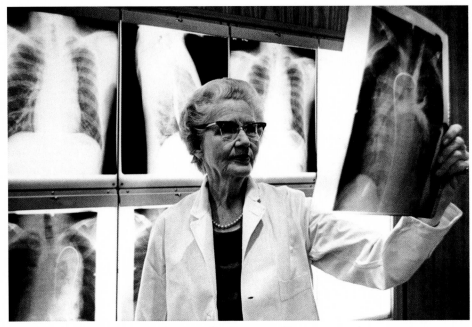

Dr. Helen Taussig, 1968
William A Smith / AP / Shutterstock

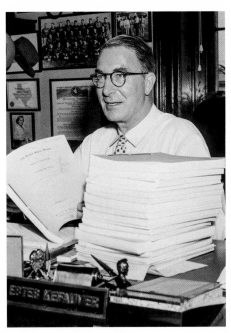

Senator Estes Kefauver, 1955
Bettmann via Getty Images

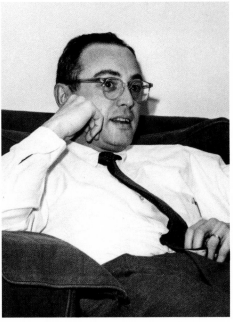

Journalist Morton Mintz, 1950s
Courtesy of the Family of Morton Mintz

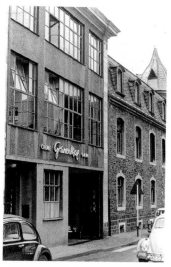

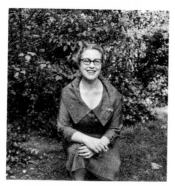

Chemie Grünenthal, circa 1960
Sepp Linckens / Hanne Linckens

Journalist Elinor Kamath
*Courtesy of the Family of Elinor
Kamath (née Kahn)*

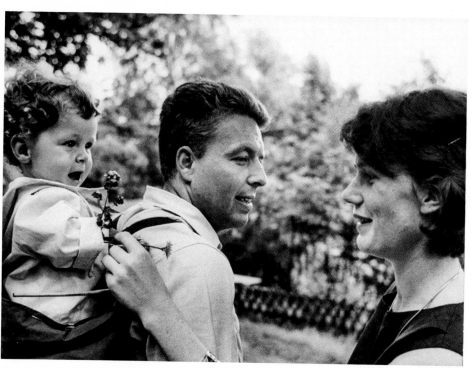

Karl Schulte-Hillen with son Jan and wife Linde, 1962
Stan Wayman / The LIFE Picture Collection / Shutterstock

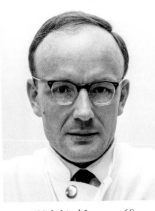

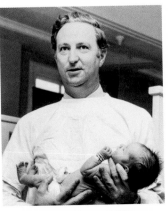

Widukind Lenz, 1968
picture alliance via Getty Images

Australian ob-gyn William
McBride, 1972
Bettmann via Getty Images

Frances's tally sheet of Merrell's clinical investigators, 1962
Courtesy of the author via Library of Congress

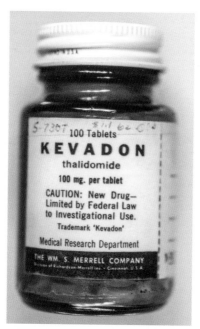

A bottle of Kevadon tablets
Courtesy of FDA

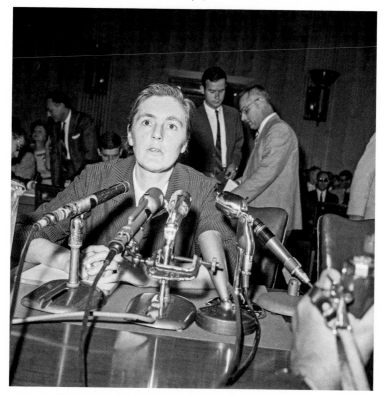

Frances testifying before the Senate subcommittee, 1962
Bettmann via Getty Images

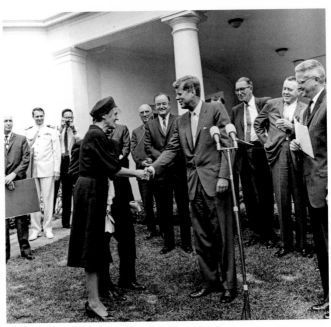

Frances receives the President's Award for Distinguished Federal
Civilian Service from President Kennedy, 1962.
Robert Knudsen, White House / John F. Kennedy Presidential Library and Museum

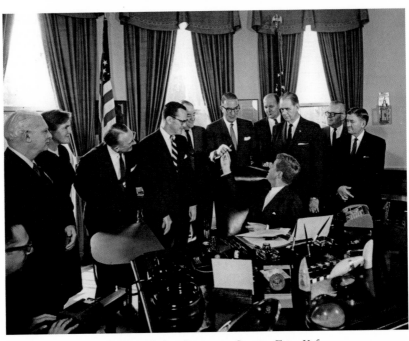

President Kennedy hands a pen to Senator Estes Kefauver
after signing the Drug Industry Act of 1962.
Abbie Rowe, White House / John F. Kennedy Presidential Library and Museum

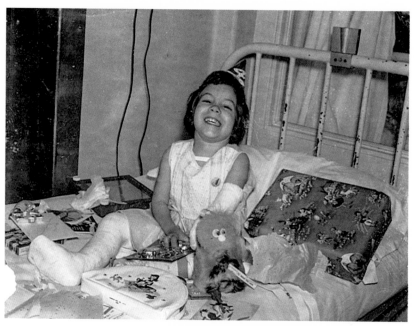

Kimberly Arndt, who may have been exposed
to thalidomide from the SKF trials, age four
Courtesy of Kimberly L. Arndt

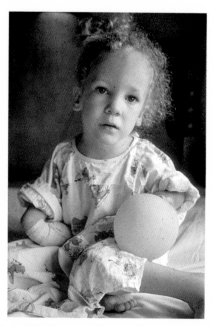

Gwen Riechmann, whose mother was a patient
of Dr. Ray O. Nulsen in Cincinnati, age four
George C. Riechmann Jr. (courtesy of Gwen Riechmann)

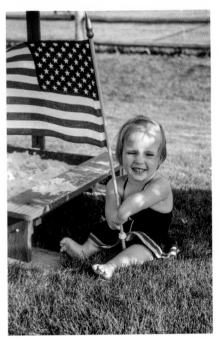

C. Jean Grover, age four
John T. Powell (courtesy of Jean Grover)

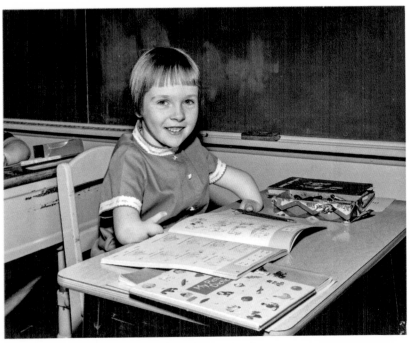

C. Jean Grover, age six
John T. Powell (courtesy of Jean Grover)

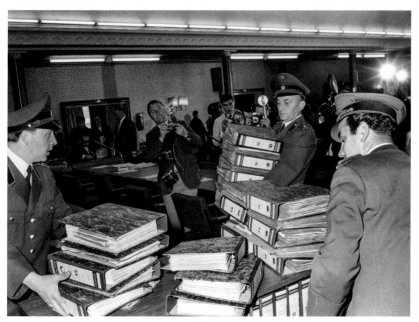

Trial against Chemie Grünenthal in Alsdorf, West Germany, 1968
picture alliance via Getty Images

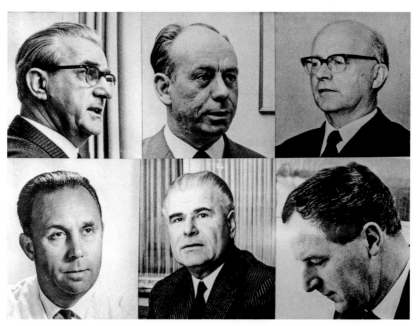

Chemie Grünenthal defendants at the Alsdorf trial. Left to right, top:
Jakob Chauvristé, Dr. Hans-Werner von Schrader-Beielstein, Klaus Wienandi.
Bottom: Dr. Heinrich Mückter, Hermann Josef Leufgens, Dr. Günther Sievers.
Bettmann via Getty Images

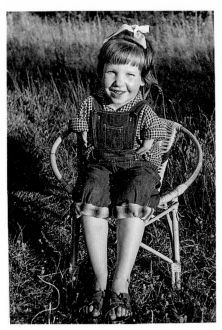

German thalidomide survivor Sabine Becker, age three
Courtesy of Sabine Becker

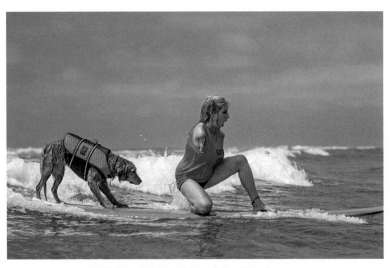

Sabine Becker with surf dog Ricochet
Robert Ochoa

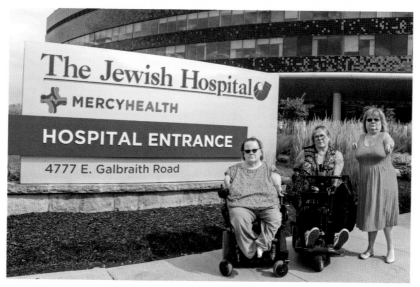

From left to right, Gwen Riechmann, C. Jean Grover, and Lori Kay Ruberg convene in 2020 outside the Jewish Hospital in Cincinnati, where they were all born in 1962.

Andrew Penner / ChooseAndy Productions

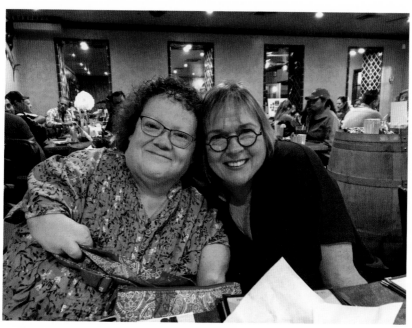

Gwen Riechmann and C. Jean Grover meet for the first time at the San Diego Convention for U.S. Thalidomide Survivors, 2019.

Courtesy of the author

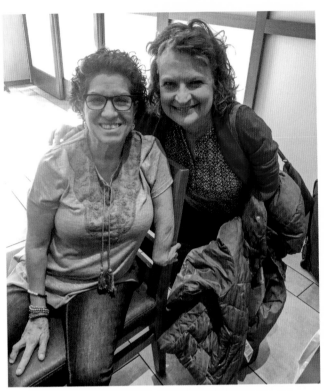

Kimberly Arndt (left) and Carolyn Sampson (right)
at the San Diego Convention for U.S. Survivors, 2019
Courtesy of the author

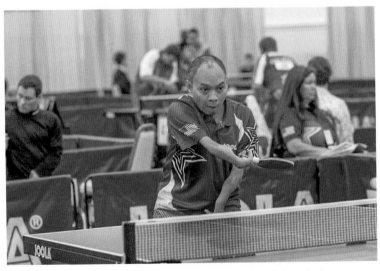

Jose (JoJo) Calora, president of the United States Thalidomide Survivors
From the collection of the Calora family

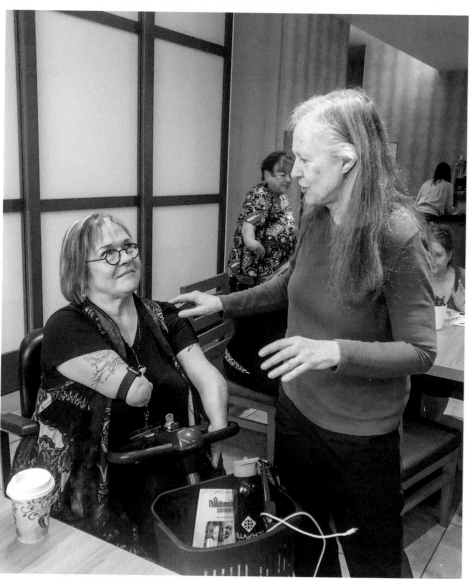

C. Jean Grover meets Frances's daughter Susan Duffield
at the San Diego convention.
Courtesy of the author

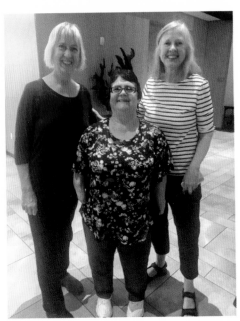

Dorothy Hunt-Honsinger, born in 1961,
with Frances's daughters: Christine Kelsey (left)
and Susan Duffield (right)
Courtesy of the author

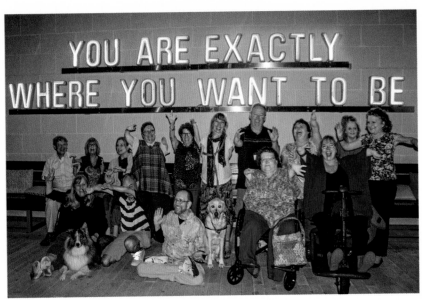

The final night of the San Diego convention, 2019. Clockwise from top left: Jeff Green,
Leslie Klein Mink, Eileen Cronin, Maria Bergner-Willig, Kimberly Arndt, Sabine
Becker, Darren Griggs, Dorothy Hunt-Honsinger, Glenda Johnson, Carolyn Sampson,
C. Jean Grover, Gwen Riechmann, Bart Joseph, Jojo Calora, and Jane Gibbons
Courtesy of the author

The slender Dr. Kelsey, who was praised by President Kennedy at his press conference last week, is a serenely calm woman with sparkling brown eyes who looks far younger than her 47 years. Short brown hair is brushed back with the casual sophistication of a thoroughbred.

—Catholic Standard,

August 1962

Our problem is this: We suspect that Richardson-Merrell may have failed to make full disclosure of adverse reactions (peripheral neuritis and/or polyneuritis, and phocomelia) associated with thalidomide in the new drug applications. . . . In other words, we think Richardson-Merrell may have had information of adverse reactions "long" before the facts were reported to FDA.

—FDA Bureau of Field Administration memorandum,

September 25, 1962

Thirty-three

Throughout the late summer of 1962, Frances bristled at the FDA's cursory investigation and its refusal to acknowledge injured babies linked to Merrell's trials.

The first case to alarm her was that of Trent Busby, a North Carolina obstetrician/gynecologist on Merrell's list of trial doctors. Back in April 1961, one of Busby's pregnant subjects had given birth to a "macerated" stillborn infant with webbed toes. Here, at last, was the smoking gun. Here was data from Merrell's own trials suggesting the drug's toxicity during pregnancy—almost a year before the firm withdrew its Kevadon application. And—most stunningly—here was an abnormal birth a month *after* Frances asked Merrell for data proving the drug was safe during pregnancy. As standard practice in a clinical trial, a patient report—detailing the stillborn's external (webbed feet) and internal (three-chambered heart) injuries—should have been submitted to the FDA. And certainly once Frances had asked for pregnancy data, Merrell should have solicited such details from trial obstetricians.

Merrell, it seemed, had shrugged off the pregnancy matter. Even after the troubling news from Germany in December 1961, Merrell hadn't warned Busby—an ob-gyn—of the suspected phocomelia link. Instead, in March they mailed him a form letter, alongside a thousand other doctors, pointing out that no conclusive evidence connected thalidomide to birth defects. Only *after* Merrell realized it would have to publicly pretend a thorough recall had been conducted did the firm telephone Busby. That was late July. Mere weeks before FDA agents knocked on his door.

Busby had leveled with FDA inspectors—he had no written record of how much thalidomide the woman had been given. He had sent Merrell a basic form about the stillborn fetus, noting that it had died at seven months but not detailing the malformations.

"What company official evaluated the qualifications of this doctor as a clinical investigator?" Frances, irate, wrote to colleagues leading the FDA's probe. Why hadn't Merrell asked for information about the condition of the dead infant? And had Busby made any effort to round up remaining pills from patients?

Frances wanted the case "investigated exhaustively."

Initially, no one at the agency shared her zeal. Busby had told the FDA that while he now believed thalidomide could cause phocomelia and he wouldn't touch it with a "ten-foot pole," he wasn't convinced the drug had harmed *his* patient's baby. He declined to share the woman's name or advise her that she had taken an experimental drug. At that, the FDA ended the inquiry.

Frances then decided to question Busby herself, wresting from him the patient's name and the baby's autopsy report. She learned that a district sales manager from Merrell—not a member of the firm's medical or scientific department—had asked Busby to test Kevadon. Busby had received a brochure and some brief patient evaluation forms. No cautions had been issued against using the drug in early pregnancy. Busby said he had never been notified of the drug's connection to peripheral neuritis and had never actually received a letter from Thomas Jones in March warning of the drug's phocomelia link. A telephone call in June or July was his first and only word from Merrell about the drug's pregnancy risk.

To Frances, this proved the firm's carelessness in recruiting clinical investigators and its lax warnings. Her dismay grew when she heard that Ray Nulsen in Cincinnati had also delivered a phocomelic baby in 1961. Frances demanded his case, as well, be investigated intensively: Had there been an autopsy? What were the baby's deformities? Most important— why hadn't the birth been reported? Frances had asked Merrell for Nulsen's patient data for a whole year.

It was now clear that at *least* two injured babies had been born to patients of Merrell's Kevadon investigators. Frances alerted her superiors: Merrell's trials blatantly violated the investigational-use provision. The doctors or the drug firm or *both* had broken the law—which required that experimental drugs only be dispensed by "an expert qualified by scientific training and experience to investigate the safety of such drug." Plus, the firm was lying. On August 6, Merrell's president had announced that the only fetal thalidomide injuries in the United States stemmed from European pills. Yet Busby had told the firm about his webbed-footed stillborn in July. The firm was actively spewing misinformation.

In late August, when the FDA released its grim findings—at least 15,000 Americans had been given the drug, 3,200 were women of childbearing age, and three babies had been injured by Merrell's pills—the agency finally sought to warn the public of stray pills. But by then, the feel-good tale of Frances sparing the country an epidemic of birth defects had proliferated so wildly that Merrell's premarket distribution of the drug—the largest in U.S. history—made little noise. Thalidomide, according to the press, was still an American success story. When *Life* published its photographs of European thalidomide victims with an article about Frances's fierce resistance of the drug application, Merrell's trials were notably downplayed.

"Some American women got the drug from European sources and from supplies of 'test pills,'" the magazine acknowledged. "Merrell had already sent the drug out to American doctors—the number eventually reached 1,200—for testing. This was standard drug firm procedure, permitted by law."

Clinical trials were standard. Twelve hundred clinical trials was not. (SKF, testing the same drug in 1956 and 1957, had sent it to only sixty-seven doctors.)

Life even published an extensive statement from Merrell's Carl Bunde, giving credence to the drug company's spin: Bunde pretended that the firm had never asked doctors to use the drug for morning sickness and claimed that Merrell's experimental thalidomide had been "for use in older patients, hospitalized patients, and in certain special situations such as orthopedic and psychiatric cases." He omitted the fact that two hundred of Merrell's trial doctors specialized in obstetrics and gynecology, and that Ray Nulsen had been specifically asked to publish a paper on thalidomide use in the third trimester. Equally misleading was Bunde's account of Merrell's response to the German news of phocomelia: "Within hours," Bunde claimed, "the firm called the FDA" and its new drug application "then became inactive." In fact, Merrell had not withdrawn its application until

March, allowing doctors—including obstetricians—to continue dispensing the drug for months after the drug was banned in Germany. Thanks to
Life, Merrell's fabricated defense reached almost seven million American
households.

The most memorable part of the *Life* spread, however, were the photographs of the afflicted children. Ask Americans of a certain age about thalidomide, and they will likely recall the *Life* magazine pictures: Bright-eyed,
lively children missing limbs. An infant girl in a romper, armless, using
her feet to hold a wristwatch. Jan Schulte-Hillen, Karl and Linde's son,
propped in a carrier on Karl's back, studying a flower held by Linde. A
British boy merrily testing out an artificial arm.

None of the children were American. And *Life*'s visuals would solidify
for readers that thalidomide was a tragedy overseas.

An exposé in the *National Enquirer* further cemented this idea. Its
story, headlined "Exclusive: First Photos, 5,000 Babies Born with 'Seal
Flippers,'" displayed nearly a dozen photographs of European children
"born into the world with horrifying and grotesque deformities." The article acknowledged Frances's feat in stopping the drug's sale in the United
States, while adding that "the manufacturer distributed the drug to physicians for trials." Again, the magazine said nothing of either the unprecedented scope or the chaotic nature of Merrell's trials. Larrick assured
Enquirer readers that "chances seem small that many American women
received the drug at what appears to be the critical time—early pregnancy," despite the fact that the FDA knew of at least two cases of malformed infants born to Kevadon trial doctors. And Merrell falsely asserted
that "little, if any, thalidomide is still in the hands of clinical investigators
and their affiliated institutions."

The FDA investigation, in fact, had established that vast quantities of
the drug had never been rounded up—to the tune of at least twenty-five
thousand pills. In the three weeks since Larrick's defense of Merrell before
Congress, the recall findings had gone from bad to worse. Merrell, it
turned out, had sent at least 2.5 million thalidomide tablets to physicians
nationwide. The drug had circulated in an array of colors—blue, yellow,
purple, tan, and white. Some versions were pure thalidomide, while others blended thalidomide with aspirin or dicyclomine—a drug used to treat
irritable bowel syndrome. The bottles in which the drug was shipped often

failed to note the words "Kevadon" or "thalidomide." The pills, in turn, had been handed to patients in envelopes and jars for an array of symptoms, including headaches, stomach aches, and menstrual cramps. Most doctors were never advised of the drug's dangers, and many had heard nothing from Merrell since first receiving the pills. A hospital in Texas had distributed hundreds of doses of thalidomide after Merrell got word from Germany of the drug's dangers.

Since many doctors had failed to alert patients as to what drug they'd been given, thousands of trial "subjects" still remained entirely in the dark. The few doctors who did reach out discovered that their patients still had heaps of thalidomide: A Nebraska doctor collected 150 tablets from his patients, and a Missouri doctor learned why it was so crucial to alert "subjects" as to the specifics of the drug they had on hand—a male patient had already innocently given his own leftover pills to his pregnant daughter. She was due in October. In late August, one New York physician who had dispensed the drug told *The New York Times* that he had called his insurance broker to reassess his professional-liability policy.

Further complicating matters, the FDA had learned that National Drug Company in Philadelphia—another Richardson-Merrell subsidiary—had also tested thalidomide, but under the name "Contergan" (or "NDR-268"). National Drug had sent the drug to more than ninety physicians but failed to notify some of them of the drug's dangers until April. Vick and Walker Laboratories, other Richardson-Merrell subsidiaries, had also distributed the drug for human testing, although Vick could not account for where the bulk of its thalidomide had gone. As the agency widened its search for those pills, FDA inspectors began finding thalidomide from the Smith, Kline & French trials *four years* earlier. Doctors with SKF #5627, it turned out, had no idea the drug they had dispensed was the sedative currently making frightening news.

While thalidomide had never been approved for "sale" in the United States, the FDA now realized that over five years, five different drug firms had shipped the drug throughout the country, under different labels and trade names, in different colors and dosages.

On August 23, the agency amended its initial report: At least 19,822 Americans had been given thalidomide, roughly 25 percent more than its first estimate. Of those, 3,760 were women of childbearing age, and 624 were pregnant. Two weeks earlier, the agency had declared that only 207 pregnant women had gotten the drug. The number had tripled.

But these women had no way of determining if they had been given the drug. The FDA, at Merrell's request, guarded the names of the Kevadon investigators as "a matter of traditional medical confidence." Merrell said it "could not in good conscience" make them public. Larrick claimed that releasing the names "would unnecessarily alarm all of their female patients who are pregnant."

Others in government passionately disagreed. Kefauver and his economist, Eppes Wayles Browne—Barbara Moulton's husband—felt that the scant information being released was "misleading to the public" and pushed the FDA to reveal all the doctors' names. But Larrick held firm.

As Frances scrambled to locate records of abnormal births, she found herself increasingly shut out of the inquiry: In August, a Philadelphia lawyer wrote to her at the FDA about a boy born with phocomelia whose mother believed she'd been given Kevadon, but the letter never reached her desk. Months later, when she got wind of the case, she telephoned the attorney, upset, determined to see the child.

She discovered that an obstetrician at Andrews Air Force base, whom she had interviewed in May, had withheld information about a baby born with phocomelia whose mother had been given Kevadon.

After their coast-to-coast inquiries, FDA agents had gathered concrete information on only twenty-one pregnant women given Kevadon. Nine of these—six of whom lived in Cincinnati—eventually did report phocomelic births. This became the FDA's official number of babies harmed by American thalidomide given in the first trimester: *nine.* All other suspect births—where a baby showed the telltale limb damage but where evidence was missing that Kevadon had been given to the mother by a trial doctor at the sensitive time—were struck from the agency's formal tally.

This erased many strange cases: In one instance, a doctor insisted he had given the mother Kevadon only in the third trimester, and the woman, whose baby was born with phocomelia, concurred. A case in New York—in which the father had worked for Merrell's New York office—eluded the count when it was decided the mother had gotten her thalidomide from Canada. (Had the agency taken better note of the baby's injuries—an inverted kidney—it might have widened the scope of its inquiry to look for injuries beyond phocomelia.)

In Baltimore, a case linked to one of Merrell's earliest trial doctors— neurologist Frank Ayd—made the count, but in a manner, the FDA believed, that exonerated both the doctor and Merrell. Ayd's male patient, being treated for alcoholism, had shared his thalidomide with his pregnant daughter. Her baby was born with a severe congenital heart malformation and shortened arms, and when thalidomide made news in August of 1962, she had the Maryland Department of Health confirm that the tablets were thalidomide. But the mother heard nothing from Merrell, and a lawyer she contacted blew her off. The FDA saw "no basis for action since the daughter took medicine dispensed to and for the treatment of her father." The case was closed.

When a Texas woman, whose nephew had been born with a truncated right arm and no right leg, asked the FDA for the names of trial doctors, the agency refused her. The FDA deemed it proper to ignore the case because the mother's doctor was not on the investigator list, even though sixty-three other doctors in Texas were, and the drug, they knew by now, had moved around freely.

Following the trail of the drug had proved near impossible for the agency. But what was first deemed medical sloppiness took on a darker hue in late August, when, at long last, the FDA strong-armed a Merrell detail man into surrendering his itinerary from the November 1960 Kevadon Clinical Hospital Program conference. The agency now saw that the Merrell sales force had been asked to sweet-talk doctors into running slap-dash "clinical trials"—without requiring data or reports. The twelve hundred doctors enlisted by Merrell to distribute the drug had no records of where it had gone because they'd been told not to keep them.

Rumors of the incriminating paperwork roiled Capitol Hill, and Senator Humphrey coaxed Larrick into sharing the document. Humphrey was in the embarrassing position of having publicly praised Merrell's conduct after the initial subcommittee hearing, praise Merrell had been widely parroting. Humphrey now leaked the confidential document to *The Washington Star*, and the paper exposed Merrell's "crash program to 'sell' thalidomide to influential doctors." Humphrey declared his about-face: This was not clinical investigation but "marketing," he told the newspaper. The manual had "extremely serious implications" and showed a "degree of carelessness" requiring investigation.

In fact, the situation was much worse than FDA reports suggested: The FDA inspection of Merrell's records had found that not only had 580 kilograms been distributed within the United States, but an additional 116 kilograms were entirely unaccounted. Further, the firm had written off a stunning 127 kilograms (58 lbs) of thalidomide to "manufacturing loss." By a conservative estimate, given that the drug was predominantly tableted in 25–100 mg amounts, at least 5 million doses of the drug had left Merrell's various facilities—double the FDA public estimate. And most of it was unaccounted for. Indeed, the FDA soon began discovering stocks of thalidomide in a "substantial" number of drugstores throughout the country. Months after the FDA recall, a concerned director of pharmacy at a large New York hospital would tell the agency that a doctor on staff was still dispensing the drug.

By late September, most of the FDA had come to suspect the sobering truth of Frances's assertion: Merrell had broken the law. The deputy director of the Bureau of Field Administration, a man who'd worked at the FDA since 1939, penned a scathing memo: The agency suspected Richardson-Merrell had "failed to make full disclosure" and had "information of adverse reactions 'long' before the facts were reported to FDA." He cited serious discrepancies in the company's paperwork, including records of Merrell's visits to Germany and Canada after the firm learned of the phocomelia link—records found in the National Drug Company files but missing from Merrell's offices. Why was Merrell hiding the visit? Merrell had clearly "gone over" files before the FDA arrived, being "less than candid" with inspectors. Further, all Merrell's telephone and interoffice memos since 1960 had seemingly vanished.

By October, FDA directors across the country had been issued a new assignment—to determine, officially, if Merrell had broken the law. Had the firm made "false and misleading assurances" to doctors? Had a promotional scheme been carried out under the banner of clinical studies? Agents were sent to interview obstetricians, gynecologists, and general practitioners who had received Kevadon.

"The investigations will require tact, persuasive powers, and finesse," headquarters warned. "Inspectors may meet with 'resistance'"—since many doctors had already been uncooperative with the FDA. The FDA also wanted—"with utmost discretion"—to find any former Merrell detail men who had attended the 1960 Kevadon conference and might say more. The mounting investigation, however, played out quietly. The public still celebrated America's escape from the thalidomide tragedy and believed Merrell to be blameless.

The *Cincinnati Enquirer* wrote that Merrell had been "catapulted unwillingly into a harsh international publicity spotlight" for merely trying to get a "seemingly supersafe" sleeping pill approved.

A nine-page spread in *The Saturday Evening Post* in October of 1962—"Exclusive: The Untold Story of the Thalidomide Babies"—featured nearly one hundred thalidomide babies in Germany and England. The sole reference to the U.S. situation was that "The United States escaped, except for a very few cases, because of the alertness of Dr. Frances O. Kelsey, the Food and Drug Administration doctor." There was no mention of the thousands of Americans receiving experimental pills or the mass of missing pills. Nothing about Merrell's fumbled recall. The article did note, however, that some German mothers had "swallowed as many as 16 different medicines while pregnant—tonics, tranquilizers, sleeping pills, tablets for headache and upset stomach"—suggesting a waywardness to the women who had taken thalidomide. "Women who are pregnant or expect to be pregnant should take no medicines which are not absolutely necessary" and "should especially avoid all new drugs," the article admonished. Mothers took more blame than the drug firms or doctors.

Merrell celebrated this public relations coup. Weeks later, Richardson-Merrell president H. Robert Marschalk and Merrell president Frank Getman told *BusinessWeek* that despite both the MER/29 and Kevadon scandals, "the reputations of both the division and the parent company seem to have come through relatively untarnished."

Q: Did you ever call on any of the physicians at any time who had previously received the drug as a result of your participation in the hospital clinical program, to warn them of the side effects of the drug?

A: Not that I remember.

—*deposition of a Merrell detail man,*

McCarrick v. Richardson-Merrell,

Superior Court of the State of California, 1971

Thirty-four

In August, right after *Life* and the *National Enquirer* ran their thalidomide stories, three out of four Americans favored stricter drug regulations. By the fall, as the House struggled to vote out a bill that aligned with what had come out of the Senate, naysayers emerged and public passion for the issue began to wane.

A *Newsweek* opinion piece claimed that no new drug laws were needed because the FDA worked so efficiently. Dr. Howard Rusk, medical columnist for *The New York Times*, decried not just the new drug bill but also the reason behind it—the "recent flurry" over thalidomide. "The thalidomide incident," Rusk wrote, "illustrated rather well that our present regulations are effective. . . . The Food and Drug Administration did keep it off the market."

In the *Medical Tribune*, Professor Louis Lasagna of Johns Hopkins went further, launching a save-thalidomide campaign. As the safest sedative discovered, Lasagna declared, thalidomide was "too valuable a drug to lose." In fact, he claimed, had it been prescribed to Marilyn Monroe instead of barbiturates, she might still be alive. Lasagna did not disclose that he had been an early Kevadon investigator for Merrell and that he had personally accompanied firm executives to the FDA a year earlier to urge Frances to fast-track the drug. Lasagna blamed "thalidomide hysteria" for prompting drug legislation that would endanger research. He especially loathed the patient-consent provision. It wasn't always "reasonable and feasible" to get informed consent from a patient, and in some instances, Lasagna thought it would be "cruel."

Helen Taussig blasted her Hopkins colleague. Would Marilyn Monroe have really tried to overdose with a *non*lethal drug? And was the life of one person ever worth the risk of a thousand children born without limbs? Rusk, who also battled with Taussig, likewise spurned advising patients they were in trials: Too much red tape would dissuade doctors from being clinical investigators.

But Taussig, knee-deep in the thalidomide backstory, would not budge on patient consent. Too many women, unsure of what drug they had been given, were now suffering dire consequences. For months, Taussig had been investigating an armless child in Connecticut whose mother had no record of what pills she'd taken. In another instance, a Texas doctor had notified Taussig of a phocomelic child whose mother likewise struggled to name her pregnancy medications.

Taussig's most alarming find was that the results of the thalidomide testing Smith, Kline & French had done in 1956–1957 had been kept quiet. Taussig later wrote confidentially to Frances:

> I am told that not only did Smith Kline and French try out thalidomide three or four years ago but that they definitely thought that they saw phocomelia resulting from women taking thalidomide in early pregnancy.

Taussig personally knew of a few other cases in New England where the birth dates aligned. And the mysterious question remained: Why would it have taken SKF a full year of human trials to determine the drug was ineffective as a sedative? Reluctant to make public accusations and be drawn into court, Taussig asked Frances:

> Do you know whether Smith, Kline and French ever told Grünenthal that they suspected that they got malformations as a result of taking thalidomide in early pregnancy? . . . If Grünenthal had received word from Smith, Kline and French three years before thalidomide was suspected, it seems to me that the drug houses had absolutely no excuse for not immediately admitting the difficulty. It does go to show how much financial investment influences what you do.

Frances, for her part, also distrusted the SKF trials. News of an "unexplained crop of deformed babies born in the same block of New York City" between 1956 and 1957, where families had all frequented the same drugstore, suggested the possibility that SKF's samples had gotten into a *pharmacy*.

Even more perplexing, at least three researchers who had worked at SKF while the firm tested and rejected thalidomide had gone on to work at Richardson-Merrell affiliates during later thalidomide trials.

Frances tried to learn more. But no paper trail from SKF's human trials existed to provide answers. She spoke to one SKF trial doctor who admitted that he had no experience testing new drugs and no special training in pharmacology. SKF had assured him that the drug had been thoroughly tested for safety, so he assumed he was simply supposed to determine if patients liked the product.

"Thoroughly tested for safety" was a bold assurance in 1956, before the drug had gone on the market in Germany, at a time when Grünenthal's early trial doctors were still voicing doubts. SKF certainly had no data to suggest the sedative was safe for pregnant women.

SKF's trials—dubbed operation "Hawk" within the firm—now looked as promotional and sloppy as Merrell's. And as secretive. After SKF quietly informed the FDA of one birth malformation potentially linked to its trials, Frances contacted the doctor, but he refused to disclose the parents' names. The mother likely had no idea she had been given thalidomide from a drug trial predating the one in the news.

The entire FDA recall effort exposed a perilous confluence of gaps in the law. Trial doctors didn't have to tell patients they were being given an experimental drug, and they didn't need to report birth abnormalities. After a drug's dangers were known, doctors had no obligation to alert patients to what drug they had been given. Plus, a doctor could thwart government follow-up by withholding the patient's identity. Names of trial doctors, forever guarded, meant that patients might never know they'd been used as guinea pigs. On all sides, the law shielded doctors, leaving patients defenseless.

In the Capitol, the thalidomide story was exposing this legal quandary. Despite drug lobbyists' angling for last-minute ground, the bill that finally came out of conference was actually *stronger* than the two that had gone in.

"The thalidomide scandal had proved that Kefauver had been right all along," a congressman explained, adding that the senator's reputation as a "strong public-interest man" helped tip the scales. "It all depends on the man's weight."

On the morning of October 10, Kefauver stood beside Frances, Commissioner Larrick, and Senator Humphrey in the sun-drenched White House Oval Office as Kennedy at long last began to sign Public Law 87-781. But Kennedy stopped midway through his signature and turned behind him, handing the pen to Kefauver.

"You played the most important part, Estes," said JFK, "so you get the first pen."

Stunned, Kefauver took the pen. "Thank you, Mr. President."

Frances stood quietly and watched, for the second time in her life, as a landmark piece of drug legislation in which she had played a role was enacted. Kennedy then also handed her a pen in congratulations. But even as these new protections were being codified into law, Frances knew something from her work on the thalidomide recall that the bill would not address. Doctors, masses of them, were lying to their patients.

My mother's doctor was the only Black doctor in Wilson, North Carolina. She trusted him. . . . She was having nausea and fainting spells during her pregnancy, so he gave her a bottle of sample pills he had. This would have been in late 1962.

I was born without arms. The doctor said I wouldn't live to be two weeks old. Then that I would never walk. That I would never have kids.

When I was eighteen years old, I came back to Wilson, North Carolina, with my mom. We were coming to get my mother's medical records. The doctor handed her only a few note cards. He looked at me and patted me on my head. "I've been waiting eighteen years to be sued for this baby," he said.

—Tawana Williams,
born May 1963

Thirty-five

The criminal exoneration of the William S. Merrell Company happened almost invisibly.

In October 1962, the FDA's investigation to determine if the firm had broken the law resulted, within weeks, in a resounding "yes." In mid-November, Frances, who was still advocating for follow-up on more cases of malformations, attended a large HEW meeting where the official findings were presented. SKF, Vick, National Drug, and Walker Labs emerged from the probe without allegation—but Merrell was resolutely denounced. The firm had distributed "false and misleading" information about Kevadon and had illegally "entered into commercialism." In essence, Merrell had put thalidomide on the market, for free, with dangerous false promises.

The question at hand: Was there enough evidence for criminal charges?

James Nakada, the FDA director overseeing the recall, took the floor and minced no words: Merrell had completely misled the agency about the content and timing of its physician warning letters and had withheld names of Kevadon investigators. Plus, the timeline of Frances's interactions with the firm showed it had withheld information on both phocomelia and peripheral neuritis.

An agency pharmacologist who'd reviewed Merrell's internal documents said that the firm had also suppressed data and submitted *false* data in its Kevadon application. Further, the FDA had statements from former Merrell detail men explaining the extensive promotional angle of the Kevadon hospital program. Multiple doctors enlisted as Kevadon investigators, including obstetricians, had signed affidavits stating that Merrell told them the drug was not experimental in the true sense, assuring them that it had already thoroughly been tested for safety.

An inspection of Merrell's offices had also turned up evidence of the company's efforts to downplay reports of side effects. Documents showed that the firm had intervened to delay publication of a research paper on thalidomide-related nerve damage in *JAMA*.

At the same time, an FDA inspector in Cincinnati had learned that Ray O. Nulsen made donations to the Children's Home of Cincinnati in the names of *twenty* dead infants during his time as a Kevadon investigator—had Nulsen's trials maimed *dozens* of babies?

The sobering HEW meeting ended with a collective decision to bring charges to a grand jury. Almost half the accusations against Merrell pertained to its "recall"—the effort Commissioner Larrick had so publicly praised before Congress. The change in tune was momentous. But the FDA's reproach did not receive notice beyond the walls of HEW.

While these marked the second set of criminal charges against Merrell—the firm was also under investigation for MER/29—the case went mysteriously silent within the FDA. "I kept inquiring about it," a perplexed Cincinnati director recalled, after recommending prosecution to the Washington headquarters, "and wasn't getting anywhere. . . . Finally I was told that the recommendation had been sent to the Department of Justice by the FDA headquarters and there it apparently died a quiet death."

In fact, the FDA's charges were filed in July of 1963. By May of the following year, Special Attorney James W. Knapp at the Justice Department asked the FDA for more information on "the reputation of the William S. Merrell Company." Someone in the agency's Bureau of Regulatory Compliance wrote back that Merrell and its parent company, Richardson-Merrell (previously Vick), had generally good reputations but had created "difficulties in our enforcement work" when the FDA tried to inspect the firm's premises. Merrell would offer up only what was explicitly spelled out in the law—nothing more.

But in September of 1964, the Justice Department declined to prosecute. Assistant Attorney General Herbert J. Miller, Jr., not one to shy away from a fight, stunned HEW with his dismissal: He didn't find the case against Merrell "sufficiently strong or clear," and criminal prosecution was "neither warranted nor desirable." Miller thought Merrell had "acted in

good faith" in construing the law at the time and seemed "innocent of intent to violate the regulations."

Miller's assessment of the facts was, of course, wildly at odds with the
FDA's findings. Miller, for some reason, thought Merrell had distributed
Kevadon "only to physicians of high professional standing." More con-
founding was Miller's claim that "as far as is known, only one malformed
baby has been born in the United States as a result of its mother's use of
Kevadon." Consequently, Miller doubted a court or jury would fault the
firm, since "it would be difficult to prove that Kevadon's distribution in the
United States resulted in grave harm."

But the number "one" seemed drawn from a hat. The FDA had already
informed Congress of nine clear-cut victims connected to Merrell's Kevadon trials. And many at the agency knew that figure was a grave undercount. Five additional cases stemmed from Kevadon that was supposedly
taken only in late pregnancy. And all the hard-to-prove cases had already
been wiped from the tally.

Further undermining Miller's odd claim of only one American Kevadon victim, by the date of his decision, at least three civil cases had been
filed against Merrell or Ray O. Nulsen by parents certain that Merrell's
thalidomide had damaged their children's limbs.

Nonetheless, Herbert Miller felt the new law would "obviate a recurrence of distribution programs such as this." The Department of Justice
was thus closing its file.

The dismissal of charges shocked many at HEW and the FDA. Frustrated scribbles by agency staff fill the margin of Miller's decision letter:
"Not correct. 10 definitely. 6 others maybe." Someone else noted making
an immediate call to clarify that "the figures for Kevadon were 9 and 5 respectively."

Having spent months gathering evidence against Merrell, the FDA
quickly regrouped. Various agency departments conferred about how to
bolster their arguments for prosecution. Even Ralph Smith, the man who
had once stormed Barbara Moulton's office to demand the immediate approval of a drug, wanted Merrell held accountable. The FDA pointed out
to the Justice Department that Merrell's Kevadon hospital plan advised
detail men that the firm *wasn't* seeking data. One of the detail men had

told them that the vice president of Merrell himself had told them at the Kevadon conference to be faithful to the firm's promotional talking points. Clearly Merrell had exploited the law's "investigational" drug exemption for commercial purposes. Further, the "one malformed baby" statement was patently false. The agency cited its nine known phocomelia cases attributable to Kevadon in early pregnancy, plus the additional five associated with late pregnancy. By this point in time, even Helen Taussig deemed Merrell's behavior "inexcusably bad."

The agency then contemplated going after Ray Nulsen. On the heels of Miller's dismissal, FDA field offices discussed prosecuting Nulsen for false statements under Title 18, Section 1001. They wanted his delivering nurses interviewed, as well as his former office assistant: "We need evidence to show that the physician intended to cover up his deformities." By that point, the Cincinnati district was investigating "some 40 infants born to Dr. Nulsen's patients which apparently are Kevadon connected."

But the Justice Department remained firm in its refusal to charge Merrell, and rumors flared. A reporter for the *Cincinnati Enquirer* heard that a "closed hearing" had been held between the DOJ and Merrell so that Merrell could make its case. Someone at the FDA heard that the DOJ felt Merrell had already "been done so much harm."

For all the media attention devoted to thalidomide in 1962, the story of the FDA's push for criminal charges and the DOJ's refusal to prosecute never entered the public conversation. And the Justice Department never corrected its misstatement that only one American baby had been harmed. What did draw interest was that in December 1963, a federal grand jury issued a twelve-count indictment against Merrell for MER/29, the firm's cholesterol drug. Also charged were three Merrell employees, including Flor Van Maanen. Van Maanen faced a five-year prison sentence for falsifying animal data, and the firm stared down $120,000 in fines.

The president of Richardson-Merrell assured the press that the company would be vindicated, but the grand jury subpoena had unearthed so much doctored data for MER/29 that in March the defendants pleaded "no contest" to eight counts (the government dropped four). Flor Van Maanen, it turned out, had routinely disposed of data that did not align with the firm's safety claims. The Merrell scientists received six months of probation and the firm was fined $80,000. This marked the first time a drug firm was convicted of misleading the government about a product.

The larger punishment, however, came from the civil suits. Fifteen hundred claims were filed in state and federal courts, marking the first-ever mass-tort drug case. The success of the joint MER/29 suits against Merrell, in fact, paved the way for the asbestos, tobacco, and Agent Orange mass-disaster litigation in the following decades.

No wave of thalidomide suits ever swept the United States. Only a handful of families ever assembled the pieces and took action.

The first American case to see a courtroom was that of David Diamond. When the thalidomide news broke in August of 1962, Joanne Diamond grew convinced she'd been given Kevadon—described to her as a "new drug"—early in her pregnancy at a Cleveland hospital while her husband was treated for chest pains. Her son, David, had been born without arms in Philadelphia in April 1961. The family had reached out to the FDA, but the mother was not a patient of an official trial doctor, so David was excluded from any agency investigation. But Joanne's brother-in-law in Cleveland still had one of the envelopes in which she'd been handed the drugs, and it showed the prescribing doctor's name. David's pediatrician sent off a query, explaining the boy's phocomelia and asking about thalidomide. "Impossible," the doctor wrote back, declaring there was no thalidomide in the hospital's pharmacy. But it came to light that an official Kevadon investigator—Dr. Charles Brown—worked at the same hospital and had a reputation for stockpiling drug samples. Dr. Brown said he had never dispensed any thalidomide yet couldn't explain what he'd done with the first seven hundred pills Merrell had shipped to him. Or the next eight hundred. Around fifteen hundred pills, it seemed, had been let loose in the Cleveland hospital, yet the doctors working there closed ranks. Perhaps Mrs. Diamond had been given a sleeping pill, they uniformly declared, but no way was it thalidomide.

After five and a half years of discovery, seventy depositions, and multiple international inquiries, the Diamond case looked precarious. The refusal of any doctor to admit Mrs. Diamond even *could* have been given thalidomide proved a hurdle for the plaintiff. Would a jury really believe that all these illustrious physicians were lying? The defense laid it on thick:

Here is a man, he is the head of the department of gastroenterology
at the Cleveland clinic, which is an institution in size comparable
with the University Hospital or the great teaching institutions in
Philadelphia, and they stand here and say that this man — everybody
is a liar.

Fortunately, the plaintiff's legal team finally tracked down the nurse
who had handed Joanne Diamond the pills. She fessed up: The drug she'd
been instructed to dispense was unequivocally Kevadon. Her deposition,
coupled with testimony from a former Merrell lab technician who said
that the firm had buried toxic results of animal experiments, revived the
plaintiff's case. Within three days of the trial's start, Merrell offered to settle with the Diamonds.

Two years later, however, the drug firm decided to chance it with a
jury.

In 1966, the family of four-year-old Peggy McCarrick brought suit
against Merrell. Shirley McCarrick was certain that the nausea pills she'd
been given in her first trimester had caused her daughter's phocomelia.
But Shirley McCarrick, like Joanne Diamond, had not gotten the drug
directly from a Kevadon investigator. The FDA had never counted or investigated her case and she was on her own. For five years, a high-powered
California firm sought to gather evidence but made little progress. As the
statute of limitations was set to run out, Richardson-Merrell offered the
family a $6,000 settlement.

But the McCarricks refused and found another firm. Jim Butler, their
new lawyer, a marine colonel and father of nine, raced the clock to mount
Peggy's case, convinced that Richardson-Merrell were "bad, bad people."

Butler quickly unearthed the paperwork showing Merrell's reckless distribution of Kevadon. He argued that a Kevadon "investigator" at the hospital, Edward Holroyd, had likely shared some of his 2,700 pills with other
attending doctors and the hospital pharmacy. Butler also grasped the visual power of Peggy: He brought her into court on her ninth birthday, in a
frilly pink dress made by her grandmother. In June 1971, after two months
and nineteen days of emotional proceedings, jurors awarded the McCarrick family $2.5 million in damages, the largest award in California

history—and $300,000 *more* than the family had sued for. One juror crossed the room to hug Peggy's lawyers.

Merrell never let another case go to trial.

By 1971, a total of thirteen civil suits had been brought on behalf of phocomelic American children, many of whom were never included in the FDA's original count. It was looking like more American children had been harmed by thalidomide than originally reported, and *The New York Times* finally acknowledged, "No one can be sure about the total number of thalidomide children in this country." The paper cited a New York epidemiologist who had seen "evidence that an 'excess' of limb deformations took place in the state in 1962."

Nonetheless, legal action for families remained cumbersome to impossible. Cases were pricey and the clock on the statute of limitations was always ticking. A condition of many previously settled cases was that litigation records were sealed. Merrell defense lawyers were always quick to point out that "no government charges of fraud have ever been brought in the thalidomide case." And the FDA—despite believing Merrell had been criminally negligent—remained uncooperative with plaintiffs' lawyers, deeming "facts developed by the FDA . . . for our exclusive use." Lawyers representing Nulsen's patients had wasted months simply trying to confirm with the agency that Nulsen was an official thalidomide "investigator." When the lawyers for the Diamond family asked the FDA for "promotional literature on Kevadon," the agency claimed to have none, refusing to share the Kevadon hospital program itinerary that was the centerpiece of the agency's own claims of Merrell's criminality. A distraught mother who believed her baby had been harmed by "blue pills in an unlabeled bottle" given to her in 1961 or 1962 asked the agency to confirm if her doctor was on the list of physicians who had "tested" thalidomide in the United States and was told that such information could "not be revealed under the law."

She was never advised that the drug had been dispensed by vast numbers of doctors who were not official investigators.

About a decade after the McCarrick verdict, another U.S. thalidomide case made headlines. In 1980, the family of Jamie Swenholt, born in April 1961 at an air force base in Alabama with malformations of all four limbs,

filed suit against Richardson-Merrell. Eleven years of negotiations with
the drug firm had gotten nowhere. Before the statute of limitations ran
out, the family enlisted Arthur Raynes—the lawyer who had represented
the Diamond family and who was sitting on the mother lode of evidence
of Merrell's misbehavior. In 1983, Merrell settled with the Swenholts.

Three years later, one last case took the spotlight. In 1986, an Ohio family begged President Ronald Reagan to lift the statute of limitations for the
Military Court of Claims to prove that Mary Lou McKenna had been
given thalidomide at the army base in Germany where her husband had
been stationed. Her son, born in December of 1960, had "flippers" for
legs.

Reagan's agreement spurred a minor flurry of publicity, and The Washington Post conjectured, "McKenna is probably the last uncompensated
thalidomide victim." But the McKenna case vanished from the headlines
when the mother couldn't name who had given her the pills thirty years
earlier. The case was dismissed.

By the mid-1980s, various experts, including Morton Mintz, predicted
that they'd seen the last of North American thalidomide suits. The National Law Journal declared the end of a "legal era." The thalidomide saga
in the United States was considered finished.

I would first like to say that I still regard the charge

as a gross injustice to me personally.

—Heinrich Mückter,

trial testimony,

Alsdorf, Germany, 1968

Thirty-six

In December 1961, within days of thalidomide's recall from the German market, public prosecutors in Aachen had begun probing criminal charges against Grünenthal. The investigation took nearly four years. Police raids were needed to procure documents from Grünenthal's secret "bunker." Evidence was seized from the home of a Grünenthal lawyer. After the preliminary indictment, it took another three years for the trial to start. But on May 27, 1968, nearly seven hundred people crowded into a vast mining company hall in Alsdorf, West Germany—the largest available space in the region—for proceedings that promised to be as thorough as those at Nuremberg.

The full bill of indictment against nine Grünenthal employees ran 972 pages. The prosecution had assembled seventy thousand pages of evidence, 351 witnesses, and twenty-nine scientific and medical experts to argue personal negligence on the part of the Grünenthal men. Five thousand case histories had been studied—of mothers with damaged babies and adults with peripheral neuritis—and four hundred coplaintiffs had signed on. The criminal and civil cases would be argued concurrently in the same trial.

While the prosecution had an arsenal of paperwork, the defense had an arsenal of lawyers—forty in total—and they constantly pushed for delays. Three of the nine Grünenthal executives were excused for health reasons and sat out the trial—including Hermann Wirtz, the firm's co-founder and head. The firm also aggressively angled to rein in bad press; five journalists would complain to the court that Grünenthal threatened retaliation over their trial coverage.

Grünenthal's overall courtroom strategy was to argue that (1) testing drugs for pregnancy safety was not standard practice at the time and (2) thalidomide did not actually cause phocomelia. An additional bold claim—emblematic of how far Grünenthal was willing to take the fight—was that thalidomide might have *saved* fetuses that would have otherwise naturally aborted. In essence, the thousands of living victims, missing arms and legs, had actually been spared from death by Grünenthal's wonder sedative.

Widukind Lenz testified and was cross-examined by eighteen defense lawyers, but as he had railed against Grünenthal so often in the press, his statements were dismissed by the court. The prosecution had hoped to call Frances Kelsey, but FDA regulations forbade her from participating in a foreign trial. Other Alsdorf witnesses, however, made strong cases: Augustin Blasiu, the doctor whose name Grünenthal had touted as having proved the drug's safety during pregnancy, testified that he'd never given the drug to a single pregnant woman. Dr. Ralf Voss described the firm's repeated attempts to silence his warnings about peripheral neuritis.

Most powerful were the thalidomide parents seated in the mining hall, watching the trial in quiet desperation as their children, attended by Red Cross nurses, played in the corridors. The outcome of these proceedings would determine their ability to afford care for their sons and daughters.

Karl Schulte-Hillen, more than anyone, grasped the stakes.

Over the past few years, he and Linde had become key community organizers for thousands of German thalidomide families. Initially concerned that parents were relegating their children to doom, Karl and Linde had resolved to prove the potential of these youngsters. They allowed newspapers to publish pictures of Jan—now thriving. The couple had taught him to lift his truncated arms by rigging a teddy bear to a typewriter, motivating him to move the bear by tapping the space bar. Imagining he might become a scientist (Jan would, in fact, become a physician), they had nurtured his curiosity and intelligence. The photographs of the flourishing Jan and loving Schulte-Hillen household elicited a flood of responses—*eight hundred* letters—from other thalidomide families. (Karl had asked newspapers to publish their home address.) One mother poignantly confessed that until she had seen the joyous photos of Karl and Jan, she had been contemplating a mercy killing: "I thank you from the bottom of my heart," she told Karl.

Karl and Linde sensed the importance of fostering community, and also of collective advocacy. They formed the Association of Parents of the Child Victims of Contergan to petition for specialized medical centers and research into artificial limbs. Linde coordinated gymnastics and writing lessons for forty-two local groups and pressed a primary academy with a pool to host swim classes. "Nothing matters," Karl told the press, "except his [Jan's] future and the future of all other handicapped children like him or even more severely handicapped."

As the start of the Alsdorf trial neared, Karl believed justice was at last at hand. Having decided to represent the other families in the civil case, he assembled a poignant photo album of one hundred thalidomide children and sent copies to the Court of Aachen, the major political parties, and the new National Ministry of Health. In addition to wanting cash settlements, Karl wanted the Grünenthal executives in jail. He also grasped that the government's criminal case was crucial to helping fund the civil suits brought by the families. But Grünenthal was so well connected, friends worried Karl was going too far; he would amass many powerful enemies. Acquaintances who had not turned away at Jan's birth now shunned Karl and Linde. And Karl was asked to resign from his father's law firm.

The trial years proved lonely and grueling for the couple. Since Karl earned no income from the case, the family barely scraped by. Karl and Linde now had two more children but lived in the same cramped third-floor apartment where they had set up as newlyweds. Movie outings, parties, and trips vanished. The children played with scraps of cloth or hand-sewn puppets. To earn money, the siblings collected bundles of old newspapers from nearby homes. Jan bought a skateboard with his savings—proving an agile daredevil like his father—and careened down the hill with other neighborhood kids. Karl, on weekends home from the exhausting court proceedings, reveled in brief outdoor adventures with Jan. Gliding through the crystal-blue sky in Karl's two-seater sailplane, Jan cheered, "Higher! Faster!"—lifting Karl's spirits.

The trial had been expected to run three years, but on December 18, 1970, the court abruptly announced its final session. The trial was "discontinued" after thirty-one months and 1.2 million feet of tape-recorded proceedings of the longest trial in West German history. Observers were shocked. But no verdict was issued.

The presiding judge officially castigated the drug firm: Grünenthal had ignored the duties of a "conscientious and careful pharmaceutical company" and had been "unethical," "obstructive," and "negligent." The court also asserted one matter was inarguable: Thalidomide was toxic and had caused the birth defects of thousands of West German infants and peripheral neuritis in hundreds of adults. But the eight accused Grünenthal executives went free (the ninth had died during the trial). And Grünenthal was neither convicted nor acquitted. The trial simply . . . ended.

The defense, it seemed, had lobbied against the length of the trial, arguing that the United Nations Declaration of Human Rights mandated a timely verdict. (The Nuremberg trials, by comparison, lasted only ten months.) More relevant: Grünenthal had offered plaintiffs a significant out-of-court settlement: $27 million for the children, plus $1.1 million for the adult peripheral neuritis victims. The firm had also agreed to cover trial costs—about $1.6 million. Grünenthal, meanwhile, suggested that a prolonged criminal trial could bankrupt the company, preventing payment of a settlement. The judge quickly ended all proceedings.

But the families felt blindsided: They had privately agreed to drop their civil suits in exchange for the settlement, but no one had told them the government would also close the criminal case. Having been adamant about wanting Grünenthal found guilty in court, the families bemoaned the outcome: Grünenthal was granted immunity from any future criminal proceedings—an irrevocable get-out-of-jail-free card the company could invoke for decades. Like Merrell, the German drug firm had now escaped the whole thalidomide debacle without a single legal penalty.

The settlement also had difficult conditions: Parents could no longer speak out against Grünenthal, and as a group, they had to accept the agreed-upon compensation. This translated to an average of $19,000 per child, or $130,000 today, depending on the severity of injury, paid in installments. The German government also contributed $29 million to the fund and administered its distribution. But the initial determined amount would have to last the child's lifetime.

This "Alsdorf Settlement" eventually supported victims in Austria, Belgium, Brazil, the Netherlands, Portugal, Syria, and Mexico—countries where Grünenthal-made thalidomide pills had been sold by foreign licensees. But this marked the extent of Grünenthal's amends to worldwide victims.

Elsewhere around the globe, families were left to battle the manufacturers and distributors in their own country. In Sweden, a four-year civil trial against Astra Pharmaceuticals spurred a $14 million settlement in 1969. The funds covered the country's one hundred thalidomide victims and eventually extended to survivors in Denmark and Norway.

In many countries, however, the courts offered no justice. In Britain, where Distillers had sold thalidomide under license since 1958, at least four hundred children had been visibly maimed by the drug. But the British government deemed Distillers blameless and the House of Commons voted down a proposed public inquiry. When a delegation of parents approached the minister of health—Enoch Powell—the man whose government agency had allowed the drug on the market in the first place, he callously rebuffed them. "I hope you're not going to sue the government," he said. He refused to meet any thalidomide children or to issue a public warning about pills still at large. Warnings of the drug's dangers had not been widely covered by the press until June of 1962, allowing mothers to unknowingly consume the toxin. In fact, the British government had decided to permit the continued use of thalidomide in hospitals, under strict conditions.

The British press, like the American press, had also gone light on the offending drug firm. *The Times* of London published an article claiming Distillers had subjected thalidomide with "great thoroughness to all the tests which any pharmacologist would have applied in the circumstances." The reporter who wrote the article retired the day after publication to take a job at Distillers.

Both the government and the press had seemingly shrugged off the idea of any culpability for thalidomide. Thus, the fate of Britain's child victims looked grim, until newspaper editor Harold Evans decided to launch a journalistic crusade for justice.

Evans had first dipped his toes into the story in 1962, as editor of the Darlington-based *Northern Echo* newspaper, when news of the drug first broke. A tall, strapping, literary wunderkind, Evans had once helped a group of wheelchair-using patients at a local hospice start a sports magazine, and the experience had deeply attuned him to the plight of disabled people. Hoping to stir up public concern for the thalidomide victims, Evans had decided to run pictures of the phocomelic babies at a Sussex rehabilitation home.

But the response stunned him. The pictures, readers angrily declared, were unfit for a family newspaper. British society seemed to disavow itself of the whole drug tragedy and the injured children.

The story continued to nag at Evans, however. A few years later, as the editor of the prestigious *Sunday Times*, he followed up. It turned out sixty-two British families had been mired in slow, costly civil proceedings against Distillers, dependent on Legal Aid funding to fight the multimillion-dollar firm. Not a single British thalidomide family had received a cent, and the government-paid lawyers, thinking the case unwinnable, were encouraging families to accept a paltry settlement. Since British law mandated a media gag order on pending lawsuits to prevent influencing of future jurors, the whole topic of thalidomide had been sealed in a "legal cocoon" since the first civil suit was filed in late 1962. The British public knew nothing of the full scandal.

Outraged, Evans took matters into his own hands and set up a "special projects" team at *The Sunday Times* to do what the British government had not—launch an investigation into Distillers' role in the disaster. The team purchased ten thousand Distillers documents from a pharmacologist who had access to the defense's internal paperwork, and three suitcases full of Grünenthal documents from one of the Swedish attorneys who had led the civil suit against Astra. Antony Terry—the dinner guest whom Elinor Kamath had pushed to file one of the first stories on the subject—was now part of the *Sunday Times* research team delegated to pore through the paperwork and conduct interviews.

The project took five years, but by 1972 Evans was ready to run the first of three front-page articles. "Our Thalidomide Children: A National Cause for Shame" laid out the drug's negligence-packed backstory and demanded "decent" compensation for the victims in particular—decrying the settlement amounts proposed by Distillers. But British courts took media silence on pending court cases seriously. Three High Court judges tried to issue an injunction and Evans was threatened with jail time. Nonetheless, Evans ran the story.

Parliament now had its first glimpse of the sordid tale. The second article in the series ran, featuring letters from victims' parents, and the opposition Labour Party called for Distillers executives to "face up to their moral responsibilities."

The High Court banned publication of the third article, but by that point the news had spread like wildfire. A public campaign erupted across London, with people pasting anti-Distillers posters on lampposts and bus stops. A nationwide retail chain declared a boycott. Even across the Atlantic, consumer advocate Ralph Nader threatened a U.S. boycott of Distillers if the company did not offer funds on par with what Peggy McCarrick had received. As the firm's stock plunged, a *Times* reporter arranged a meeting between thalidomide families and key Distillers shareholders. Soon, an emergency company shareholder vote authorized a £28.4 million victims' fund, covering the 62 families who had sued, plus an additional 341 families. The Court of Appeals then lifted the ban on the final *Sunday Times* article, only to have the five Law Lords (Britain's Supreme Court) reinstate the ban. Evans had to take his appeal to the European Commission in France to get the House of Lords to back down and permit publication of the final installment on June 27, 1976.

The team aggregated its findings in the 1979 *Suffer the Children*, one of two authoritative books on the subject published in the twentieth century—showing that both Grünenthal and Distillers had ignored key reports on side effects and had bypassed essential research. Putting to rest the myth that no drug firms at the time were doing reproductive testing on animals, Evans and his team had confirmed with Hoffman–La Roche, Lederle, Pfizer, Burroughs Wellcome, and other large pharmaceutical companies that reproductive testing had been standard product research since the 1940s. Sedatives like Miltown and Librium, for example, had been specifically studied in animals for pregnancy safety. It had taken almost twenty years since the drug hit the market to show that what was first spun as an unforeseeable tragedy by the offending firms was in fact the culmination of cut corners and reckless promotion. The Insight Team's tome laid the groundwork for those seeking justice in the following decades.

By 1962, thalidomide was thought to have damaged approximately ten thousand babies in West Germany alone, about half dying shortly after birth. Since that time, estimates for the drug's worldwide victims have risen as high as 150,000, accounting for unreported miscarriages and internal organ damage not initially recognized as thalidomide damage.

Those who survived fought tooth and nail for compensation in legal suits that spanned decades. In addition to going after the manufacturers and distributors, victims' families appealed to their respective governments. More than forty-five nations had, after all, green-lit a drug that the FDA's Frances Kelsey had suspected and refused. But some nations shirked responsibility, and others were abysmally slow to meet the needs of victims.

In Japan, where thalidomide had been sold under fifteen different names, it wasn't until January 1963 that the drug was fully pulled from shelves. Approximately three hundred babies had been harmed. The victims eventually sued two Japanese manufacturers and the country's Ministry of Health and Welfare—the proceedings took five years to begin and then another year for all three defending parties to admit liability.

Spain, which had only halted thalidomide sales in May of 1962, six months after the German recall, without a single public announcement about the drug's dangers, only accepted responsibility and compensated its survivors in 2010—almost a half century after their injuries.

Italy was similarly negligent. Some versions of the drug had remained on shelves for nine months after the German recall, and an estimated two thousand babies were harmed. Yet it wasn't until 2008 that the government granted the known 350 Italian survivors a pension.

Amid these worldwide legal battles with health authorities and drug distributors, Grünenthal remained untouchable. The Alsdorf nonverdict—painted by the firm as an exoneration—allowed the drug firm to continually dodge liability claims. But as victims reached adulthood and their medical needs increased, the Alsdorf settlement funds fell short of costs. Appeals to Grünenthal for additional assistance were for decades rebuffed. Only in 2008, after an aggressive media campaign to shame the company, did Grünenthal grant a one-time top-off to the German trust.

Grünenthal's proclaimed immunity stirs anger within the thalidomide community—which still numbers in the thousands. Victims, now in their early sixties and grappling with prematurely aging bodies, speak of a drug company that got away with murder. To this day, the Wirtz family still helms Grünenthal. The son of Hermann Wirtz, Dr. Michael Wirtz, serves as the firm's chief executive, and the Wirtzes have maintained stunning wealth and political influence in Germany despite their well-documented wrongdoing and a sizable body count from their products.

In addition to thalidomide, Grünenthal's painkiller tramadol—created in 1962 by former SS doctor Ernst-Günther Schenck—sparked a decades-long global opioid crisis before it was classified as a Schedule IV controlled substance in 2014.

Billing itself "a global leader in pain management," Grünenthal currently generates approximately $1.4 billion annually, about half of that from sales of painkillers. Rumors abound that the family would like to sell the firm to an international conglomerate—a Roche or a Sanofi. But the thalidomide legacy remains a dark stain, a worrisome liability for a potential parent company. Despite Grünenthal's legal evasions, the firm is routinely embarrassed by victim memoirs, documentary films, and picketing of its Stolberg offices.

In the last few years, Grünenthal has made several clumsy efforts to recast its reputation. After decades of stony silence, in 2012, as though hoping to present a more compassionate face, the firm issued an unexpected "apology." Harald Stock, chief executive of the Grünenthal Group, stood outside the company's Stolberg's headquarters on a crisp September day at the unveiling of a statue to honor victims and said:

> Thalidomide is and will always be part of our company's history. We have a responsibility and we face it openly. On behalf of Grünenthal with its shareholders and all employees, I would like to take the opportunity at this moment of remembrance today to express our sincere regrets about the consequences of Thalidomide and our deep sympathy for all those affected, their mothers and their families. We see both the physical hardship and the emotional stress that the affected, their families and particularly their mothers, had to suffer because of Thalidomide and still have to endure day by day. We also apologize for the fact that we have not found the way to you from person to person for almost 50 years. Instead, we have been silent and we are very sorry for that.

It was, on the surface, a surprising about-face for a firm that spent the whole Alsdorf trial denying any causal connection between thalidomide and birth defects, brazenly arguing that the drug had actually saved doomed babies. But the company held tight to its denial of wrongdoing, and the "apology" came with zero financial support. A memorial statue of a thalidomide survivor that the firm helped fund—depicting the plight of being born without arms—did not win fans. Nobody needed a bronze statue. Everyone needed help with medical bills.

"Put your money where your mouth is," victims worldwide railed.

"A lie wrapped in an apology is still a lie," said Harold Evans, who had continued over the decades to track emerging evidence of Grünenthal's deception.

In fact, within a few years of the apology, even more evidence came to light suggesting malfeasance by Grünenthal. A class-action suit in Australia on behalf of formerly unrecognized thalidomide survivors uncovered a stash of documents in a German state archive indicating that Grünenthal had secretly orchestrated the end of the Alsdorf trial. A private meeting in late 1970 between Grünenthal's upper echelons—including seventy-one-year-old Hermann Wirtz—and the federal health ministry seemed to have prompted federal ministries to stop the criminal proceedings. And one of the state prosecutors, it turned out, had been Hermann Wirtz's personal defense attorney up until two years before the trial.

The archives also housed evidence never shown at trial: Chemistry grad student Dr. Günter von Waldeyer-Hartz had sent prosecutors a statement that he had seen "a packaging unit for Contergan-Thalidomide with the sticker NOT FOR PREGNANT WOMEN" at the Grünenthal factory six weeks before the drug was withdrawn, but his statement was never presented at the proceedings.

Grünenthal dismisses analysts of the decades-old documents as "conspiracy theorists," and adamantly denies back-channeling: "The government and the prosecution were not parties to that settlement."

But in 2018, a heavily researched book subsidized by the UK Thalidomide Trust, *The Thalidomide Catastrophe*, meticulously detailed Grünenthal's dismissals of early warnings about the drug's toxicity, making the firm's assertion of total innocence increasingly hard to sustain.

In response, Grünenthal launched a website—www.thalidomide
-tragedy.com—to put forth its own version of story. The site celebrates the
German Contergan Foundation, funded by the 1970 Alsdorf settlement
and enhanced in 2009 with the firm's voluntary contribution of an additional fifty million euros. The foundation, they say, supports victims in
Germany and the thirty-seven countries where Grünenthal's licensees distributed the product. In countries where thalidomide was sold without
Grünenthal's permission, such as in Italy and Spain, victims are "generally
supported" by their country. (Italian and Spanish survivors received government support only recently.) In countries where licensee firms sold
their own thalidomide—such as the UK, Australia, New Zealand, and
Sweden—those companies, along with the respective governments, provide financial support.

"Financial support programmes have been established in all of the
countries where Thalidomide was marketed by Grünenthal or by its licensing partners at that time," Grünenthal boasts. Absent in Grünenthal's
narrative of support for international victims is any mention of thalidomide survivors in the United States. The firm assures the public that in the
United States, "Thalidomide was not sold because the FDA did not issue
an approval."

Is anyone here from the United States?

—*Carolyn Sampson,*

post on "Stop the Tears,"

international thalidomide survivors Facebook group, 2011

HELLO: MY NAME IS GLENDA JOHNSON AND I WAS BORN IN 1962 AS A THALIDOMIDE VICTIM WHEN MY MOM WAS GIVEN THE DRUG WHICH CAUSED ME TO HAVE NUMEROUS BIRTH DEFECTS. I HAVE HALF A RIGHT ARM WITH ONLY FOUR FINGERS AND MY LEFT HAND IS DEFORMED AS WELL ALONG WITH OTHER BIRTH DEFECTS. MY HEART REALLY GOES OUT TO THE MANY OTHER VICTIMS, ALSO I LIVE IN THE UNITED STATES AND WOULD LOVE TO HEAR FROM OTHER VICTIMS AS WELL. I ALSO HAVE NEVER RECEIVED ANY COMPENSATION AT ALL AND IF THEIRS SOME-ONE THAT CAN HELP ME OR GIVE ME SOME INPUT PLEASE CALL ME OR E-MAIL ME AS POSSIBLE AS I SEARCHED ENDLESSELY AND I REALLY NEED HELP. IT WOULD BE SO APPRECIATED. . . . THANK YOU AND

MAY GOD BLESS: GLENDA

—2010 *comment on* "*Thalidomide Victims Seek $6.3 Billion,*" Insurance Journal (*online*)

Thirty-seven

In 1987, an aspiring author in her late twenties published an op-ed in *The Washington Post* entitled "I Would Choose My Life."

Eileen Cronin, a beautiful dark blonde who could pass for the sister of Mariel and Margaux Hemingway, was born in Cincinnati in 1960 without legs. For years, her large Catholic family told her that her condition was God's will.

But in the early 1980s, thalidomide had begun making news again: Found to slow tumor growth, the drug seemed poised for a revival in the fight against cancer. Also, the Merrell Company, then Merrell Dow, was in court on account of another drug—Bendectin, Raymond Pogge's morning sickness concoction from the 1950s. After three decades on the market, Bendectin, like thalidomide, was being accused of causing birth defects. Around this time, the narrative pinning Eileen's disability on "God's will" suffered a blow. Learning that her mother had been given a nausea pill while on an airplane to Germany, Eileen suspected thalidomide.

After some digging, she confirmed that the drug had made its way into the hands of some American women. In her *Washington Post* essay, she sought to correct the widespread misconception that thalidomide was never used in the United States. "It did make its way into this country through one company," she wrote, citing the twenty or so known cases of American phocomelia.

No new investigations came from the article, but Cronin's suspicion that thalidomide had caused her injuries was an emotional turning point in her life. When Eileen married and wanted to have children, she decided to figure out, once and for all, if her legs had been harmed by something genetic or something environmental. Reading a copy of *Suffer the Children,* she learned that the American company distributing Kevadon had actually been based in her own hometown. For so long she'd assumed that the pills her mother took on the international flight had come from Germany. Now a whole new set of suspicions emerged. Stunned by the vast number of Merrell's clinical investigators and the mass of pills distributed, Cronin sensed there was much more to the long-buried story. After all, she had never been counted as one of the FDA's American victims.

Cronin accepted that she was likely a thalidomide survivor. She eventually became a mother to a healthy baby girl and, while working as a clinical psychologist, penned a powerful memoir of her long journey to navigate her relationship with her family—she has ten siblings and a complicated relationship with her mother—and the trauma of trying to understand the source of her injuries. After the publication of *Mermaid: A Memoir of Resilience* in 2014, strangers around the country reached out to her claiming to be or to know of other American thalidomide victims. Cronin's worst suspicions were quickly confirmed. One letter, in particular, devastated her: A Dominican nun who had worked in Kentucky in the 1970s described a care home where she had seen numerous children, without legs, stranded in cribs. The nun recalled the couple running the home telling her that the mothers had taken thalidomide and abandoned their babies.

Cronin sensed that vast parts of the story had gone unreported, and in a 2014 *HuffPost* op-ed, she urged "deeper coverage of the truth about thalidomide and its U.S. victims." But the media didn't bite.

A law firm in Seattle, however, was in the midst of digging deeper. On the heels of a promising class-action suit in Australia and New Zealand, Hagens Berman, a Seattle firm known for squeezing multibillion-dollar settlements out of Philip Morris, Visa and Mastercard, and Volkswagen, probed the possibility of unrecognized American thalidomide victims. Scouring internet message boards, running ads in newspaper classified sections, and speaking to lawyers around the country, the firm launched a nationwide search for survivors. By 2011, Hagens Berman had filed its first lawsuit on behalf of approximately forty-five plaintiffs.

One of these was Carolyn Sampson, a no-nonsense Minnesotan who runs a web design company. Born in 1962 with a shortened arm and missing fingers, Carolyn, like most of the plaintiffs, had spent most of her life oblivious to what had caused her injuries until, at age seventeen, a stranger on a bus asked: "Are you a thalidomide baby?"

Carolyn questioned her mother, who admitted she had taken a packet of headache pills given to her by her doctor during pregnancy. Miraculously, one pill was left. Carolyn reached out to a lawyer, but when lab analysis of the pill proved inconclusive, the attorney assured Carolyn that thalidomide had never been approved in the United States.

As decades passed, Carolyn was passed over for basic jobs—cash register work, fast-food kitchens—because of her misshapen hand. She married at nineteen, had two girls, and was divorced by age twenty-three. Meanwhile, the pain in her arms intensified and she tried to conceal her limitations, even from her family: hiding the way she had to contort her arm behind her neck to simply put on earrings. She eventually sought occupational and physical therapy to deal with her arm. Then, as she was nearing fifty, a co-worker congratulated Carolyn on how surprisingly confident she'd been as she gave a presentation, "considering . . . ," and then trailed off. It was only then that Carolyn realized that, like it or not, others saw her as "disabled," and she conceded the label.

But the word "thalidomide" still nagged at her, and one feverish late-night Google session landed her on a *Time* magazine article from August 1962, mentioning that 1,231 doctors had distributed Kevadon in the United States. Carolyn knew the name of her mother's doctor, so she wrote to the FDA, invoking the Freedom of Information Act, and demanded the names of the trial doctors. Her mother's doctor was not on the list. But the FDA did not tell her what it had known since 1962—that the "list" was a red herring, because the drug had been passed frequently from investigators to other doctors. This part of the narrative remained buried in thousands of FDA documents.

Carolyn still had a nagging sense that thalidomide played a role in her story. She joined a Facebook group for international thalidomide survivors and posted a query: "Is anyone here from the United States?" A Canadian activist told her about the American lawsuit, and Carolyn signed on. It was the Hagens Berman lawyers who, according to Carolyn, finally told her the full truth: Merrell's so-called trials were sloppy, sample pills were handed out in unmarked envelopes and shared between doctors, and women had no idea they were taking something "experimental."

Carolyn was enraged by what seemed a decades-long cover-up. A born organizer with a talent for public relations, she launched a Facebook group specifically for U.S. survivors and created a spreadsheet with everyone's birth date, birth city, hospital, and doctor. A thalidomide survivor from Oregon named JoJo Calora soon connected with her online and the two fast became friends. JoJo, a married father of two who works in IT, also had the organizational bug. They decided the group should meet and planned a small gathering in Atlanta in 2018 for the members to devise a plan of action. They launched a nonprofit to correct the erroneous information still widely circulating—that only nine American babies were affected by U.S. thalidomide. The lawsuit had amassed more than fifty plaintiffs; Carolyn and JoJo suspected the number of victims might top one hundred.

For a year, Carolyn worked feverishly, chasing every lead on survivors around the country, interviewing potential group members on the phone. Most of the victims named in the lawsuit had never met or spoken—they knew one another only as names on shared court filings. Hagens Berman had cautioned plaintiffs against being in touch or posting anything publicly—the strategy likely being to keep them in the dark as long as possible to hammer home for the court how little the plaintiffs knew about thalidomide. The firm had even advised them not to conduct any research of their own. But after decades of misinformation and isolation, the survivors were eager to take control of their futures, and desperate for community.

Carolyn invited me to her home in Minneapolis in 2018 after I had reached out to her about a blog post she had written describing her journey to find the cause of her injuries. We sat for hours on her living room couch, her dog Ellie frequently bounding in to break up the intense conversation. Carolyn's stunning crystal-blue eyes and long, dark lashes reminded me that she had told me she had once been a Mary Kay cosmetics consultant—among her many jobs. Carolyn was warm and self-possessed as she waded through the painful backstory of her thwarted efforts to learn the source of her injuries. Two law firms before Hagens Berman had egregiously misled her, going so far as to lose her paperwork. A journalist in Minnesota had promised Carolyn to write about her story in 2013, but then abandoned the piece. The Hagens Berman lawsuit was moving glacially. It seemed any glimmer of hope for justice or financial support might be going dark once again.

I told Carolyn what I had discovered in FDA records and legal archives. There was a trove of information, I said, seemingly ignored for decades, showing that the FDA knew the drug had been spread far beyond the trial doctors. The agency knew many more babies than publicly noted were likely harmed by thalidomide but had kept quiet about cases not easily traced to a named clinical investigator. The paperwork indicated that mothers had no idea they were given experimental pills, and that no one had told them after the fact. Trial records of the few cases that made it to court showed doctors uniformly lying. The deck had been stacked overwhelmingly against any American victims. I was amazed they had found one another.

Carolyn, tired of waiting on lawyers, decided she would probe the FDA records herself. She wanted to know what had happened and to empower her newly formed group. She now had the names of scores of Americans who believed they had been harmed by thalidomide and felt they all deserved to understand the drug's full history. Carolyn planned to hold a conference the following year to connect members from around the country and to determine a plan for finally getting justice.

In November 2019, Jean Grover and her fourteen-year-old daughter left their upstate New York house in the morning's bitter cold. They were headed to San Diego, California, to meet a group of thalidomide survivors. Jean is an artsy dynamo of a woman who sports cobalt-blue glasses and purple-streaked short hair. Colorful floral tattoos adorn her upper arms. She channels a strong hippie vibe. "That's cool" is one of her favorite expressions, and her voice is melodic and soothing. Nothing in her relaxed, joyous demeanor suggests she was once given up for dead, or that as far as the government is concerned, she doesn't exist.

Jean, the daughter of Ann Morris, was the Cincinnati baby whose parents sent her to foster care. For most of her first year, Jean's mother did not lay eyes on her. But her father snuck visits, and when he finally confessed this to Ann, he told her that Jean was cute. Having been warned about

Jean's missing limbs, Ann had pictured her as a mere torso of a child. But when she finally visited and saw Jean scuttle around the floor, Ann thought, "That's not so bad!" The next day, Ann and Doug took Jean home.

Jean's official diagnosis was proximal femoral focal deficiency. Practically speaking, her legs were about half length, and her feet jutted out at an odd rotation. One of her arms was only elbow length, and her hands, also attached at strange angles, had only one and two fingers, respectively.

But Jean continued to astonish her parents. "They were amazed that I lived, and then they were amazed that I was able to achieve potential," says Jean, now sixty.

The family moved to Kentucky, where Jean spent time in a rehabilitation hospital and got prosthetic legs. In 1971, they all settled permanently in Rochester, New York. There, Jean was soon "mainstreamed," attending regular school. But by her midteens, she had befriended a small group of kids with disabilities, and the group elders—a boy with spina bifida and another with injuries similar to Jean's—were driving cars using hand controls. Jean was mesmerized. "I'm like: *I can do that!*" She told her mother she would like to learn to drive and found a vocational rehabilitation school.

Jean's thirst for independence only grew. With her prosthetic legs, she could walk a quarter mile. Using both hands and her few fingers to hold a pencil, she discovered her tremendous talent for drawing. After high school, she attended the Rochester Institute of Technology, majoring in graphic design and communications, with a minor in creative writing. She graduated in 1984 with highest honors.

Jean's personal life, too, defied expectations. She had been anxious about losing her virginity. Would she get crushed under the guy's weight? Would he be unable to perform because of her disability? But when the time came, Jean found it surprisingly natural: "I liked sex and it became an important part of my life." In college, Jean had a series of healthy romantic relationships with able-bodied boyfriends who hoped to marry her. She likes to point out that she broke many hearts.

Eventually she did marry, and on her thirty-third birthday she gave birth to twin boys, Jake and Andy. When the Rochester paper interviewed her for a Mother's Day feature, Jean quipped, "It's a strange irony that God would give me half the arms and double the babies." The quote ran in bold letters across her photo, and Jean laughed, realizing readers were likely horrified. She was over the moon.

Jean resolved to shower her sons with affection, aware that her own bond with her mother suffered from the year she was in foster care. (Jean—not prone to anger—gets visibly angry when discussing her birth hospital's prediction of her imminent death.) With her sons, the connection was strong from the start. One story in particular makes Jean tear up.

When she arrived at a Mother's Day luncheon at her sons' preschool for her first-ever school "appearance," the other kids erupted with questions: *Who's that? What happened to her arm?* Jean was horrified, but four-year-old Jake—her oldest by two minutes—lifted his hand to quiet the crowd. "Everyone, this is my mom," he announced. "Her arms are like this because she was born like this. But she can eat by herself, and she can draw pictures." Soon, Jean was making drawings for all the kids at Jake's request. The day was transformative for Jean. Jake had set the tone for her feeling like a regular mom.

At thirty-seven, Jean became a mother again—this time, through adoption. Jean had heard of a young girl in India with arthrogryposis, a congenital immobility of the joints. Priya's legs had been stuck in a crossed position since birth, and at four weeks old she had been surrendered to an orphanage. By age three, no one had adopted her. The story of this girl halfway around the world nagged at Jean, who eventually arranged to have Priya flown to the United States to join her family.

Jean and Priya bonded fast. Jean knew the importance of nurturing Priya's independence and problem-solving skills. At age fifteen, when Priya got a summer job in another town and needed wheelchair-friendly transportation, she sorted out the four-hour daily commute on her own with multiple bus transfers. She became highly organized and driven. After Jean took her to a disability-rights rally, Priya became a community organizer, and attended Syracuse University on a full scholarship.

At age forty-two, Jean gave birth to a fourth child, Sarah, with her second husband, Keith. Sarah, at first glance, looks like a typical hair-flipping, selfie-taking teenager, except for the deep maturity in her eyes. She boasts of the independence she developed from having a mom who couldn't help her dress or manage household chores.

Sarah also grew up watching the world watch her mother: "All my life

I've been used to people staring." But she forgives this impulse. "Human eyes are attracted to difference," she explains. She even relishes a few funny memories, such as the time at the mall when a group of crying kids suddenly fell silent as Jean whizzed by on her electric scooter. It's Sarah who has joined her mom on this San Diego adventure. Flying in separately are Jean's son Andy and his friend Yasin, who are filming a documentary about Jean's first meeting with American thalidomide survivors.

Only recently did Jean begin to identify as a thalidomide victim, though of all the stories of misled and gaslit victims across the United States, Jean's is the most shocking. The Jewish Hospital in Cincinnati had witnessed at *least* four phocomelic births in the two years before Jean was born, a stunning statistic. This information was never shared with Jean's mother, and Jean's birth may never have been reported to the FDA or state and local health authorities. Given her birth date, her mother had likely taken thalidomide after the German recall in November of 1961—meaning Jean's birth was perilous for the hospital and Merrell, and people might have had an interest in making her "case" disappear.

Ann went through life telling people that Jean's abnormality was "just one of those things," but Jean had nurtured a quiet curiosity about it. Throughout her childhood, doctors would ask if her limb deficiency was caused by thalidomide, and Jean always said no. But in a rehabilitation facility in Kentucky, Jean had met a girl with identical injuries who'd been born near Cincinnati the same year Jean was. At the time they met, neither girl imagined her condition had anything to do with prenatal drug exposure. But Jean always considered it odd that she and her friend, who had such stunningly similar injuries, had been born mere months apart.

Life as a working mother kept Jean on the go and distracted. But when she became a mentor for the International Child Amputee Network in 1996, she came across pictures of thalidomide survivors who looked hauntingly like her. In 2014, curiosity got the best of her, and she friended someone in a UK thalidomide support group on Facebook. The friend gave Jean a primer on Grünenthal and Merrell. He also told her about the Hagens Berman lawsuit.

Jean signed on. Even though her mother still insisted she hadn't taken thalidomide, she did recall the unmarked bottle of "vitamins" for morning sickness. The fact that Jean's mother never suggested she had taken thalidomide was a boon to Jean's case. It explained why, for decades, Jean had brought no legal action. But the lawsuit moved slowly, and plaintiffs were counseled not to speak to one another. So isolated did plaintiffs remain that it wasn't until I interviewed Jean in her upstate New York home in 2018 that she learned—from me—that Merrell had been headquartered in her hometown and that several "thalidomide babies" had been born in the same hospital as her.

In fact, I had just been in Cincinnati to meet two of them, both of whom had received settlements from Merrell decades earlier. Their cases had been somewhat straightforward, since their mothers had been patients of Dr. Nulsen—on the official investigator list—and both mothers were adamant that he had given them Kevadon.

Between Nulsen's delivering multiple phocomelic babies, publishing the ghostwritten research paper, and swapping Kevadon for Bendectin, his behavior was likely problematic enough that Merrell offered settlements to both girls in 1968. The two ended up meeting in kindergarten at a Cincinnati public school for the disabled, but they assumed they were the only living U.S. thalidomide victims.

One of the women, whose parents are still living, won't speak about her settlement for fear of jeopardizing her funds. The other, Gwen Riechmann, a former Girl Scout leader, is all fire and defiance. She wants to stick it to Merrell. "I didn't sign anything!" she proudly declares. (Her parents, who signed nondisclosure papers, are both dead.) Gwen is happy to share her story, her settlement papers, and the swollen folder of press clippings her father kept. She is also happy to announce, as a badge of honor, that she is one of the "original" thalidomide babies officially counted by the FDA.

When I met them both at Gwen's house in Cincinnati in 2018, I gave them a rundown of Nulsen's misconduct. To them he had been only a name on a birth certificate. But I explained that Nulsen was the big bad wolf of Merrell's trials. The information shocked them. Growing up, they knew little about what their parents had faced in their attempt to find justice. Connecting with other American survivors brought them a new understanding of the larger story in which they played a key role.

Gwen decided to fly to San Diego from Cincinnati for the conference after a travel mishap on the way to the Atlanta gathering a year earlier had left her stranded on the side of I-75 for five hours. ("I will never put a toe on a Greyhound bus again," she declares.) A former high school newspaper editor and 4.0 student, Gwen has a commanding presence. She makes powerful eye contact and does not mince words. She owns two shelties and two cats, and in addition to leading Girl Scouts, she worked for years as a special education teacher. But she has not held a job since 2001.

She is one of the most physically afflicted U.S. thalidomiders. Both of her legs and arms are severely truncated. She never used prosthetics of any kind and can navigate the world outside her house only in a wheelchair. (Inside, she maneuvers across her floor as needed on very calloused knees.) But there is no fragility in her demeanor. Gwen has a distinct "don't fuck with me" vibe—which makes sense given her family history. Her mother suffered a nervous breakdown after Gwen's birth, and the family grew secretive about everything that had happened. Gwen was never told that thalidomide caused her injuries until, after a sex-ed class in middle school, Gwen asked her parents what would happen if she had children.

Her father, a General Electric chemist who spearheaded the family lawsuit, took a tough-love approach to raising Gwen. Once, as he let Gwen flail on the floor while trying to put on a hat, a visiting relative exploded, "Bud, help her!" But Gwen's father wouldn't budge: Gwen had to learn to manage on her own. In 2010, after her mother's death, Gwen moved back to Cincinnati to care for her father, who was suffering from early dementia. Thanks to her father's deliberate parenting, Gwen manages exceptionally well on her own.

For the San Diego gathering, she arrives in her power wheelchair with her college friend Deb. Another survivor has rented a van to fetch people from the airport, so upon Gwen's arrival, five of us bound out of the vehicle to greet her near baggage claim and shepherd her back to the hotel.

As Gwen finally zooms into the Homewood Suites lobby with her entourage, she looks exhausted from travel. But at the sight of Jean—her "Cincinnati sister"—she lights up. The two women recently spoke on the phone, and the excitement as they lay eyes on each other is palpable. Of the whole group of thalidomide survivors, their injuries look the most similar, but their personalities are like night and day. Gwen's hard stare is a sharp contrast to Jean's soft gaze and trail of blue chiffon scarves. But when Jean throws her tattooed arms around Gwen, Gwen melts.

By sunset, about twenty survivors plus their partners and children congregate by the hotel bar, a boisterous gaggle of exuberant new friends with atypically shaped arms, legs, and hands. Someone makes a liquor store run for vodka and bourbon while others pile happy-hour meatballs onto hotel plates and settle companionably onto cushioned benches. So intense is everyone's joy that no one minds the curious glances of other hotel guests. The stares are kind, born of fascination, as if the great mystery is simply why all these people are so wildly happy.

The "US Thalidomide Survivors Conference: Silent No More; Setting Our Story Straight" is packed with roundtable conversations, presentations, group meals, late-night karaoke, and impromptu ping-pong. There are official tote bags and printed programs. I present on my research. Eileen Cronin reads from her memoir. There are standard hotel conference snafus—a three-hour wait for sandwiches, people oversleeping and straggling in late, tech glitches, personality clashes—but also friendships forged in lobby booths.

In the daily group discussions, common themes emerge. Most survivors had highly fraught relationships with their mothers. "Lack of affection" comes up as a frequent complaint, and one woman rises in a session to tearfully describe how in her teens she found a letter revealing that her mother planned to give her up, but her father threatened divorce, a fact her mother refuses to discuss. Thalidomide mothers are generally reluctant to revisit the past. One mother rescheduled my phone interview so many times I finally gave up. After several phone calls with Linde Schulte-Hillen, her children asked me to back off—the topic was too painful.

But a record exists of the trauma these women suffered in the days and months after giving birth. In 1966, Ethel Roskies, a Canadian professor of psychology, launched a five-year study at the Rehabilitation Institute of Montreal to look at how thalidomide mothers were coping. The results were bleak. "The maternity described here is not a pretty one," she confessed in the preface of her 1972 book, *Abnormality and Normality: The Mothering of Thalidomide Children.* "But if this record does not present a mother-child relationship neatly tied with pink or blue ribbons, it does contain much that is beautiful and even heroic."

Roskies spoke to twenty mothers to document the harrowing delivery-room experience: Mothers awoke to see their doctor crying and nurses acting strangely. They were told everything was fine, yet they were not shown the baby. Odd questions about hereditary abnormalities ensued. Visitors looked sad; nurses avoided eye contact. Finally, some combination of doctor, priest, and husband arrived to draw a curtain. The behavior was so unsettling that many mothers assumed they were dying.

Then the blow would come. One doctor simply motioned with his hands to indicate that the woman had delivered half a child. Another doctor told the father that the baby could be helped to die. A nun offered to swap a phocomelic baby for a normal one. The stunned mothers occasionally hemorrhaged.

Leaving the hospital proved no easier. Few mothers were referred to any kind of rehabilitation specialist. Some had no experience as mothers; some had to care for other children. Most of the women were left on their own. Baby items prepared at home before the birth had vanished.

Then came the deception. Many Canadian victims were born in 1963, well after the drug's dangers were known, but the mothers were not alerted by their doctors about what they'd been given. One doctor simply changed the mother's prescription. Another doctor left town. When asked if the thalidomide in the news was the same medicine he'd prescribed for her, a woman's doctor flatly denied it.

In the most unsettling account, a doctor denied prescribing thalidomide to the mother of a deformed child. But months later, his dogs bore limb-deficient puppies—as if he had been testing to see if the drug was a teratogen.

While the public fixated on the missteps of drug companies and regulatory agencies, the quiet, unchecked deceit by doctors went unremarked. The medical community stonewalled victims. Even in Canada, where the drug had been government approved, when families filed lawsuits against drug firms, the doctors refused, under oath, to admit giving thalidomide to the mothers.

In America, most doctors never told women after the fact that they'd been given thalidomide. And American mothers, reading news of America's great escape from the German drug, did not know to ask if they had been "experimental subjects." This left most American survivors without a

The sheer number of newly self-identifying victims (there are scores as of the publication of this book) would seem to prove the essential point needed to sidestep the statute of limitations—how difficult it was for these families to learn the truth. One of the plaintiffs in the Hagens Berman case, Philip Yeatts, is the phocomelic boy born in 1962 whose aunt begged the FDA for information about Texas doctors who may have given out Kevadon. FDA records show a swift dismissal of her query once the agency determined that the doctor who had tended the boy's mother was not an "official" investigator. In sixty years, the FDA has never once advised the public that thalidomide was frequently passed along to other doctors by trial investigators. Or that masses of the drug—likely millions of pills— remained unaccounted for after its investigation. Yet every plaintiff's case rests on this fact.

The FDA investigated what it could of the drug's official distribution. But it was the drug's shadow distribution—the vast, undocumented, casual circulation of pills—that injured the most American babies. Doctors, un- willing to admit their role, seemingly made sure that families remained in the dark.

Extensions of the statute of limitations have, at times, been granted. In cases where children were the victims of sex crimes, state legislators have been lobbied to "do the right thing." American thalidomide survivors hope not just to amend the law for their own cases but to bring about acknowl- edgment that other injuries to children may require a prolonged clock. After all, what legal challenges might arise down the road from in vitro genetic modifications? Or new medicines used during pregnancy? If an injury so visible, from a drug so notorious, could be swept under the rug for more than a half century, what else could be hidden from view—long past the legal statute? And does the law's expectation for "reasonable care" account for disparities in class, education, and access to lawyers?

On top of the litigation quagmire, survivors are irate that the FDA still insists they don't exist. The agency's reported nine victims included two stillborn babies and one child who died shortly after birth—which means only six American survivors were supposed to exist. In sixty years, the agency has never amended its victim count. As recently as 2010, during an FDA ceremony at which government luminaries celebrated Frances's re- fusal to approve thalidomide, no mention was made of any Americans

harmed by the drug, or even of the drug's vast trials. The FDA acknowl-
edges that "how many were actually affected may never be known" but
suggests that any undercount would be attributable to stillbirths or effects
other than phocomelia. For the survivors, this erasure from history seems
a cruel irony for people prevented, in many ways, from fading into the
background.

And it highlights the dilemma facing American victims: Both the FDA
and the Department of Justice effectively claimed, decades ago, that their
injuries were *not* from thalidomide. Sixty years later, the law now penal-
izes these same victims for not being savvy enough to know the U.S. government was wrong. To this day, the FDA refuses—despite multiple
appeals to the Freedom of Information Act—to make public the names of
the SKF thalidomide investigators. To my request, the FDA replied—after
almost three years—that "release of the requested information could lead
to identification of the patients or their offspring" and "lead to the patients
and their offspring receiving unwanted contact." This despite the wildly
improbable logic—that anyone could track down a doctor's patients, sixty
years later, by merely having a doctor's *name*. Worse, the agency routinely
withheld information about the SKF trials from inquiring families: An attorney retained by the family of a "malformed child" born in 1959 was
simply told the birth occurred some "four or five months prior to the first
shipment of the drug to any area doctors." Likewise, the agency closely
guarded the Merrell investigator list for decades. Doctors—who by the
hundreds had blatantly violated the investigational-use provision of the
law—were shielded by the FDA for over a half century while American
women and children exposed to the drug were left to untangle the story on
their own. Further, the FDA never alerted the public to the drug's other
side effect—peripheral neuritis.

To this day, the United States remains the world's sole developed nation to refuse support to a single thalidomide victim. Canada, Britain,
Spain, Ireland, Germany, Sweden, Denmark, Australia, New Zealand,
Japan, Italy . . . Every other country where the drug was distributed has
subsidized survivors' care costs. The U.S. government absolved Merrell of
any criminal accountability and essentially dodges any responsibility of its
own on a technicality: The millions of offending tablets were given out for
free, not sold.

Advocates around the world decry the U.S. government's apathy toward its victims. British activist Guy Tweedy—an outspoken thalidomide survivor who zips around England in a "Grünenthal are Nazis" van—has promised to assist them in pressing for government compensation. Researcher Trent Stephens, who penned a book in 2000 about thalidomide's revival as a treatment for cancer and leprosy, has volunteered to medically assess the injuries of any possible survivor. And Scotland-based developmental biologist Neil Vargesson—a highly respected thalidomide researcher—now discusses their plight when he lectures.

Vargesson played an important role in untangling how thalidomide damages embryos. Since the 1960s, dozens of theories had competed to explain the mechanism by which thalidomide shortened limbs. Some thought the drug hurt DNA; some thought it attacked the nervous system. Some thought it affected blood vessels, while others posited that the bones themselves were directly impacted. By the late 1990s, nerve damage was the front-running theory. But Vargesson, who had grown up knowing someone injured by the drug, wanted a definitive answer.

Working with a pharmacologist at the NIH, Dr. W. Douglas Figg, Vargesson essentially tested different types of thalidomide: one targeting blood vessels, one targeting the inflammatory systems and another that targeted them all. In no time, chicken-embryo experiments showed that thalidomide impairs developing limbs by blocking the formation of blood vessels, depriving the growing tissue of oxygenated blood. Tissue died or limbs stopped growing. (This is why thalidomide was found effective at stopping tumor growth.)

Further lab experiments also showed that limb damage can vary widely. This contradicted an assumption made in the 1960s: that thalidomide babies displayed a very specific phocomelia. Even Widukind Lenz had been called to testify against various North American victims, acknowledging that their phocomelia did not appear textbook. Recent research has indicated that animal litters exposed to the drug in utero can show an array of injuries, and when thalidomide-exposed mothers bear twins, the damage is not identical. This new evidence has broadened the scope of identified victims. Many Australians in the recent class-action suit had not, at birth, been deemed thalidomide victims. Americans Jane and Carolyn—whose limb damage is asymmetrical—might have been overlooked in the 1960s.

But recent science indicates their symptoms fall well within the range of injuries.

At the San Diego gathering, the vast range of thalidomide's effects are visible. Jean and Gwen use wheelchairs; Sabine can run marathons but lacks arms. JoJo, Carolyn, and Jane are noticeably afflicted only in their arms and hands. And a Californian named Bart, though he suffers internal organ damage only, believes it stems from thalidomide exposure.

What unifies them is their mission: to make public the long-lost details of the distribution of thalidomide in America. They want the public to know there are many American thalidomide victims. At the 2019 conference, the group agrees to build a website, to make maps showing the locations of trial doctors, to make a documentary film . . . anything to get the word out.

For too long the narrative has focused on Frances Kelsey—the heroine who "blocked" a drug already, it turns out, in wide use. Frances still looms as a patron saint for thalidomide survivors worldwide—she alone suspected the drug's risks, and she undeniably spared thousands of American babies from harm. For this, the American survivors are grateful. They celebrate her brilliance, her courage. But there is a whiff of envy that she became the American face of the story, while they remained invisible. Her name hovers over every public account of thalidomide. And to the survivors, she seems a larger-than-life, unreachable figure.

This accounts for the gasps and double-takes in the conference room when, on day two of the San Diego gathering, two surprise guests enter: Frances's daughters, Susan and Christine, now in their early seventies, have come to say hi.

At age one hundred, Frances returned to Canada to live with Christine and her husband, John, in London, Ontario. Frances had fallen at home. And even though she had methodically written out instructions for the mailman to call for assistance, which she slipped beneath the front door, her daughters thought it time their mom had family supervision.

This was in 2005. Until then, Frances had lived in the same Chevy Chase house where letters of thanks from across the country had once arrived.

Until 2005, when she was ninety, Frances continued to work at the FDA.

After the 1962 Kefauver-Harris bill, Frances was tapped to direct the agency's Investigational Drug Branch. Four years later, she helmed the new Office of Scientific Investigations, a position she held until 1995 when she began work at the FDA's Center for Drug Evaluation and Research. The hallmark of her time there was creating institutional review boards to approve the how, who, and where of clinical trials *before* they started. The FDA would eventually create an award for Drug Safety Excellence in her honor. The horrors of thalidomide never left her, and she is rightly credited with revamping the process of drug testing to ensure patient consent and protection.

She was also honored long after her White House medal. In late 1962, the widow of Harvey Wiley—the crusading chemist who first led the FDA—presented Frances with a citation from the D.C. Federation of Women's clubs. By December, Frances ranked number eight on Gallup's "Year's Most Admired Women" list—just below Madame Chiang Kai-shek. In the 1963 *Who's Who of American Women*, Frances was cited alongside Katherine Anne Porter and Rachel Carson. She was featured prominently in civil service recruitment films. Both a Canadian high school and an asteroid were named in her honor.

As her star rose, however, she met resistance. Dr. James Lee Goddard, who succeeded George Larrick as FDA commissioner in 1966, loathed Frances. "Frances became a Presidential Gold Medal award winner and a heroine because she procrastinated," Goddard said in his agency oral history. "Frances couldn't make her mind up and just sat on the material. . . . My appraisal of her is that if it were raining, she'd drown before she could make her mind up that she ought to go indoors. . . . President Kennedy wanted to pin a medal on somebody and that somebody happened to be Frances Kelsey. So that was basically how Frances came to become a sacred cow in FDA."

Goddard didn't even meet Frances until 1966. But his retrospective rant serves as a reminder that "America's sweetheart" was still a female scientist in a very male agency. Goddard likewise smeared Moulton: He spoke of "trouble developing if Barbara came back" and blocked her return to the FDA. "Frances Kelsey was frankly enough trouble on the staff without bringing Barbara back," he ranted.

Those close to Frances acknowledge a "backlash" to her fame. Frances's parking spot was moved farther away from the agency building as a "message." People trying to call Frances at the FDA were told she no longer worked there. Frances got the "bare-desk" treatment—she was ignored by colleagues and given little to do. Her morale plummeted.

Frances also suffered the loss of her closest allies. In August of 1963, Kefauver had a heart attack on the Senate floor while submitting an amendment to an appropriations bill. Two days later, he died. Three months later, President Kennedy was assassinated in Texas. And in 1966, Frances suffered the greatest blow of her life: Her husband, Ellis, died suddenly of a heart attack. She found herself unable to function or even speak of the loss for weeks. Soon after, Professor Geiling began to suffer from Alzheimer's. Frances cared for him as his legal guardian until his death in 1971.

Solitude turned Frances into an even greater workaholic. After her daughters left for university, she lived alone in Chevy Chase, making the daily commute to the FDA, unwinding in the evening with crossword puzzles, biographies, and her ritual old-fashioned. Barbara Moulton remained a confidante until Alzheimer's rendered conversation with her impossible. Moulton died in 1996 at age eighty, her role in the overhaul of U.S. drug laws entirely forgotten.

The thalidomide story, too, faded from American headlines, until, in 1975, the FDA approved thalidomide as a treatment for leprosy. Israeli physician Jacob Sheskin, undeterred by the worldwide thalidomide recall, still had some on his shelves at Hadassah University Hospital, and when a male leprosy patient came in, suffering from incurable insomnia, Sheskin gave him thalidomide. The drug not only cured the patient's insomnia but also alleviated his leprosy. This was 1964. By 1975, the U.S. Public Health Service had begun importing the drug from Germany for use in leprosy patients.

By the 1980s, thalidomide was piquing the interest of researchers in other medical subspecialties. If the drug stopped leprous growths, what else could it stop? The FDA formed the Thalidomide Working Group, and by 1998, the drug was approved for a host of ailments, including AIDS and multiple myeloma.

News on the subject always noted the drug's tragic history, and Frances followed each development closely, clipping articles. She also tracked news of the afflicted children and their fight for justice. One major story she followed near the end of her life concerned the "Right the Wrong" campaign launched in Canada in 2014 by an alliance of lawyers, lobbyists, journalists, and thalidomide victims. A series of heart-wrenching portraits of thalidomide survivors in *The Globe and Mail* helped spur Parliament to grant the country's survivors additional funds. The Canadian government's delay in recalling the drug—months after the German recall—showed negligence. And Frances's suspicions of the Kevadon paperwork made Canada's Food and Drug Directorate approval of the drug look remiss. On December 1, 2014, the House of Commons voted unanimously to recognize the urgent needs of thalidomide victims and the government's duty to support them.

The following year, the lieutenant governor of Ontario, Elizabeth Dowdeswell, heard that Frances was nearing death. She traveled to London, Ontario, where Frances was living with her daughter, to bestow on Frances the Order of Canada award. On a Thursday in August, Dowdeswell arrived at Christine Kelsey's house in the afternoon. The small ground-floor bedroom in which Frances, 101, lay sleeping overflowed with crossword puzzles and books. Frances wore light-blue pajamas on a bed of red sheets; her gray hair was at chin length, as it had been throughout her life. A cat nestled nearby. Across from her hung two pictures of her childhood home, Balgonie—one of the house her father had built, the other the view from its front porch, showing the woods she had wandered so happily and curiously as a child.

Christine stood beside her frail mother as Dowdeswell explained Frances's act of heroism for the thalidomide community. The slumbering Frances grew alert and animated as Dowdeswell placed the medal in her hand. She tried to speak but could not. Still, she smiled, and a longtime family friend played "Goodnight, Irene" and "O Canada" on the piano as Frances, speechless, conducted. That night, Frances died peacefully in her sleep.

Susan, a retired high school science teacher, lives on a sprawling rural property in Shelton, Washington, with her husband, Tom. Christine, a retired physiotherapist, still lives in Ontario with her husband, John. The sisters are fiercely close and honor their mother's legacy with great seriousness. As teenagers, the thalidomide story meant little to them beyond their mom being on TV or the radio, or her giving a speech at their high school. But after Ellis's death, the girls grew closer to their mother. And as adults, they came to grasp her role in the saga.

Before she died, Frances donated her papers to the Library of Congress so they could be available to the public. The sisters have since assisted any and all researchers—including high school students—wanting to understand Frances and her work. Both Susan and Christine hosted me in their homes for long visits, sharing private letters, photographs, home movies, childhood journals, and amusing recollections—far beyond what was available in the Library of Congress.

I grew fond of these women, who embody their mother's intelligence, humility, and moral scrupulousness—the qualities that first drew me to the story. At some point, while we were all sipping Manhattans in honor of their mom, I told them what I had discovered—that there were actually dozens, maybe scores, of American thalidomiders never counted by the FDA. Somehow Frances's higher-ups at the agency had botched the investigation, and the trial doctors had all lied. It was a somber piece of news to drop on two women who for most of their lives believed the official FDA version—that the United States had mostly been spared from thalidomide.

When I told them that I was attending the survivor gathering in San Diego, both sisters wanted to come.

When they are formally introduced at the group session, they shrug off the gasps and get right down to chatting with everyone, trying to get to know the group. They grew up in contact with thalidomide survivors, mostly Canadians, who regularly befriended Frances. For Susan and Christine, this meeting with American thalidomiders is particularly emotional. They sense that their mother would want them here.

Sabine, though German born, always discusses Frances in her motivational speeches and is especially thrilled by this encounter. Photos are taken. Hugs exchanged. And Susan and Christine do seem to conjure their mother's fun, low-key spirit. They wear their hair gray and straight. There is no trace of makeup on their faces. They both stand tall in clogs, wrapped in a combination of flannel and fleece, exuding curiosity and warmth. They are quick to laugh. They, too, enjoy a strong cocktail.

After the presentations on Saturday, both women join the group at a nearby Mexican restaurant that serves absurdly large margaritas. Along the massive, warmly lit table, the weight of the day's emotional confessions has lifted. Talk of the stalled lawsuit is set aside, and everyone revels in their new community. An Australian survivor named Jeff cracks jokes about where he does and doesn't need the extra inches. JoJo starts rallying the crew for a late-night karaoke session, determined to belt out "My Way." Jean sits beside Gwen, her Cincinnati "sister." Carolyn, who brought the whole group together, sits with her daughter Angie, marveling at how far things have come since her tentative Facebook post eight years earlier in "Stop the Tears," the international thalidomide survivors group.

Gathered side by side, nothing about their bodies seems out of place. And yet they now know their bodies are the ground on which the country built its legal safeguards. They hope the country will help them in return.

FDA does not have a more recent number than what has been publicly reported for many decades, which has not changed: about 10 children suffered phocomelia from the domestic distribution of investigational thalidomide, and an additional 7 children had the same result due to thalidomide obtained from other countries.

—*FDA press officer, 2020*

Dear Ms. Vanderbes:

This responds to your Freedom of Information Act request dated July 9, 2019, and received in this Office on July 9, 2019, for Criminal Division records concerning a U.S. Department of Justice investigation of William S. Merrell Company pertaining to Kevadon.

Please be advised that Criminal Division personnel searched the sections most likely to maintain records and no responsive records subject to the FOIA were located. . . .

—*letter from FOIA/PA Unit, Criminal Division, Department of Justice, May 14, 2021*

Epilogue

In 2004, Darren Griggs, a licensed practical nurse, was working on the skilled nursing floor at Boone Hospital in Columbia, Missouri, when his supervisor alerted him that he was needed to administer a special medicine to a cancer patient. The other nurses—all young women—were forbidden from touching the drug. Darren, who had been a nurse for over a decade, did as instructed and brought the capsules to the patient. He thought nothing more of it. Only later did he realize—with horror—that the drug was essentially thalidomide, the very drug his mother had taken in late 1961, the drug that had maimed him in utero. In fact, having lived in Missouri his entire life, Darren had dispensed thalidomide in the same hospital in which he'd been born.

The reason Darren did not immediately know the drug was a thalidomide derivative is that the current version is sold under two names: "Thalomid," which hints at the drug's origins but is not marked by name on the capsules, and "Revlimid," which bears no trace of the drug's early name. Both are made by Celgene Corporation, a New Jersey pharmaceutical company, which was granted exclusive permission by the FDA in 1998 to finally put the notorious "orphan drug" on the American market—at that time, to treat leprosy.

Getting the potentially toxic product approved by the FDA was no easy task. Celgene had to work in tandem with the federal agency to create a system that would ensure the drug never fell into the hands of pregnant women. For this, Celgene also grasped the importance of speaking to actual thalidomide survivors. Likely unaware of the large number of Americans harmed by the drug, Celgene executives reached out to a Canadian

group. The Thalidomide Victims Association of Canada, terrified of a re-
surgence of harmed babies, knew that controlled sale of the drug was safer
than underground distribution. The two groups met in person, trust grew,
and eventually Celgene enlisted Canadian "thalidomiders" to sit on an
oversight committee and provide video and written testimonials for patients contemplating taking the drug.

Celgene's resulting System for Thalidomide Education and Prescribing Safety (STEPS) had multiple components: Physicians prescribing thalidomide and their patients had to register in a national database. Female
patients had to show two negative pregnancy tests—the first, ten to fourteen days before treatment, and another within twenty-four hours of taking
the drug; pregnancy tests had to be retaken monthly. Women would also
have to prove they were using two forms of contraception. Men using thalidomide must use a condom during intercourse. (As far back as 1967, research suggested that thalidomide in sperm might negatively affect
reproduction.) The product would eventually bear a "Category X" FDA
label, reserved for drugs known to cause fetal deformities and whose risks
or undesired effects outweigh possible medical benefits.

At first, it wasn't clear that thalidomide stood to generate meaning-
ful profits for Celgene. Its use was highly restricted and the drug was
approved only to treat erythema nodosum leprosum (a debilitating condition associated with leprosy)—which afflicted only seven thousand
Americans (though the international market was larger). Further, since
the drug was decades old, Celgene didn't own any patents on the medication itself. But Celgene spun the drug's dangers to its advantage; the firm
patented its *safety protocol* for thalidomide. The FDA requires a Risk Evaluation and Mitigation System (REMS) for all potentially dangerous drugs,
and Celgene scored fourteen patents for its thalidomide safety protocol.
This effectively gave Celgene the exclusive right to sell thalidomide for
twenty years.

That gave the firm ample time to find its audience. And the leprosy
patients, it turned out, were only a gateway to a larger target.

As early as 1962, the Merrell Company had probed the drug's ability to
slow tumor growth. It seems that when the firm realized that thalidomide,
like aminopterin, caused fetal damage, researchers wondered if the com-

pound might similarly thwart tumor growth. But in 1965, doctors at the National Cancer Institute and NIH testing thalidomide on seventy-one cancer patients found the drug ineffective. Radiation and other remedies looked more promising. Leprosy, then, remained the drug's sole viable target. But in 1989, a Rockefeller University research team dusted off the drug once again, reporting that new experiments suggested thalidomide could suppress tumor necrosis and help regulate immune response. Excited scientists began testing the drug for a host of conditions from AIDS to lupus—with apparent success. In particular, thalidomide seemed to help reverse mouth ulcers and severe weight loss associated with AIDS.

When word got out that thalidomide was, after all these years, an *actual* "wonder drug," buyers' clubs of the day—groups that smuggled promising but FDA-*un*approved therapies back to the United States—scrambled to secure the product. This wasn't hard, since the drug had been distributed abroad, for free, as a "compassionate care" treatment for leprosy patients since the 1970s. "It works like magic," declared Dr. Robert C. Hastings, head of the National Hansen's Disease Center's laboratory research branch in Carville, Louisiana—a stone's throw from the Carville prison where Merrell's Raymond Pogge had crafted his own leprosy cure a half century earlier.

This underground distribution rattled the FDA, and the agency pressed Celgene and other firms to investigate safe uses for the drug so it could be approved and tracked. Celgene ran a formal study on seventeen leprosy patients in the Philippines, then applied for FDA approval.

This time around, the thalidomide NDA advanced swiftly. By July of 1998, the FDA determined that Celgene had "met its scientific obligation in showing that the benefits outweigh the risks" in treating leprosy and granted approval.

But Celgene, from the start, was clear that it intended to broaden the drug's approved uses. "Our hope," said Bruce Williams, Celgene's vice president for marketing, "is that E.N.L. [erythema nodosum leprosum, that debilitating condition associated with leprosy] will not be the only indication for long." In fact, the company had proposed a trade name—"Synavir"—rejected by the FDA for its dangerous similarity to AIDS antiviral treatments.

The firm, however, did not wait for official clearance for additional uses. The FDA immediately got wind that Celgene detail men—now known as "sales reps"—had been telling oncologists that the highly restricted drug could treat bone marrow and other cancers. At an investors' meeting, Celgene purportedly assured shareholders that "off-label" uses would be encouraged—thus increasing sales. Celgene's promotional materials also seemed to downplay the drug's risks. The FDA sent a warning. Then another.

Celgene's claims that thalidomide could help with other ailments was not far-fetched. The firm had been actively researching the drug's use against myeloma and other cancers—but the FDA had not yet approved the firm's clinical data. The agency, it seemed, was taking its cautious time with the world's most infamous teratogen.

But in 2003, Celgene's Thalomid suffered a massive blow. The World Health Organization seemingly revoked its support for thalidomide as a leprosy treatment. In fact, the organization found, the original research on the drug's efficacy for the condition seemed murky. Prednisone and clofazimine, they claimed, showed much better clinical results. And thalidomide was proving too risky—a new generation of "thalidomide babies" had grown up in Brazil, a country with a large leprosy population. Further, more than 90 percent of Thalomid sales were now for off-label use to treat multiple myeloma and other blood cancers and tumors. Leprosy, in retrospect, seemed like a bogus entry point to revive the product on the world market.

But demand for thalidomide for other ailments was so high, and the prospect of an underground market so perilous, that in 2006 the FDA at last gave Celgene the nod to sell thalidomide for multiple myeloma. It also approved Revlimid (lenalidomide)—a slightly tweaked version of Thalomid; Celgene had removed an oxygen atom from thalidomide and added a nitrogen atom, and this change endowed the new drug with additional years of patent protection.

Even though multiple myeloma is a fairly uncommon cancer—about thirty thousand new cases are diagnosed per year in the United States—Celgene began raking in wild profits. In the late 1950s and early '60s, thalidomide was sold as a cheap drug for daily use. But in 2006, multiple myeloma patients paid $6,195 for twenty-one capsules of Revlimid, a month's supply. By November 2010, the price was about $8,000 a month. By 2018, the monthly cost had hit almost $17,000. The drug was earning Celgene more than $9 billion in annual revenue. But the price hikes had been so dramatic—everyone knew the R&D costs on a sixty-year-old drug were minimal—that they drew the attention of the House Committee on Oversight and Reform. Kefauver's concerns from sixty years earlier had found a new champion—Congressman Elijah E. Cummings. He alerted his House colleagues:

> We have seen time after time that drug companies make money hand over fist by raising the prices of their drugs—often without justification, and sometimes overnight—while patients are left holding the bill.

With competition, Celgene's prices would have dropped naturally at some point. The firm holds no patent on thalidomide; and while the drug firm does hold four patents for Revlimid itself (which began to expire in 2019), the bulk of its other Revlimid patents pertain to its distribution system. Here the drug's dangers wrapped Celgene in a cocoon of market exclusivity. Any other company wishing to sell thalidomide or a thalidomide derivative had to also make sure it was kept away from pregnant women. Celgene's STEPS program—with its fourteen patents—made it nearly impossible for any other company to propose a non-infringing risk evaluation and management system.

Pharmaceutical company Mylan finally sued, claiming Celgene's fourteen patents never should have been granted. After all: How innovative is the idea that a female patient should take a pregnancy test before using a teratogenic drug? How much research and development did that require?

Further, Celgene allegedly prevented competitors from even getting their hands on enough of the drug to conduct studies. To bring a generic version to market, a drug firm has to show the FDA that its product is identical to the brand-name version—same chemical compound, absorbed by the body in the same way. This would require upward of two thousand doses of the Celgene version. According to the lawsuit filed by Mylan,

Celgene, behind the shield of its safety protocol, had refused to sell samples of thalidomide to Mylan. In response, Celgene told a New Jersey federal court that it wished to ensure "that the product was going to be used safely, that patients' health was going to be maintained, and safe conditions [were maintained] not only for the people involved in the test but the personnel who were administering the test." But patent disputes were eventually settled, and in early 2022, generic Revlimid (lenalidomide) hit the market. But the agreements with Celgene, now owned by Bristol Myers Squibb, stipulated only a limited volume of lenalidomide in the market, and some myeloma patients quickly complained that the sticker price and copays for their "badly needed medication" were barely affected by the limited supply of these generics.

The American survivors are adamant that thalidomide and any teratogenic derivatives must remain strictly controlled. But Jean Grover feels that if something good can come of the drug—if lives can be saved—then good should come of it. From her home in Fairport, New York, surrounded by her children, the sixty-year-old woman who was never expected to live more than a few months says, "I hope that the fact that I tested this with my body and my life can benefit someone positively in the future."

In fact, her husband, Keith, who recently died, had suffered from both a meningioma—a primary central nervous system tumor—and Lewy body dementia. Jean served as his primary caretaker for seven years. "If thalidomide could have cured his brain tumor or alleviated his symptoms," says Jean, "I would have given it to him myself."

Timeline

September 1960
Merrell submits FDA application to sell thalidomide in U.S., assigned to medical reviewer Frances Kelsey.

May 1961
Frances Kelsey asks Merrell for proof that thalidomide is safe during pregnancy.

May 1961
Australian ob-gyn William McBride begins investigation into possible thalidomide-phocomelia link.

November 1961
Geneticist Widukind Lenz declares thalidomide the likely cause of the phocomelia outbreak in Germany; thalidomide is recalled in Germany and the UK.

1954
Chemie Grünenthal files the first thalidomide patent in Germany, begins human testing soon after.

1938
Food, Drug, and Cosmetics Act in the U.S.

November 1956
Smith, Kline & French (SKF) begins human testing of thalidomide in the U.S.

December 1956
First thalidomide-affected baby is born in Germany to Chemie Grünenthal employee.

March 1962
Merrell withdraws its FDA application to sell thalidomide in U.S.

July 1962
Morton Mintz publishes a *Washington Post* story on Frances Kelsey, the first major U.S. news story on thalidomide.

August 1962
FDA begins investigating Merrell's thalidomide clinical trials in the U.S.

October 1962
Kefauver-Harris Amendment (Drug Efficacy Amendment) is signed by President John F. Kennedy.

February 1959
Cincinnati-based William S. Merrell Company begins human testing of thalidomide in the U.S.

September 1964
U.S. Department of Justice declines the FDA's recommendation to prosecute Merrell, cites only one victim of American thalidomide.

1968–1970
Trial against Chemie Grünenthal
in Alsdorf, West Germany.

1971
McCarrick v. Richardson-Merrell in the U.S., jury
awards victim $2.5
million in damages.

2011
Law firm Hagens
Berman files a civil
suit on behalf of
alleged unrecognized
American
thalidomide survivors,
eventually naming
over fifty plaintiffs.

1972–1976
Harold Evans at
The Sunday Times
in England runs a
four-part series on
thalidomide.

1987
Cincinnati native
Eileen Cronin publishes
an essay in *The
Washington Post*
declaring herself an
American thalidomide
survivor.

2019
United States
Thalidomide
Survivors non-profit
launches, hosts a
convention in San
Diego for U.S.
survivors.

Acknowledgments

This book would not exist without early support from the Sloan Foundation and the National Endowment for the Humanities. I am endlessly grateful for being granted the time and funds to pursue the research needed to tell this story properly.

I am fortunate to have Hilary Redmon as an editor and friend. She was the first person to cheer me on when I casually mentioned I was considering writing a non-fiction book about this long-lost saga and she remained unwavering in her support—even as the project *entirely* changed from the book she agreed to publish and it took twice as long as expected. Her keen eye for structure helped find the narrative in the early unwieldy pages. Her feedback sharpened the prose and quickened the pacing. She is truly the editor all writers dream of. Also at Random House, a million thanks to: Windy Dorresteyn, Benjamin Dreyer, Lucas Heinrich, Miriam Khanukaev, Matthew Martin (a saint!), Steve Messina, Fritz Metsch, Tom Perry, Monica Stanton, Stacey Stein, and Andy Ward. It was an extraordinary blessing that this book found its way to Random House under publisher Susan Kamil—the editor of my first novel so many years ago. I wish she were here to see the final product, as it bears the stamp of much of what she taught me about storytelling.

At WME, I'm eternally grateful to my team: the ever-fierce Dorian Karchmar, Anna DeRoy, Fiona Baird, James Munro, Lauren Szurgot, Niki Montazaran, and Susan Weaving. At Harper Collins UK, thanks to Imogen Gordon Clark.

Several early readers offered invaluable feedback: Olivia Gentile, Eric Katz, Aryn Kyle, Leila Hatch (who has been roped into reading my drafts since we were college roommates!), Tom Perriello, Janet Bloom, and Sarah Funke Butler.

This project began as a book about Frances Kelsey, and I was blessed, from start to finish, with the extraordinary kindness and historical acumen of Frances's daughters: Susan Duffield and Christine Kelsey. At opposite sides of the North American continent, they took turns housing me, feeding me, sharing childhood journals, home movies, and family letters. It is an act of supreme trust to let a stranger sift through your life, and I hope I have done right by you both. Thank you also to Tom (here's how you make a Manhattan, Jennifer!) Duffield and John Broeze—great husbands in the tradition of Ellis Kelsey.

Morton Mintz was ninety-five when I met him in his Washington, D.C., home and questioned him about events from half a century ago. His lifelong passion for reporting and zeal for the truth afforded him the grace to endure my repeated visits. Thank you to Margaret Mintz, his daughter, for letting me prowl in the basement storage locker—what I now call the "Mintz Archive."

I was lucky to locate Brucie Moulton, Barbara Moulton, and Warren Senders, who all generously shared the anecdotes, photographs, and letters that helped bring to life the long-neglected story of their aunt and friend, Barbara Moulton Wayles.

History is fortunate that Chris Kahn, nephew of Elinor Kamath, preserved her thalidomide research papers. Kamath's name has never before been mentioned in association with this story, even though she was the first American to urge the international press to cover this news. Further, she single-handedly orchestrated the dispatch sent from the American Embassy in Bonn to the U.S. State Department detailing Widikund Lenz's research about thalidomide's dangers. When Kamath moved back to the United States, she spent decades collecting statements from the key players in the international story and I am indebted to her investigative work.

Helen Taussig's 1961 meeting with Frances Kelsey and John Nestor has long been noted in the basic timeline of this saga. But Taussig's yearslong independent study of thalidomide's impact overseas and her advocacy for victims had been egregiously overlooked. Taussig's archives were an unexpected gift.

I am deeply indebted to Linde Schulte-Hillen, one of the few mothers who agreed to speak on the record, and to her son, Jan Schulte-Hillen, for sharing his medical, legal, and personal knowledge of the thalidomide story. Donald Firestone, who passed away before this book could be published, kindly shared his experiences as a father of an injured child. Mary Ferguson Polhemus, Ann Morris, and Delia Galvez Calora kindly entrusted me with their experiences being given the drug while pregnant, and Sarah Grover graciously opened up about her life as the daughter of a survivor.

In the process of my research, I spoke to scores of people who identify as thalidomide survivors. Many shared deeply personal information and I am forever grateful for their trust. Their collective determination to trumpet this long-buried story remains a constant inspiration. For their patience, kindness, and willingness to participate in this book, a heartfelt shout-out to: Kimberly Arndt, Eric Barrett, Sabine Becker, Jojo Calora, Eileen Cronin, Gus Economides, Jan Garrett, Jane Gibbons, Jeff Green, Darren Griggs, C. Jean Grover, Dorothy Hunt-Honsinger, Glenda Johnson, Bart Joseph, Peggy Martz Smith, Lori Kay Ruberg, Gwen Riechmann, Carolyn Sampson, Tawana Williams, and Philip Yeatts. I wish I could have featured all of the amazing survivors I interviewed, as each one has a story worthy of a book. (Eileen Cronin and Tawana Williams have already published memoirs.) Please visit www.usthalidomide.org—the website of the United States Thalidomide Survivors non-profit—to learn more about the American survivors and to offer support.

Archival visits were essential to this project, and the wonderful staffs at the Library of Congress, National Archives, Harvard Countway Library, and the Chesney Archives at Johns Hopkins were of invaluable assistance.

For pesky questions along the way, FDA historian John Swann was a vital resource. Guy Tweedy and Angie Mason in the UK generously shared information about their research into the drug's origins. Benjamin Zipursky gave me a delightful Zoom lesson in product liability law and Michael Dan shared memories from his time as second chair in the Peggy McCarrick trial. Lawyer Stephen Raynes, who was crucial to advocating for support for Canadian thalidomide victims, offered useful context from start to finish.

On the science front: Developmental biologist and thalidomide researcher Neil Vargesson generously gave of his time to review this material and Professor Alessandra Leri kindly assisted with all chemistry questions.

I am not the first writer to tackle thalidomide, and I owe a debt of gratitude to my predecessors. *Suffer the Children* by *Sunday Times* Insight Team and *Thalidomide and the Power of the Drug Companies* by Henning Sjostrom and Robert Nilsson, both published in the 1970s, were the first books I encountered on this subject, and they laid key groundwork for all subsequent researchers. Michael Magazanik, a plaintiff's lawyer in the successful 2012 Australian lawsuit, later penned *Silent Shock*, which cited many Grünenthal documents not known about in the 1970s. *The Thalidomide Catastrophe* by Martin Johnson, Raymond Stokes, and Tobias Arndt impeccably details the early days of Grünenthal and lays out the various theories for the "creation" of thalidomide. Martin Johnson graciously read portions of my manuscript. A shout-out to Katie Thomas at *The New York Times*, who, after being contacted by the survivors several years ago, delved into this history.

For helping to ensure that the facts, source citations, and permissions for this book were in order, many thanks to Dale Brauner, Holly Van Leuven, Reid Singer, and Lydia Weintraub.

Much of this book was written during the pandemic while caring for my children and my parents. Friends were essential to keeping me on track during that time, especially Abby Santamaria, Justin Cronin, Gina Gionfriddo, Rena Ningham, and Gabrielle Stanton. My dear "Bookies"— Alex Horowitz, Sally Koslow, Betsy Carter, Lauren Belfer, Elizabeth Kadetsky, Aryn Kyle, and Patricia Morrisroe—always reminded me of the importance of books. And the group I refer to as "Brooklyn Writers," helmed by Nell Freudenberger and Julie Orringer, offered time and space to talk through various project challenges—thank you for always allowing an interloper from across the river! My gratitude goes out to Ann Kao, Elizabeth Balfour, and Erik Dopman for providing rooms to crash in and for facilitating access to documents.

Last, but never least, my amazing daughters: Annika, you were born a year before this project began and have never known life without hundreds of overflowing file folders around the house! I missed a lot of time with you, but I hope when you are old enough to read this, you will understand why. Thank you for your daily "Go, Mom!" Ellery, you immediately grasped the importance of this story and have been an unwavering cheerleader at every step. I could not be prouder, or more grateful, for you both.

Dear Mom and Dad, the answer to the six-year question—"Are you done with that book?"—is, at last, yes.

Notes

Prologue

xiii **Ann Morris felt her first:** Author interview with Ann Morris (pseudonym).

xiv **"the safest thing":** Statement by Dr. John Chewning, Merrell Co. spokesman, quoted in "Thalidomide Study: Prevent Monsters," *Daily Iowan*, Aug. 9, 1962.

xiv **"single largest holocaust":** Allan C. Barnes, "Our Uncomfortable Glass House," *American Journal of Obstetrics and Gynecology* 84, no. 3 (Aug. 1962): 411.

xvi **largest criminal trial:** "Code K17," *Der Spiegel*, June 3, 1968.

xvi **As the only country:** East Germany would decline to approve the drug in 1961, after news of its link to peripheral neuritis was public.

PART ONE: THE ROOKIE
One

3 **"The human being who would not":** Morton Mintz, *At Any Cost: Corporate Greed, Women, and the Dalkon Shield* (New York: Pantheon, 1985), xv.

6 **"Lemmon Patients Are Treated":** *The Lemmon Leader*, Sept. 26, 1957.

6 **"hectic series of crises":** Letter from Frances to Geiling, Oct. 3, 1957, Eugene M. K. Geiling Collection, Alan Chesney Medical Archives (hereafter Geiling Archives).

7 **"This is a desolate area":** Letter from Ellis Kelsey to Geiling, Sept. 13, 1956, Geiling Archives.

7 **"left out in the cold":** Letter from Frances to Geiling, Dec. 27, 1956, Geiling Archives.

7 **"a man with a PhD":** Letter from Ralph G. Smith to F. Ellis Kelsey, Jan. 22, 1957, Frances Kelsey Papers, Library of Congress (hereafter Frances Kelsey Papers).

8 **barely dented:** The pharmaceutical industry was ranked at no. 16, according to Ralph C. Epstein, "Industrial Profits in the United States," *National Bureau of Economic Research*, 1984.

8 **$2.7 billion:** Hearings Before the Subcommittee on Antitrust and Monopoly of the Committee on the Judiciary, U.S. Senate, Sept. 28–30, 1959.

8 **regional offices and inspectors:** "Larrick, Career Employee, Heads FDA as Crawford Retires . . . Big Case Load and Limited Budget Are Major Problems," *Journal of Agricultural and Food Chemistry* 2, no. 16 (1954): 840.

8 **fewer than nine hundred employees:** Ibid.

8 **369 applications:** "Tabulation of New Drug Applications" table, "Summary of NDA Approvals & Receipts, 1938 to the Present," Food and Drug Administration, available at fda.gov/about-fda/histories-product-regulation/summary-nda-approvals-receipts-1938-present.

8 "**highly encouraging**": Martin Towler report included in "Kevadon: A New, Safe, Sleep-Inducing Agent" in New Drug Application 12-611, FDA Archives.

10 "**Frankie's conduct**": Report card, St. George's School for Girls, Victoria, B.C., Dec. 16, 1927, Frances Kelsey Papers.

10 "**Frankie has improved greatly**": Report card, St. Margaret's School, Victoria, B.C., June 28, 1929, Frances Kelsey Papers.

11 "**greatly enriched**": Frances Kelsey Oral History, FDA Oral History Interview, 5.

11 "**master gland**": Ibid., 9.

11 "**Don't be ridiculous**": Ibid., 12.

11 **Frances telegrammed**: Writings & Editorials, ca. 1940s, Frances Kelsey Papers.

12 "**It was a pretty slimy trip**": "Screwy News," *The New Yorker*, May 31, 1941.

13 "**The comparison of turning over**": Ruth DeForest Lamb, *American Chamber of Horrors: The Truth About Food and Drugs* (New York: Farrar & Rinehart, 1936), 9.

13 "**Crusading Chemist**": "The Good Fight," *Evansville Courier and Press*, July 3, 1930.

13 "**defeated by a durable alliance**": Morton Mintz, *The Therapeutic Nightmare: A Report on the Roles of the United States Food and Drug Administration, the American Medical Association, Pharmaceutical Manufacturers, and Others in Connection with the Irrational and Massive Use of Prescription Drugs That May Be Worthless, Injurious, or Even Lethal* (Boston: Houghton Mifflin, 1965), 41.

13 "**embalmed beef**": "Old Time Farm Crime: The Embalmed Beef Scandal of 1898," *Modern Farmer*, Nov. 8, 2013.

13 "**to investigate the character**": "National Control of Food Products," *Journal of Proceedings of the Annual Convention of the National Association of State Dairy and Food Departments* (Herman B. Meyers, 1903), 43.

14 "**Poison Squad**": Bruce Watson, "The Poison Squad: An Incredible History," *Esquire*, June 27, 2013.

14 "**false *and* fraudulent**": *Public Health Reports*, Jan. 21, 1916, 137.

15 "**Since B&M has been tested**": Lamb, *American Chamber of Horrors*, 45.

14 **pilfered letterhead**: Ibid., 46.

15 **The FDA's case**: Ibid., 53.

15 "**I have brought my authorities**": Ibid., 55.

15 **jury sided with the FDA**: Ibid., 58.

15 **knowing Geiling doubted**: "He really did not hold too much with women as scientists." Frances Kelsey Oral History, FDA Oral History Interview, 13.

15 **his first PhD student**: Author interview with Christine Kelsey.

17 "**Dr. Geiling immediately set up**": Frances Kelsey Oral History, 22.

17 "**not once could have foreseen**": Carol Ballentine, "Taste of Raspberries, Taste of Death: The 1937 Elixir Sulfanilamide Incident," *FDA Consumer*, June 1981.

18 "**Chamber of Horrors**": Lamb, *American Chamber of Horrors*, 296.

18 "**All that is left to us**": Letter reprinted in "Taste of Raspberries, Taste of Death: The 1937 Elixir Sulfanilamide Incident," *FDA Consumer*, June 1981.

18 **University of Chicago's first PhD**: "Notes and Comment," *Medical Alumni Bulletin, University of Chicago*, 1962, Frances Kelsey Papers.

Two

19 "**1. The voluntary consent**": Evelyne Shuster, "Fifty Years Later: The Significance of the Nuremberg Code," *New England Journal of Medicine*, Nov. 13, 1997.

22 **world's first synthetic drug**: Alan Wayne Jones, "Early Drug Discovery and the Rise of Pharmaceutical Chemistry," *Drug Testing and Analysis* 3, no. 6 (June 2011).

22 **world's first pharmaceutical firm**: "Merck, the Oldest Pharma Company Turns 350," *Deutsche Welle*, July 16, 2018.

22 **world's first blockbuster drug:** Jones, "Early Drug Discovery."

23 **first successful nonbarbiturate epilepsy treatment:** Emmanouil Magiorkinis et al., "Highlights in the History of Epilepsy: The Last 200 Years," *Epilepsy Research and Treatment*, 2014, 582039.

23 **some eight hundred drug injections:** Norman Ohler, *Blitzed* (Boston: Houghton Mifflin Harcourt, 2017), 108.

23 **In one instance, two Allied soldiers:** "Secrets by the Thousands," *Harper's Magazine*, Oct. 1946.

24 **total value of the plunder:** Douglas M. O'Reagan, *Taking Nazi Technology: Allied Exploitation of German Science After the Second World War* (Baltimore: Johns Hopkins University Press, 2021), 37.

24 **United States indicted:** F. López-Muñoz, P. García-García, and C. Alamo, "The Pharmaceutical Industry and the German National Socialist Regime: I. G. Farben and Pharmacological Research," *Journal of Clinical Pharmacology and Therapeutics* 31, no. 1 (Feb. 2009): 67–77.

24 **chief donor to Hitler's election campaign:** Jacques R. Pauwels, *Big Business and Hitler* (Toronto: Lorimer, 2017), 72.

24 **at least thirty thousand prisoners:** Jonathan B. Tucker, *War of Nerves: Chemical Warfare from World War I to Al-Qaeda* (New York: Anchor, 2007), 88.

24 **Zyklon B gas:** "German Firm Is Cited as Top Producer of Death Camp Gas," *Los Angeles Times*, Dec. 4, 1998.

25 **"new sleep-inducing drug":** Patricia Posner, *The Pharmacist of Auschwitz: The Untold Story* (Surrey, UK: Crux Publishing, 2017), 61.

25 **"Please prepare for us":** Correspondence between Auschwitz camp commander and Bayer headquarters quoted in ibid., 62.

25 **All 150 women died:** Ibid., 61.

25 **200 women with strep throat:** Ibid., 62.

25 **discovered she was sterile:** Ibid., 64.

25 **"I am only a chemist":** Ibid., 114.

25 **"These IG Farben criminals":** Telford Taylor quoted in Scott Christianson, *Fatal Airs: The Deadly History and Apocalyptic Future of Lethal Gases* (New York: Praeger Press, 2010), 70.

25 **"If the guilt of these criminals":** Ibid.

25 **"disregard of basic human rights":** *The United States of America Against Carl Krauch et al.*, Military Tribunal, No. VI, C.A. No. 6, Paul M. Hebert, Dissenting Opinion, *Nuremberg Trials Documents* (1948).

26 **ardent Nazi enthusiasts:** "The Nazis and Thalidomide: The Worst Drug Scandal of All Time," *Newsweek*, Sept. 10, 2012.

26 **several hundred slave laborers:** Martin Johnson, Raymond G. Stokes, and Tobias Arndt, *The Thalidomide Catastrophe: How It Happened, Who Was Responsible, and Why the Search for Justice Continues After More Than Six Decades* (London: Onwards and Upwards, 2018), 72.

27 **arranged for typhus:** "The Nazis and Thalidomide: The Worst Drug Scandal of All Time," *Newsweek*, Sept. 10, 2012.

27 **known to be arrogant:** Interview with Christian Wagemann, conducted by Monika Eisenberg and Martin Johnson, Achen, Germany, July 2009, shared with author.

27 **"completely cut off":** "Code K17," *Der Spiegel*, June 3, 1968.

28 **some would accuse:** "This story taxes credibility to the breaking point!" Johnson, Stokes, and Arndt, *Thalidomide Catastrophe*, 77–78.

28 **firm's investment grew sixfold:** Johnson, Stokes, and Arndt, *Thalidomide Catastrophe*, 79.

28 **a hundred times more often:** Ibid., 80.

28 "used in man": Wichmann, Koch, and Heiss, *Zeitschrift für Klinische Medizin* (1956), cited in Johnson, Stokes, and Arndt, *Thalidomide Catastrophe*, 80.

29 bonus of 1 percent: "He was also a shrewd businessman; shrewd enough to have a contract which gave him 1 per cent of Grünenthal's turnover as a bonus over and above his salary." United States Congress, Congressional Record: Proceedings and Debates. . . . (Washington, D.C.: U.S. Government Printing Office, 1969), 14553.

29 "sleep is distinguished": *Sunday Times* Insight Team, *Suffer the Children: The Story of Thalidomide* (London: Andre Deutsch, 1979), 28.

30 "The products of the invention": U.S. Patent # 2830991 and UK Patent # 768821, cited in Johnson, Stokes, and Arndt, *Thalidomide Catastrophe*, 85.

31 official human trials: Affidavit of Michael Magazanik as to the Plaintiff's Case Against the First Defendant, *Lynette Suzanne Rowe v. Grünenthal GmbH*, in the Supreme Court of Victoria at Melbourne, Common Law Division, Major Torts List, document prepared July 13, 2012, cites GRT.0001.00010.0172, a letter from Dr. Ferdinand Piacenza to Dr. Mückter, March 25, 1956, which refers to a patient who received the drug on Nov. 25, 1955. Mückter's reply on April 3, 1956, GRT.0001.00010.0181, states that "we have been testing k17 in many clinics and various sanatoriums for about two years . . ." (hereafter *Rowe v. Grünenthal* Affidavit).

31 methodology was shoddy: Johnson, Stokes, and Arndt, *Thalidomide Catastrophe*, 82.

31 "no undesirable side effect": *Sunday Times* Insight Team, *Suffer the Children*, 42.

32 "absolute intolerability": Letter from Dr. Ferdinand Piacenza to Dr. Mückter, March 25, 1956, GRT.0001.00010.0172, *Rowe v. Grünenthal* Affidavit.

32 "We have never had": Letter from Mückter to Piacenza, April 3, 1956, GRT.0001.00010.0181, *Rowe v. Grünenthal* Affidavit.

32 "K17 is such a strong": Ibid. Translated elsewhere as "I believe that you were a little over-enthusiastic with regard to the dosage."

Three

33 "The better known thalidomide becomes": *Sunday Times* Insight Team, *Suffer the Children*, 100; Report for the month of March 1959 (Dr. Michael), GRT.0001.00053.0079, *Rowe v. Grünenthal* Affidavit.

35 "somewhere north": Author interview with Susan Duffield and Christine Kelsey.

36 "vials": Frances Kelsey Oral History, FDA Oral History Interview, 27.

37 "I don't think a woman": Letter from Roger Stanier to Frances Oldham, March 14, 1943, Frances Kelsey Papers.

37 "I'm very fond of you": Letter from Roger Stanier to Frances Oldham, July 31, 1943, Frances Kelsey Papers.

38 contracted to enlist inmates: Frances's personal notebooks, Kelsey Family Archives, Shelton, Washington (hereafter Kelsey Family Archives).

38 An initial call for 200 prisoners: Nathaniel Comfort, "The Prisoner as Model Organism: Malaria Research at Stateville Penitentiary," *Studies in History and Philosophy of Biological and Biomedical Sciences* 40, no. 3 (Sept. 2009).

38 she met Nathan Leopold: Frances's personal notebooks, Kelsey Family Archives.

38 "I forgot to tell you": Letter from Ellis to Frances Kelsey, undated, 1944, Kelsey Family Archives.

38 "Remember the offspring": Letter from Ellis to Frances Kelsey, Sept. 6, 1944, Kelsey Family Archives.

Four

41 **"I was my mother's seventh child"**: Author interview with Eileen Cronin.

43 **"opulent"**: Letter, Dec. 5, 1961, Frances Kelsey Archives.

44 **She saw right away**: Letter from Frances to the Merrell Co., Nov. 10, 1960, FDA Archives.

44 **"no significant symptoms"**: "The Experimental Toxicology and Pathology of Kevadon (Thalidomide.)," New Drug Application 12-611, 44, FDA Archives.

44 **"In the various species"**: Ibid., 45.

45 **animal data in the brochure**: Letter from Frances Kelsey to the Wm. S. Merrell Company, Nov. 10, 1960, FDA Archives.

45 **"investigators"**: Nov. 14, 1960 report from Frances indicates that the first application showed reports from "17 American investigators," FDA Archives; letter from Frances Kelsey to Dr. R. G. Smith, "The original submission concerned reports of 37 investigators covering 1,589 patients," May 31, 1962, FDA Archives.

46 **"The objections raised by the authors"**: Memo to Dr. Smith, May 18, 1953, Frances Kelsey Papers.

47 **pleaded with her**: Letter from Dr. Austin Smith to Frances, March 23, 1956, Frances Kelsey Papers.

47 **reprinting *JAMA* articles**: Letter from Frances Kelsey to Dr. Smith, March 27, 1956, Frances Kelsey Papers.

47 **"aggressive selling"**: "Drug Promotion," JAMA, Oct. 12, 1957, Frances Kelsey Papers.

48 **"understanding of mutual problems"**: *Therapeutic Nightmare*, 181.

48 **had openly orchestrated**: Philip Hilts, *Protecting America's Health: The FDA, Business, and One Hundred Years of Regulation* (Chapel Hill: University of North Carolina Press, 2004), 120.

48 **"one of sweetness and light"**: *Drug Trade News*, vol. 34, no. 13, June 29, 1959.

48 **"very warm spot"**: Winton Rankin quoted in Hilts, *Protecting America's Health*, 120.

49 **equally troubled by the paperwork**: Frances Kelsey Oral History, 51.

49 **filled with errors**: Ibid.

49 **Oyama took a sunnier view**: Oyama's assessment of Kevadon, New Drug Application 12-611, Oct. 25, 1960, FDA Archives.

49 **Frances decided to find her**: It has been incorrectly reported that Frances watched Moulton testify. Frances was not in Washington, D.C., at the time. She heard about Moulton's testimony through Ellis, who sent her a clipping.

Five

51 **"We have sufficient raw material"**: "Kevadon—Hospital Clinical Program," Inter-Department Memo, Merrell, Oct. 10, 1960, Plaintiff's exhibit 298A, *McCarrick v. Richardson-Merrell*.

52 **My parents were dairy farmers**: Author interview with Eric Barrett.

53 **"hardships, hopes, pleasures"**: Mary C. Moulton, *True Stories of Pioneer Life* (Detroit, 1924), dedication page.

54 **"policy of friendliness with industry"**: Testimony of Barbara Moulton, Hearings Before the Subcommittee on Antitrust and Monopoly of the Committee on the Judiciary, U.S. Senate, June 2, 1960 (hereafter Moulton Testimony).

54 **New Drug Branch stepped in**: Ibid.

55 **crushing the Republican incumbent**: "Sullivan, Leonor Kretzer," "History, Art, and Archives" section, United States House of Representatives website, available at history.house.gov/People/Detail/22444.

55 "non-partisan": United States Information Service, USIS Feature, United States Department of State, 1952.

55 "ten most admired men": Kefauver made Roper polling agency's list of the ten most-admired men in America. U.S. Senate's web page for Special Committee on Organized Crime in Interstate Commerce.

55 "flashes of promise": Jack Anderson and Fred Blumenthal, *The Kefauver Story* (New York: Dial Press, 1956), 22.

55 "like twins": Ibid., 20.

55 **Kefauver graciously signed:** Richard Harris, *The Real Voice* (New York: Macmillan, 1964), 49.

56 "one of the finest men": Anderson and Blumenthal, *Kefauver Story*, 6.

56 **Dr. Irene Till:** Harris, *Real Voice*, 14.

56 **net revenues of drug firms:** "Blair was amazed to find that its profit came to 18.9 percent of invested capital after taxes." Ibid., 17.

56 "My God": Ibid.

57 **Wholesale pharmaceuticals had raked in:** Ibid., 21.

57 **among the country's top fifty companies:** "Administered Prices, Drugs": Report of the Committee on the Judiciary, Subcommittee on Antitrust and Monopoly, U.S. Senate, Eighty-seventh Congress, First Session (Washington, D.C.: U.S. Government Printing Office, 1961), 54.

57 **an elderly man in line:** Harris, *Real Voice*, 36–37.

57 "How in the world": Ibid., 37.

57 **found paperwork:** Ibid., 36.

57 **$2.37 per gram:** Ibid., 38.

58 "clean out the rats": Ibid., 42.

58 **five days' worth:** Ibid., 43.

58 **Other doctors offered:** Ibid., 44.

58 "no worrisome side effects": "Administered Prices, Drugs: Report of the Committee on the Judiciary, United States Senate, Made by Its Subcommittee on Antitrust and Monopoly, Pursuant to S. Res. 52, Eighty-seventh Congress, First Session," 209.

58 **fabricated the names:** John Lear, "Taking the Miracle Out of the Miracle Drugs," *Saturday Review*, Jan. 3, 1959, 42.

58 **a series of charts:** "Charge Drug Price Hiked over 7000 Percent," *Chicago Daily Tribune*, Dec. 7, 1959.

58 "put two sick people": "Administered Prices: Hearings Before the Subcommittee on Antitrust and Monopoly of the Committee on the Judiciary, United States Senate, Eighty-sixth Congress, First Session" (Washington, D.C.: U.S. Government Printing Office, 1960), 7888.

59 "fixing": Harris, *Real Voice*, 80.

59 "perverted marketing attitudes": Martin Seidell's testimony quoted in "The High Price of Drugs," *Washington Post*, Feb. 26, 1960.

59 "almost complete absence": Harris, *Real Voice*, 96.

59 **Drug firms now spent:** Ibid., 88–89.

59 "it would take two railroad cars": Ibid., 89.

59 "I wonder if any member": "Administered Prices: Hearings Before the Subcommittee on Antitrust and Monopoly of the Committee on the Judiciary, United States Senate, Eighty-fifth Congress, First Session" (Washington, D.C.: U.S. Government Printing Office, 1960), 10616.

59 **He also noted:** Harris, *Real Voice*, 113.

59 "honorariums": "U.S. Drug Aide Got $287,142 on Side," *New York Times*, May 19, 1960.

59 **a jaw-dropping $287,142:** Ibid.

60 **"third great new era"**: Henry Welch, opening remarks, Fourth Annual Antibiotics Symposium, *Antibiotics Annual, 1956–1957.*

60 **"blessings"**: Ibid.

60 **participants were stunned**: "Drug Makers and the Government: Who Makes the Decisions," *The Saturday Review,* July 2, 1960.

60 **"added luster"**: R. E. McFadyen, "The FDA's Regulation and Control of Antibiotics in the 1950s: The Henry Welch Scandal, Félix Martí-Ibáñez, and Charles Pfizer & Co," *Bulletin of the History of Medicine* 53, no. 2 (Summer 1979).

60 **"little dynasty"**: "Investigation of Food and Drug Agency Planned," *Port Angeles Evening News,* June 1960.

60 **"argue the case"**: Moulton Testimony.

60 **"a mere service bureau for industry"**: Ibid.

60 **"a man with neither legal nor scientific training"**: Ibid.

61 **"No drug is 'safe'"**: Ibid.

61 **"lady doctor"**: "Ex-FDA Aide Asks Agency Shake-Up," *Baltimore Evening Sun,* June 2, 1960.

61 **"I have jeopardized"**: Harris, *Real Voice,* 107.

61 **quickly blacklisted**: Ibid.

61 **to rejoin the FDA**: James Lee Goddard Oral History, National Library of Medicine, 1969, 306.

Six

63 **"Kevadon: A New Hypnotic"**: Elinor Kamath papers, Harvard Medical Library, Francis A. Countway Library of Medicine, Boston (hereafter Kamath Papers).

65 **immediately called to protest**: "Murray called to say he had received the letter on Kevadon and was 'distressed' at its contents." "Summary of Substance of Contact," Nov. 15, 1960, FDA Archives.

65 **manufacturing Kevadon in Pennsylvania**: Letter from Murray to Frances, Dec. 9, 1960, NDA 12-611, vol. 3, FDA Archives.

66 **"personal information"**: Account of Dec. 29, 1960, in "Chronology of transactions with the William S. Merrell Company regarding 'Kevadon' (thalidomide)," April 17, 1962, FDA Archives.

66 **"None of these data"**: Memo from Ellis Kelsey to Frances Kelsey, Dec. 30, 1960, Frances Kelsey Papers; Kevadon NDA, 12-611, vol. 3, 240, FDA Archives.

PART TWO: THE DRUG

Seven

69 **"I want to emphasize"**: Congressional Record, Proceedings and Debates of the 90th Congress, Second Session, vol. 114, part 2, May 22, 1968, 14495.

71 **"non-hazardous"**: Michael Magazanik, *Silent Shock: The Men Behind the Thalidomide Scandal and an Australian Family's Long Road to Justice* (Melbourne: Text Publishing, 2015), 66.

71 **"examine"**: Ibid.

71 **"Grippex"**: *Sunday Times* Insight Team, *Suffer the Children,* 45.

71 **fifty advertisements**: Leonard Gross, "The Thalidomide Tragedy: A Preview of a New Horror Trial," *Look,* May 28, 1968.

72 **"the atoxicity proved"**: Ibid.

72 **"side effects were not observed"**: Excerpt from Blasiu's paper in *Medizinische Klinik,* May 2, 1958, printed in *Sunday Times* Insight Team, *Suffer the Children,* 68.

72 **"sleeplessness, unrest and tension"**: Grünenthal's letter printed in Gross, "Thalidomide Tragedy."

72 **"Blasiu has given many patients"**: Congressional Record: Proceedings and Debates of the 90th Congress Second Session (Washington, D.C.: U.S. Government Printing Office, 1968), 14553.

72 **The erroneous belief**: Johnson, Stokes, and Arndt, *Thalidomide Catastrophe*, 115.

73 **"If all the details"**: *Sunday Times* Insight Team, *Suffer the Children*, 62.

73 **one million Britons**: Ibid., 63.

73 **"sedative"**: Magazanik, *Silent Shock*, 120.

73 **"large number"**: Ibid., 120.

73 **"unjustifiable"**: *Sunday Times* Insight Team, *Suffer the Children*, 79.

74 **Murdoch conceded**: Ibid., 80.

74 **Somers couldn't replicate**: Ibid., 36–37.

74 **"no known toxicity"**: Ibid., 66.

74 **"avoiding prolonged administration"**: Ibid., 83.

74 **"limited clinical trials"**: Letter from Walter A. Munns, Smith, Kline & French Laboratories, to Commissioner Larrick, July 31, 1962, FDA Archives.

75 **an apparent "lack of efficacy"**: Ibid.

75 **"The material was not of interest"**: Ibid.

75 **Grünenthal approached**: *Sunday Times* Insight Team, *Suffer the Children*, 90.

75 **known, since 1952**: Johnson, Stokes, and Arndt, *Thalidomide Catastrophe*, 121.

76 **"Pogge Cure-All Cocktail"**: Pam Fessler, *Carville's Cure: Leprosy, Stigma, and the Fight for Justice* (New York: Liveright, 2020), 136.

76 **untapped market**: Memorandum from Dr. Raymond Pogge to Merrell president Frank Getman, Oct. 26, 1953.

76 **ingredients could behave**: Michael D. Green, *Bendectin and Birth Defects: The Challenges of Mass Toxic Substances Litigation* (Philadelphia: University of Pennsylvania Press, 1996), 90.

76 **only one clinical study**: Betty Mekdeci, Executive Director, Birth Defect Research for Children, "Bendectin: How a Commonly Used Drug Caused Birth Defects, Part One," Birthdefects.org.

76 **garnered sales**: Andrea Tone, *The Age of Anxiety: A History of America's Turbulent Affair with Tranquilizers* (New York: Basic Books, 2009), 54.

77 **Soon Ayd was dispensing**: Raymond C. Pogge to Frank J. Ayd, "Since your series is now up to about one hundred cases, . . ." March 14, 1960, Kamath Papers.

77 **penned by Pogge**: Ray O. Nulsen, "Bendectin in the Treatment of Nausea in Pregnancy," *Ohio Medical Journal* 53, no. 665 (1957). In a 1983 deposition in the Bendectin litigation, Pogge admitted to "ghost-writing" this paper. Green, *Bendectin and Birth Defects*, 176, 179. See also *Raynor v. Richardson-Merrell, Inc.*, 643 F. Supp. 238 (D.D.C. 1986), Aug. 8, 1986.

77 **His office did not track**: Deposition of Ray O. Nulsen, *Soroka v. Richardson-Merrell*, Civil Action No. 75-962, Nov. 15, 1976, 53–54 (hereafter Nulsen Deposition).

77 **"impressions"**: Ibid., 43, 46.

78 **The editor promptly wrote**: Ibid., 112.

78 **"There is no danger"**: Ibid., 121.

78 **"There is a difference"**: Deposition of Thomas Jones, *Diamond v. William S. Merrell Co. and Richardson-Merrell, Inc.*, Eastern District of Pennsylvania, CV 62-0032132, filed Oct. 4 1962, deposition taken May 11, 1966 (hereafter Jones Deposition), 38.

Eight

79 **"RAYMOND POGGE: The Nulsen studies"**: Direct Examination of Raymond Pogge, *Diamond v. William S. Merrell Co. and Richardson-Merrell, Inc.*, Eastern

District of Pennsylvania, CV 62-0032132, filed Oct. 4, 1962 (hereafter Pogge Deposition).

80 **"I was reassured"**: Nulsen Deposition, 30–31.

81 **Merrell's three categories**: Ralph Adam Fine, *The Great Drug Deception: Lessons from MER/29 for Today's Statin and Drug Consumers — What Your Doctor May Not Know* (New York: Stein and Day, 2012), 122.

82 **"Hospital Clinical Program"**: "Kevadon Hospital Clinical Program: Meeting Agenda & Job Description," 1960, FDA Archives.

82 **"Appeal to the doctor's ego"**: Ibid.

83 **"Special Kevadon Representatives"**: Ibid.

83 **"I feel that you would"**: Ibid.

83 **"clinical trials"**: Ibid.

83 **"Bear in mind"**: Ibid.

83 **large, inexperienced team**: Ibid.

84 **"Only emergency requirements"**: Ibid.

85 **"Kevadon is so safe"**: Ibid.

85 **In experiment 1257-40**: Deposition of Evert Florus Van Maanen, *McCarrick v. Richardson-Merrell*, No. 882 426, Superior Court of California, Los Angeles, Feb. 27, 1971, 14, 24 (hereafter Van Maanen Deposition).

85 **All the experimental animals**: Van Maanen Deposition, 111.

85 **the dog was dead**: *Sunday Times* Insight Team, *Suffer the Children*, 97.

86 **Merrell withheld the dead-rat**: Van Maanen acknowledged that Experiment Number 1257-40 was dated June 28, 1960, over two months before Merrell's FDA application for Kevadon was submitted and that within the chain of command it was his responsibility to report such findings to the FDA. Van Maanen Deposition, 16, 17, 21.

86 **"specific human safety data"**: Plaintiff's Exhibit E, Feb. 27, 1959, letter from Raymond Pogge, read aloud in the Jones Deposition, 38.

86 **One doctor had submitted**: F. Jos. Murray to Dr. R. C. Pogge, Inter-Department Memo, March 16, 1960, Kamath Papers.

87 **blind eyes and concessions**: Murray describes Epstein as being responsible for many past "concessions" and claims Epstein offered to "intercede" to assist the MER/29 application. Memos cited in Fine, *Great Drug Deception*, 200.

87 **"READ AND DESTROY"**: Fine, *Great Drug Deception*, 46.

87 **within a day he wrested**: Ibid., 47.

87 **"irrespective of diet"**: *Sunday Times* Insight Team, *Suffer the Children*, 92.

88 **"SHOW MORE ENTHUSIASM"**: Fine, *Great Drug Deception*, 133–34.

88 **"even if you know"**: Ibid., 141.

88 **$42 million a month**: Ibid., 136. Fine cites "Campaign Strategy," a publication for the Merrell sales force, and calculates annual sales for MER/29 at $400 million. *Sunday Times* Insight Team, *Suffer the Children*, 92, cites possible sales for MER/29 at $4.25 billion annually. I've used $500 million annual sales.

88 **They had secured**: "Kevadon — Hospital Clinical Program," Inter-Department Memo, Merrell, R. H. Woodward to G. L. Christenson, Oct. 10, 1960.

88 **"agency superior"**: "The Feminine Conscience of the FDA: Dr. Frances Oldham Kelsey," *Saturday Review*, Sept. 1, 1962.

Nine

89 **"As a sleep-inducing agent"**: Kevadon brochure, 1960, Plaintiff's Exhibit, *McCarrick v. Richardson-Merrell*, Superior Court of California, Los Angeles.

90 **WILLIAM S. MERRELL CO. INTERDEPARTMENT MEMO**: Reprinted in Interagency

Coordination in Drug Research and Regulation, Hearings Before the Subcommittee on Reorganization and International Organizations of the Committee on Government Operations, U.S. Senate, Agency Coordination Study, Government Operations, Aug. 1 and 9, 1962.

91 **Cohen wanted $4,000:** Letter from Sidney Cohen to Thomas Jones, Nov. 5, 1960, Exhibit 22-A, Jones Deposition.

91 **$3,000 and $3,600:** Keith Ditman to Thomas Jones, December 28, 1960, and Thomas Jones to Charles Freed to Merrell, Nov. 22, 1960, Exhibit 16-F, Jones Deposition.

91 **an additional 762 trials:** "Kevadon Clippings: Quota Exceeded," November 29, 1960. Reprinted in Interagency Coordination in Drug Research and Regulation, Hearings Before the Subcommittee on Reorganization and International Organizations of the Committee on Government Operations, U.S. Senate, Agency Coordination Study, Government Operations, Aug. 1 and 9, 1962.

91 **More than twenty-nine thousand Americans:** Ibid.

92 **"It has not been established":** Thomas L. Jones to E. B. Linton, Acuff Clinic, letter, Dec. 5, 1960. Ibid, 273.

Ten

93 **"Sooner or later":** *Sunday Times* Insight Team, *Suffer the Children*, 68.

95 **ninety thousand packets:** Magazanik, *Silent Shock*, 63.

95 **250,000 more brochures:** *Sunday Times* Insight Team, *Suffer the Children*, 46.

95 **"a negative effect on the circulation":** Report of Grünenthal sales representative Zila of a visit to a pharmacist in Düsseldorf, July 14, 1959, GRT.0001.00021.0151, *Rowe v. Grünenthal* Affidavit.

95 **"severe side effects":** Letter from Pharmacolor AG, Switzerland, to Grünenthal, Aug. 27, 1959, GRT.0001.00021.0272, *Rowe v. Grünenthal* Affidavit.

95 **"Do you know anything":** Letter from Dr. Ralf Voss to Grünenthal, Oct. 7, 1959, GRT.0001.00022.0013, *Rowe v. Grünenthal* Affidavit.

96 **"Happily we can tell you":** *Sunday Times* Insight Team, *Suffer the Children*, 48–49.

96 **"sensory disturbances":** Sales report to Management, Oct. 15, 1959, GRT .0001.00022.0055, *Rowe v. Grünenthal* Affidavit.

96 **"vitamin B deficiencies":** Letter from Grünenthal to doctor in Iserlohn, Oct. 26, 1959, GRT.0001.00022.0056, *Rowe v. Grünenthal* Affidavit.

96 **"We have no idea how":** Letter from Grünenthal to Dr. Ralf Voss, Dec. 17, 1959, GRT.0001.00022.0169, *Rowe v. Grünenthal* Affidavit.

96 **"severe circulatory disruptions":** Grünenthal report by sales rep Zila, Dec. 17, 1959, GRT.0001.00022.0167 at 0168, *Rowe v. Grünenthal* Affidavit.

96 **"a causal connection":** Letter from Grünenthal to Dr. Grafe von Schroder, Dec. 30, 1959, *Rowe v. Grünenthal* Affidavit.

96 **"heard or seen anything":** Ibid.

96 **about twenty thousand meetings:** *Sunday Times* Insight Team, *Suffer the Children*, 49.

96 **"harmless even over a long period":** Ibid.

96 **Germany's most popular sleep aid:** Magazanik, *Silent Shock*, 95.

96 **"paraesthesias and hypoaesthesias":** Letter from Grünenthal to surgeon, March 11, 1960, GRT.001.00024.0021, *Rowe v. Grünenthal* Affidavit.

96 **"We have received":** Ibid.

97 **"severity of side effects":** Magazanik, *Silent Shock*, 72.

97 **"Everything":** Rock Brynner and Trent Stephens, *Dark Remedy: The Impact of Thalidomide and Its Revival as a Vital Medicine* (New York: Basic Books, 2001), 22.

97 "no pathological changes": Dr. Mückter report for the month of July 1960, GRT.0001.00026.0128, *Rowe v. Grünenthal* Affidavit.

97 "a quick publication": *Sunday Times* Insight Team, *Suffer the Children*, 52.

97 megadoses of thalidomide: Ibid., 34.

97 ten to twenty times: Ibid.

97 "Contergan could be described": Ibid., 52.

97 "friendly connection": Ibid., 53.

97 "atoxicity": Ibid.

97 "We intend to fight": Ibid.

97 "As with most drugs": Ibid.

98 "greater and greater intensity": Situation Report from Düsseldorf Sales Area, Dec. 7, 1960, GRT.0001.00029.0129, *Rowe v. Grünenthal* Affidavit.

98 "We should be briefed": Ibid.

Eleven

99 "IS THALIDOMIDE TO BLAME?": A. Leslie Florence, "Is Thalidomide to Blame?" *British Medical Journal*, Dec. 1960.

100 "Q: You also made no investigation": *Soroka v. Richardson-Merrell*, Civil Action No. C C75-962, Nov. 15, 1976, 148.

101 Murray accused her: Joseph Murray to Dr. Harold W. Werner, "Kevadon ND— Report of FDA Visit," Inter-Department Memo, Merrell, April 4, 1961, Kamath Papers.

102 names of all trial doctors: Letter from Frances Kelsey to Merrell, Feb. 23, 1961, Kamath Papers.

102 she got her list: Ibid.

102 "any comments": Letter from Joseph Murray to Denis Burley Distillers, Feb. 15, 1961.

103 "I do not think": Letter from Leslie Florence to Chief Medical Officer, Distillers, Feb. 17, 1959, Kamath Papers.

103 "unable to ascribe": Letter from D. M. Burley, Distillers, to Dr. Florence, Feb. 25, 1959, Kamath Papers.

103 "in the last year": Letter from Distillers to Dr. Mückter, Grünenthal, Nov. 1960, Frances Kelsey Papers.

104 "pins and needles": "Alexander Leslie Florence," *British Medical Journal*, May 4, 2018.

104 *all* his lab mice: *Sunday Times* Insight Team, *Suffer the Children*, 83.

104 "a very real danger": Ibid., 59.

104 "got out of perspective": Ibid.

105 thalidomide sales in Germany: Magazanik, *Silent Shock*, 95.

105 told Grünenthal to remove it: Letter from Dr. Eckerle to Grünenthal, Nov. 2, 1961, *Rowe v. Grünenthal* Affidavit.

105 The director of a nerve clinic: Letter from Lauberntha to Scheid, director of the Universität Nerve Clinic, Oct. 30, 1961, *Rowe v. Grünenthal* Affidavit.

105 "foster confusion": Sales letter from Dr. Goden to Sievers, Feb. 23, 1961, GRT.0001.00031.0256, *Rowe v. Grünenthal* Affidavit.

105 complaints reached four hundred: Magazanik, *Silent Shock*, 72.

105 "for a large percentage": Letter from Grünenthal to Franz Wirtz in U.S., Feb. 23, 1961, GRT.0001.00031.0253, *Rowe v. Grünenthal* Affidavit.

106 "any complications": D. Burley, "Is Thalidomide to Blame?," *British Medical Journal* (Jan. 14, 1961).

106 Dr. Michael Winzreid: Dr. D. M. Burley, "Thalidomide and Peripheral Neuritis: A Report on the Joint Discussions with representatives of Chemie Grünenthal,

Stolberg-in-Rheinland and Wm. Merrell Limited, Cincinnati, Ohio with notes on visit to West Germany," March 1961, Kamath Papers.

106 **Another psychiatrist in Düren:** Ibid.

106 **Two doctors at the University of Cologne:** Ibid.

106 **vitamin B, deficiencies:** Ibid.

106 **cases of peripheral neuritis:** Ibid. "There are approximately one hundred and fifty known cases of peripheral neuritis attributed to thalidomide in Great Britain and West Germany combined. It can be presumed that there are others so far unreported."

Twelve

107 **"I agree with you":** Letter from Thomas Jones, Merrell, to Denis Burley, April 28, 1961, Kamath Papers.

109 **tracked milking patterns:** Memo to John Swann, 1998, Frances Kelsey Papers.

109 **her search for government work:** Harris, *Real Voice*, 107.

109 **Murray put forth:** "Kevadon NDA—Report of FDA Visit," Inter-Department Memo, April 4, 1961, Kamath Papers.

110 **"Pins and needles":** F. Joseph Murray to Frances Kelsey, March 29, 1961, Kamath Papers.

110 **"instructions from above":** Routing and Transmittal slip from Frances Kelsey to FDA Historian John Swann re: handwritten notes from Ralph Smith, Nov. 24, 1995, Frances Kelsey Papers.

110 **"damage suits":** Fine, *Great Drug Deception*, 64.

110 **"really angry" . . . "drastic measures":** Letter from Franz Wirtz to Dr. von Schrader describing "the atmosphere at R&M," May 7, 1961, GRT.0001.00037.0116, *Rowe v. Grünenthal* Affidavit.

110 **His language grew threatening:** "Chronology of transactions with the William S. Merrell Company regarding 'Kevadon' (thalidomide)," April 17, 1962, FDA Archives.

110 **"yes or no":** Ibid.

111 **"Abandon any idea":** Draft of letter from Frances to Merrell, April 26, 1961, Frances Kelsey Papers.

111 **a hearing to determine:** "Chronology of transactions with the William S. Merrell Company regarding 'Kevadon' (thalidomide)," April 19, 1961, FDA Archives.

111 **"incomplete":** Letter from Frances Kesley to Merrell, May 5, 1961, FDA Archives.

111 **"make a frank disclosure":** Ibid.

111 **"libelous":** Memo of telephone interview, Ralph Smith, FDA, and Joseph Murray, Merrell, May 9, 1961, FDA Archives.

111 **"failure of communication":** Notes on meeting between Frances Kelsey, R. G. Smith, J. Archer, and Joseph Murray, May 11, 1961, Frances Kelsey Papers.

111 **"expedite":** Ibid.

111 **Frances demanded to see evidence:** Ibid.

PART THREE: THE FIGHT
Thirteen

115 **"Upper and lower extremities":** Memo from Cincinnati District to Bureau of Field Administration, Aug. 21, 1962, FDA Archives.

116 **"On April 5, 1961":** American Trial Lawyers Association, Midwinter Meeting, 1969, San Francisco, California, 654.

117 **"When I was born":** Author interview with Dorothy Hunt-Honsinger.

119 **"knights":** Dan G. McNamara et al., "Historical Milestones: Helen Brooke Taussig, 1898 to 1986," *Journal of the American College of Cardiology* 10, no. 3 (Sept. 1987): 662–71.

119 **"elfin faces":** Jesús De Rubens Figueroa et al., "Cardiovascular Spectrum in

Williams-Beuren Syndrome: The Mexican Experience in 40 Patients," *Texas Heart Institute Journal* 35, no. 3 (2008): 279–85.

119 **"seal limbs":** "The Unfolding Tragedy of Drug Deformed Babies," *Maclean's*, May 19, 1962.

120 **"What is more":** Letter from Helen B. Taussig to Ms. Elinor Kamath, June 23, 1976, Helen B. Taussig Collection, Alan Mason Chesney Medical Archives, Baltimore, Maryland (hereafter Taussig Collection).

121 **"Professor Taussig's daughter":** Gerri Lynn Goodman, "A Gentle Heart: The Life of Helen Taussig," thesis, Yale University School of Medicine, New Haven, Connecticut, 1983, 4.

122 **An amplified stethoscope:** Joyce Baldwin, *To Heal the Heart of a Child* (New York: Walker & Company, 1992), 39.

122 **So Helen taught herself:** "Learn to listen with your fingers" is widely attributed to Taussig. See J. Van Robays, "Helen B. Taussig (1898–1986)," *Facts, Views & Vision in ObGyn* 8(3) (Sept. 2016): 183–87, published online Dec. 5, 2016.

123 **the first woman elected:** McNamara et al., "Historical Milestones."

123 **secured a $1,000 travel grant:** Letter from Taussig to Dr. Leonard Sherlis, Maryland Heart Association, Feb. 6, 1962, Taussig Collection.

123 **agreed to meet with Helen:** Letter from Prof. Dr. Med. Gerhard Joppich to Taussig, Jan. 29, 1962, Taussig Collection.

123 **"congenital absence of the upper arm":** Laurence Urdang, *Bantam Medical Dictionary*, 5th ed. (New York: Random House, 2009).

123 **The doctors had no idea:** Magazanik, *Silent Shock*, 94.

123 **the number had risen:** Helen B. Taussig, "A Study of the German Outbreak of Phocomelia: The Thalidomide Syndrome," *JAMA* 180 (June 30, 1962).

Fourteen

125 **"It would be an understatement":** K. H. Schulte-Hillen, "My Search to Find the Drug That Crippled My Baby," *Good Housekeeping*, May 1963, 95.

127 **Labor progressed slowly:** Ibid.

128 **Nazi regime had targeted:** "People with Disabilities," annotated bibliography, United States Holocaust Museum, available at ushmm.org/collections/bibliography/people-with-disabilities.

129 **Karl wandered the cobbled streets:** Magazanik, *Silent Shock*, 98.

130 **"Things are not always":** Schulte-Hillen, "My Search," 96.

130 **The doctor issued:** Author interview with Linde Schulte-Hillen.

130 **"He isn't telling":** Ibid.

131 **As if her own arms:** Ibid.

131 **"This means telling":** Schulte-Hillen, "My Search," 96.

131 **"face things squarely":** Ibid.

Fifteen

133 **"I would find it":** Internal GRT memo re Contergan Situation by Dr. Michael, May 10, 1961, GRT.0001.0037.0141, *Rowe v. Grünenthal* Affidavit.

136 **hands that seemed to sprout:** *Sunday Times* Insight Team, *Suffer the Children*, 7.

136 **"It seems quite normal otherwise":** William McBride, *Killing the Messenger* (Cremorne, Australia: Eldorado, 1994), 53.

136 **McBride was rattled:** McBride's "start date" as an obstetrician was more or less in 1954. "Doctor Who Alerted the World to the Dangers of Thalidomide," *Sydney Morning Herald*, July 18, 2018.

137 **"For God's sake, Bill":** Bill Nicol, *McBride: Behind the Myth*, ABC Enterprises for the Australian Broadcasting Corp, Jan. 1, 1989, 16.

137 On September 16, 1960: Magazanik, *Silent Shock*, 241.

137 he was peddling: Ibid., 6.

137 McBride gave Hodgetts: *Sunday Times* Insight Team, *Suffer the Children*, 6.

137 akin to pure *cyanide*: McBride, *Killing the Messenger*, 9.

138 "extremely efficient": Magazanik, *Silent Shock*, 243.

138 "I would be only too pleased": McBride, *Killing the Messenger*, 58.

138 "We are in receipt": Ibid., 59.

138 After swallowing twenty-one: Ibid., 61.

139 "Thalidomide is derived from glutamic acid": McBride, *Killing the Messenger*, 61.

139 ability to metabolize glutamine: H. Eagle, "Nutrition Needs of Mammalian Cells in Tissue Culture," *Science* 122, no. 3168 (1955): 501–14.

139 McBride telephoned the Distillers office: This is the person McBride believes he spoke with. No confirmation exists.

140 It was June 1961: "Obstetrician's Decisive Action on Thalidomide Helped Spare Many," *Sydney Morning Herald*, Sept. 8, 2015.

Sixteen

141 "If you have one man": Lenz quoted in Nicol, *McBride*, 27.

143 a dozen cases like Jan's: Schulte-Hillen, "My Search," 96.

143 did not share a water source: Ibid., 97.

144 "There is one man in Germany": Ibid., 98.

144 "sterilization of all the unfit": Horst Biesold, *Crying Hands: Eugenics and Deaf People in Nazi Germany* (Washington, D.C.: Gallaudet University Press, 2004), 18.

144 "central mission of all politics": Henry Friedlander, *The Origins of Nazi Genocide: From Euthanasia to the Final Solution* (Chapel Hill: University of North Carolina Press, 1995), 12.

144 "We doctors are constantly": Schulte-Hillen, "My Search," 98.

145 to confirm about ten cases: Dr. W. Lenz, "Thalidomide Embryopathy in Germany, 1960–1961," paper presented at the 91st Annual Meeting of the American Public Health Association, Kansas City, Missouri, Nov. 1963, 2 (hereafter 1963 Lenz Paper).

145 fifteen recent cases in Münster: Ibid.

145 "It's as if we were": Schulte-Hillen, "My Search," 98.

145 "You can't give up!": Ibid.

145 a nurse in Hamburg: Ibid.

146 The grandfather soon passed along: Author interview with Linde Schulte-Hillen.

146 Worried what a household: In 1962, Suzanne Vandeput of Belgium would stand trial—and be acquitted—for killing her armless infant.

147 Lenz read a research paper: 1963 Lenz Paper, 5.

147 she immediately blamed the drug: Ibid, 11.

147 "I think it is Contergan": Ibid., 12.

147 By November 15: Helen B. Taussig, "Thalidomide and Phocomelia," *Pediatrics* 30, no. 4 (October 1962): 656.

148 "The beginning of July": Schulte-Hillen, "My Search," 100.

148 "You little idiot!": Ibid.

148 "Linde!": Ibid.

Seventeen

149 "If I were a doctor": Heinrich Mückter quoted in Henning Sjöström and Robert Nilsson, *Thalidomide and the Power of the Drug Companies* (Harmondsworth, UK: Penguin, 1972), 88.

150 "All of us have eaten": 1963 Lenz Paper, 21.
151 Privately, the German firm: June 1961 report, GRT.0001.00040.0034, *Rowe v. Grünenthal* Affidavit.
151 "difficult psychologically to promote": Staff Meeting report (Hamburg office), May 12, 1961, GRT.0001.00037.0145, *Rowe v. Grünenthal* Affidavit.
151 Grünenthal's inner circle: Note re: Contergan, by Grünenthal's legal department, July 10, 1961, GRT.0001.00225.0282, *Rowe v. Grünenthal* Affidavit.
151 The Gerling Group: Memo on Liability, July 5, 1961, GRT.0001.00042.0078, *Rowe v. Grünenthal* Affidavit.
151 "the extent and severity": Ibid.
151 "negligence": Ibid.
151 Grünenthal's lawyers told: Note re: Contergan, by Grünenthal's legal department, July 10, 1961, GRT.0001.00225.0282, *Rowe v. Grünenthal* Affidavit.
152 "inadequately informed": Magazanik, *Silent Shock*, 59.
152 "If I were a doctor": Sjöström and Nilsson, *Thalidomide and the Power of the Drug Companies*, 88.
152 "Take only as directed": Internal memo, Oct. 1, 1961, GRT.0001.00211.0239, *Rowe v. Grünenthal* Affidavit.
152 Not until August 1, 1961: Sjöström and Nilsson, *Thalidomide and the Power of the Drug Companies*, 91.
152 even when *Der Spiegel*: Memo, Aug. 16, 1961, GRT.0001.00225.0276, *Rowe v. Grünenthal* Affidavit.
152 "we would not now": Memo, Aug. 16, 1961, GRT.0001.00225.0276, *Rowe v. Grünenthal* Affidavit.
152 "There are dozens of us": Letter, Sept. 15, 1961, GRT.0001.00048.0142, *Rowe v. Grünenthal* Affidavit.
152 "Get rid of Contergan!": Ibid.
152 "I am appalled": Letter from Dr. Raschow to Dr. Sievers, Oct. 10, 1961, GRT.0001.00050.0157, *Rowe v. Grünenthal* Affidavit.
152 "Medical practitioners are not": "File memo Dr. Helbig," Nov. 17, 1961, GRT.0001.00055.0202, *Rowe v. Grünenthal* Affidavit.
153 "symptoms would disappear": Letter from Laubenthal to Scheid, director of the University Nerve Clinic, Oct. 30, 1961, GRT.0001.00050.0427, *Rowe v. Grünenthal* Affidavit.
153 "This is just not true": Ibid.
153 "downright horrified": Letter to Grünenthal from an associate of Dr. Kalvelage, Nov. 7, 1961, GRT.0001.00050.0207, *Rowe v. Grünenthal* Affidavit.
153 Soon eighty-nine lawsuits: "To date 89 recourse claims have been lodged," internal memo re Contergan, Oct. 1, 1961, GRT.0001.00211.0239, *Rowe v. Grünenthal* Affidavit.
153 its first reimbursement request: "On 19 Sept. 1961, we received the first written request to date for reimbursement of costs for Contergan damage by a statutory health insurance fund, namely the Leipziger Varein-Barmenia head office." Ibid.
153 "unleash an avalanche": Ibid.
153 the company knew of 2,400: "At a meeting at Stolberg in Sept. 1961, Grünenthal told its licensees from Britain, the United States and Sweden about the risks and seriousness of peripheral neuritis but concealed the fact that it now knew of 2,400 cases in Germany alone." *Sunday Times* Insight Team, *Suffer the Children*, 60.
153 "Improbable": Magazanik, *Silent Shock*, 90.
153 "teratogenic effects": Johnson, Stokes, and Arndt, *Thalidomide Catastrophe*, 115.
153 Grünenthal sent no reply: Ibid., 115.
154 "based on all observations": Magazanik, *Silent Shock*, 74–75.
154 "empirical knowledge": Grünenthal to Dr. von Rosenstiel, National Drug Co., March 23, 1961, GRT.0001.00031.0252, *Rowe v. Grünenthal* Affidavit.

154 **"might be useful":** Ibid.

154 **"Everything is done":** Magazanik, *Silent Shock*, 95.

154 **A doctor who had delivered:** Ibid., 92.

154 **the firm stayed silent:** Ibid., 92–93.

154 **Mückter's research department:** Resignation of Dr. Schuppius described in *Rowe v. Grünenthal* Affidavit; and Hagens Berman Notice to plead—COMPLAINT 006185-11 627962 V1, 82.

154 **A team from Stolberg:** This was four months after Frances Kelsey asked Merrell for evidence that the drug was safe during pregnancy.

154 **pregnancy made the agenda:** On October 3, 1961, the National Drug Company, one of Richardson-Merrell's subsidiaries, wrote to Grünenthal saying the FDA was asking specifically whether Contergan was transferred to the fetus. Letter from W. H. Rosenstiel to Dr. von Schrader, Oct. 3, 1961, Frances Kelsey Papers.

154 **Jones wrote to three obstetricians:** Thomas Jones letters to Dr. Ray O. Nulsen, Dr. Edward Holyroyd, and Dr. James Seiver, all dated Sept. 12, 1961.

154 **"The question has been raised":** Thomas Jones letter to Edward Holyroyd, head of obstetrics, Rio Hondo Memorial Hospital, Downey, California, Sept. 12, 1962.

154 **he asked about "fetal abnormalities":** FDA agents would later find a copy of Jones's letter to Nulsen. Memo from Ralph Weilerstein, MD, to Bureau of Medicine, Sept. 4, 1962, FDA Archives.

155 **at least two babies:** Nulsen Deposition, 144–48. Nulsen would later claim he didn't even consider the possibility that the baby's condition was linked to thalidomide.

155 **"experiences and problems":** Letter from F. H. Wadey, managing director, the Wm. S. Merrell Company, to Dr. H. W. von Schrader, Chemie Grünenthal GmbH, Stolberg im Rheinland, Germany, Sept. 27, 1961, Frances Kelsey Papers.

155 **Kemper guessed:** "Dr. Michael's report of visit to Dr. Kemper," Oct. 24, 1961, GRT.0001.00050.0207, *Rowe v. Grünenthal* Affidavit.

155 **to study thalidomide's effect:** Magazanik, *Silent Shock*, 81.

155 **"NOT FOR PREGNANT WOMEN":** Ibid., 91–92. In 1969, Dr. Günter von Waldeyer-Hartz wrote to the German government stating what he had seen in October 1961.

Eighteen

157 **"Q: In September of 1961":** "Deposition of Evert Florus Van Maanen," *McCarrick v. Richardson-Merrell*, Superior Court of California, Los Angeles, Feb. 27, 1971, 62.

158 **"The pharmacologic properties of drugs":** "Committee on Fetus and Newborn; Statement by Committee on Fetus and Newborn: Effect of Drugs upon the Fetus and the Infant," *Pediatrics* 28, no. 4 (Oct. 1961): 678.

159 **I was born in Melbourne, Australia:** Author interview with Jeff Green.

161 **"We've had a report":** Magazanik, *Silent Shock*, 261.

161 **Bishop was particularly rattled:** *Sunday Times* Insight Team, *Suffer the Children*, 121–22.

162 **though many would acknowledge:** Magazanik, *Silent Shock*, 254.

162 **routinely drank whiskey together:** Ibid., 255.

162 **Hodgetts would storm the German embassy:** Magazanik, *Silent Shock*, 239.

162 *The Lancet* **rejected his paper:** Nicol, *McBride*, 72. The editor of *The Lancet* at that time, Dr. Ian Munro, denies receiving or rejecting this paper, arguing that no record of McBride's paper appears in the journal's submission ledger. Ian Munro, "Thalidomide and the Lancet," *British Medical Journal*, June 16, 1979. But a 1972 letter from the medical superintendent of Crown Street Women's Hospital claims that the assistant editor of *The Lancet* rejected the paper on July 13, 1961.

163 **a fourth phocomelic baby:** McBride, *Killing the Messenger*, 73.
163 **"IATROGENIC DISEASES OF THE NEWBORN":** S. A. Doxiadis et al., "Iatrogenic Diseases of the Newborn," *The Lancet*, Sept. 30, 1961, 753–54.
163 **"It is with absolute safety":** Magazanik, *Silent Shock*, 126.
163 **McBride immediately fumed:** McBride, *Killing the Messenger*, 75–76.
164 **"We are most concerned":** Letter to McBride from Denis Burley, Distillers UK, Nov. 29, 1961, reprinted in McBride, *Killing the Messenger*, 77.

Nineteen

165 **"We've asked these":** Schulte-Hillen, "My Search," 95.
167 **he at last had telephoned:** Ibid., 100.
167 **the very first he'd heard:** *Sunday Times* Insight Team, *Suffer the Children*, 134.
167 **"In view of the incalculable human":** 1963 Lenz Paper, 15.
167 **fourteen detailed, incriminating:** Ibid., 17.
168 **"I'm going to speak":** Schulte-Hillen, "My Search," 100.
168 **conferring with a professor of pediatrics:** 1963 Lenz Paper, 16.
168 **"As a man and a citizen":** Ibid., 17.
168 **"Each month's delay":** Ibid., 18.
168 **Lenz confided to the man:** John Clymer, "The Untold Story of the Thalidomide Babies," *Saturday Evening Post*, Oct. 20, 1962.
169 **A ministry official condemned:** *Sunday Times* Insight Team, *Suffer the Children*, 136.
169 **"unjustified attack":** Ibid.
169 **they asked the drug firm representatives:** Leonard Gross, "The Tragedy of Thalidomide Babies: Preview of a New German Horror Trial," *Look*, May 28, 1968, 52.
169 **so worried the ministry officials:** Ibid.
169 **They privately told the ministry:** *Sunday Times* Insight Team, *Suffer the Children*, 138.
170 **threatened legal action:** Ibid., 138.
170 **"We have had a rather":** Letter reprinted in *Sunday Times* Insight Team, *Suffer the Children*, 139.
170 **Mückter's sole concession:** Ibid., 139–40.
170 ***Welt am Sonntag:*** "Missgeburten Durch Tabletten?," *Welt am Sonntag*, Nov. 26, 1961.
171 **"WE ARE TAKING CONTERGAN OUT":** Telegram reprinted in *Sunday Times* Insight Team, *Suffer the Children*, 40.
171 **"Because press reports have undermined":** Letter reprinted in *Sunday Times* Insight Team, *Suffer the Children*, 141.

Twenty

173 **"December 6, 1961":** Letter from Max Sien to Elinor Kamath, Dec. 6, 1961, Kamath Papers.
175 **A drug called Contergan:** "Missgeburten Durch Tabletten?"
175 **a fraught story:** Kamath, "Echo of Silence: The Causes and Consequences of the Thalidomide Disaster," unpublished manuscript, Kamath Papers.
176 **"Have you seen":** Ibid.
176 **"I don't know who":** Ibid.
176 **spurned the story:** Kamath claims that Sydney Gruson later said, "She handed me the story on a platter." Ibid., 14.
177 **first article to appear in England:** Ibid., 13–14.

177   **The embassy immediately reached out:** Telegram from Chemie Grünenthal to
      Merrell, Dec. 22, 1961, Frances Kelsey Papers.
177   *Medical Tribune:* "Sedative Drug Is Withdrawn by British, German Makers,"
      Medical Tribune, Dec. 25, 1961.
178   **"academic interest":** Letter from Kamath to Mr. Fritz Silber, Physicians News
      Service, June 7, 1963, Kamath Papers.

Twenty-one

179   **"My name is Sabine Becker":** Author interview with Sabine Becker.
181   **In July, Norman Orentreich:** Letter from Norman Orentreich, MD, to Thomas
      L. Jones, Associate Director of Clinical Research, Merrell, July 14, 1961, Kamath
      Papers.
181   **"numbness, tingling":** Letter from Ralph L. Byron to Thomas Jones, Depart-
      ment of Medical Research, Merrell, Aug. 28, 1961, Kamath Papers. (Jones wrote
      back to Byron on Sept. 12, 1961, that he was "puzzled" by Byron's results.)
181   **Jones asked him to delay:** Letter from Thomas L. Jones to Sidney Cohen, MD,
      April 13, 1961.
181   **asked him to downplay:** Letter from Thomas Jones, Associate Director of Clini-
      cal Research, Merrell, to Frank J. Ayd, MD, Aug. 18, 1961, Kamath Papers.
181   **on more than 150 alcoholics:** Letter from Joseph Murray to Frances Kelsey,
      Aug. 21, 1961, Kamath Papers.
181   **urged to tell the FDA:** Letter from Thomas Jones to Sidney Cohen, Aug. 28, 1961,
      Kamath Papers.
182   **more than a dozen men:** "Conference of Sept. 7th. Frances O. Kelsey," undated,
      FDA Archives.
182   **drug recommended for chronic use:** Frances Kelsey, memo of telephone inter-
      view with Dr. Donald Tower, Chief of Clinical Neurochemistry Laboratory, Insti-
      tute of Neurological Diseases and Blindness, June 28, 1961, Frances Kelsey Papers.
182   **the drug's effect on the fetus:** "On inquiry the group said they had no knowledge
      of what this drug might do to the fetus if used in pregnant women." "Conference
      of Sept. 7th. Frances O. Kelsey," undated, FDA Archives.
182   **A week after the presentations:** Frances Kelsey to Wm. S. Merrell Company,
      Sept. 13, 1961, Kamath Papers.
182   **peak sedative season:** Frances Kelsey Oral History, 62.
182   **He'd write it down:** Dr. Murray and Frances Kelsey, "Memo of (Telephone) In-
      terview," Sept. 26, 1961, Frances Kelsey Papers.
182   **a quick "OK":** Ibid.
182   **Frances reminded him:** Ibid.
183   **Murray was anxious:** Ibid.
183   **"the safety of thalidomide":** Letter from Joseph Murray to Frances Kelsey,
      Sept. 28, 1961, Kamath Papers.

Twenty-two

185   **"My mom became pregnant":** Author interview with Gwen Riechmann.
186   **"Dear Tom":** Plaintiff's Exhibit in *Diamond v. William S. Merrell Co. and
      Richardson-Merrell, Inc.,* Eastern District of Pennsylvania, Case CV 62-0032132.
187   **"I was born at the University Hospital":** Author interview with Gus Economides.
189   **The Mayo Clinic reported:** Fine, *Great Drug Deception,* 73.
189   **customers began returning:** Ibid., 71–72.
189   **"false sense of security":** Ibid., 75.
189   **Nestor stormed:** Ibid., 112.
189   **avoiding the word:** Ibid., 88.

189 **"major promotional revision"**: Ibid., 105.

189 **"an example before"**: Getman's quote appears in ibid., 90.

189 **liability claims would ensue**: Ibid., 91.

189 **"all-out fight"**: Ibid., 89.

190 **"pose a threat"**: Ibid., 90.

190 **Though more than sixteen thousand**: In September 1961, Merrell told Grünenthal the total number of patients receiving Kevadon in the United States was 16,821. Letter from Thomas Jones to H. W. von Schrader-Beielstein, Dec. 29, 1961.

190 **"Wheeled Avenger of the Beltway"**: Curt Suplee, "John Nestor: Strife in the Fast Lane," *Washington Post*, Nov. 21, 1984.

191 **Despite the mass of complaints**: Fine, *Great Drug Deception*, 93.

191 **Merrell ran ads**: Ibid., 108.

191 **Compelling Merrell to issue a warning**: Ibid., 95–96.

191 **pressured Wallace & Tiernan**: "Memorandum," Office of Commissioner to Bureau of Medicine, Nov. 7. 1961, Frances Kelsey Papers.

191 **relay bizarre news**: Joseph Murray and Frances Kelsey, memo of telephone call, Nov. 30, 1961, Frances Kelsey Papers.

191 **FDA application under consideration**: Merrell officially withdrew its Kevadon New Drug Application in March 1962.

191 **"hazard to the fetus"**: Reference to telephone call between Frances and Dr. Miller J. Sullivan in letter from Frances to National Drug Company, Oct. 4, 1961, FDA Archives.

192 **"the reports are of such"**: Letter from Distillers to Herr H. Leufgens, Grünenthal, Nov. 29, 1961, Frances Kelsey Papers.

Twenty-three

193 **"My friends call me JoJo"**: Author interview with Jose Calora.

194 **"I was born in Oklahoma City"**: Author interview with Jan Taylor Garrett.

195 **"My mother was sedated"**: Author interview with Carolyn Farmer Sampson.

197 **Frances had heard nothing more**: Merrell had sent two representatives overseas to investigate, but had relayed no update. *Medical World News* ran a small story on the matter Feb. 2, 1962. Frances was then called by a *Time* magazine reporter for background on the drug and referred the reporter to Merrell. Frances Kelsey and Jean Franklin, memo of telephone conversation, Frances Kelsey Archives; *Time* ran its story Feb. 13, 1962.

197 **found its way**: Reference to a "Foreign Service Dispatch" about thalidomide appears in a memo from Ralph Smith, Division of New Drugs, FDA, to Mr. F. D. Clark, Office of the Commissioner, Jan. 12, 1962, FDA Archives. Letter from Herman I. Chinn, Deputy Scientific Attaché, Foreign Service, to Elinor Kamath, June 11, 1963, Kamath Papers. "His [Larrick's] statement that no reports were seen prior to the publication in the *Medical World News* on February 2, 1962 is difficult to understand. Both your reports and mine antedated this by six weeks or so."

197 **Merrell finally requested to withdraw** : Letter from Harold W. Werner to Frances Kelsey, FDA, March 5, 1962.

197 **the firm pulled the drug**: Letter from C. A. Morrell to Joseph Murray, March 2, 1962, Frances Kelsey Papers.

197 **"that these birth defects can accurately"**: National Drug Company "Dear Doctor" letter, Jan. 11, 1962, FDA Archives.

197 **demanded a thalidomide recall**: Letter from C. A. Morrell to Joseph Murray, March 2, 1962, Frances Kelsey Papers.

198 **"This step was taken"**: Letter from Robert H. Woodward to Dr. H. W. v. Schrader-Beielstein, March 12, 1962, Frances Kelsey Papers.

198 **patients of Ray O. Nulsen**: "Dr. Jones stated that he had first seen the two letters

in question sometime in March of 1962. These letters were dated Feb. 14, 1962 and January, 1962, and related to four cases of abnormal children born to patients of Dr. Nulsen." Memo from Ralph Weilerstein, MD, to Bureau of Medicine, Subject: Kevadon (brand of thalidomide), visit to William S. Merrell Division, Sept. 4, 1962, FDA Archives.

198 *seven* **injured babies:** Memorandum of Conference: Helen Taussig, Frances Kelsey, and John Nestor, April 6, 1962, FDA Archives.

198 **were the children of doctors:** Ibid.

198 **two cases of babies:** Ibid.

198 **upward of fifty such children:** Ibid.

198 **Yet Grünenthal had swiftly managed:** Letter from Taussig to Dr. von Schrader Beielstein, Grünenthal, April 9, 1962, Taussig Collection.

198 **had been smeared:** Magazanik, *Silent Shock*, 102.

199 **Lenz decided to vilify:** Letter from Widukind Lenz to Helen Taussig, April 4, 1962, Taussig Collection.

199 **Lenz thought Grünenthal was:** "Most people in this country thought it wiser to hush up the matter, especially as the firm is affiliated with rather big business." Letter from Lenz to Taussig, Jan. 31, 1962, Taussig Collection. And, later, "the pressure against truth which has been so conspicuous in the beginning of the affair, continues to be unabated." Letter from Lenz to Taussig, Aug. 19, 1964, Taussig Collection.

199 **"behaved disgracefully":** "Reminisces of Helen Brooke Taussig: Oral History," 1975, 42, Columbia Center for Oral History, Columbia University.

199 **German medical community:** Letter from Lenz to Taussig, Aug. 19, 1964, Taussig Collection.

199 **undertaken her own probe:** See Taussig's extensive correspondence with German medical authorities throughout April 1962. Taussig Collection.

199 **the clinics saw 302:** "Heroine of FDA Keeps Bad Drug Off Market," *Washington Post*, July 15, 1962.

199 **not a single incident:** Taussig to Colonel Immon, MD, April 19, 1962, Taussig Collection.

199 **asking them to come over:** Dick Smithells, "Teratoserendipity," *Issues and Reviews in Teratology* 7 (1994): 1–36.

199 **He'd given the mother thalidomide:** A few months before that, Somers had proven that thalidomide reduced litter size and increased stillbirths in rats. Magazanik, *Silent Shock*, 232.

199 **short article in a February edition:** "Sleeping Pill Nightmare," *Time*, Feb. 23, 1962.

199 **"the most ghastly thing":** "Deformed Babies Traced to a Drug," *New York Times*, April 12, 1962.

199 **"because officials were suspicious":** Ibid.

200 **she demanded a complete list:** "Medical Analysis of BFA Information on Kevadon Investigational Drug Recall," Frances O. Kelsey, May 31, 1962, FDA Archives.

200 **monkey harmed by MER/29:** Knightley et al., *Suffer the Children*, 93; and "The Mer/29 Investigation," Bureau of Enforcement, June 5, 1962, FDA Archives.

200 **troves of falsified data:** Ibid.

200 **"out of an abundance of caution":** "Richardson-Merrell Is Withdrawing Drug Used on Heart Patients: Side Effects Cited," *Wall Street Journal*, April 17, 1962.

200 **"thorough verification":** Memo from William Kessenich, May 7, 1962, FDA Archives.

200 **"investigators then active with Kevadon":** "Medical Analysis of BFA Information on Kevadon Investigational Drug Recall," Frances O. Kelsey, May 31, 1962, FDA Archives.

201 **"as well as others":** Ibid.

200 **"no positive proof"**: John M. Premi, Medical Director, Merrell "Dear Doctor" letter, Feb. 21, 1962, FDA Archives.

201 **pregnant rats given thalidomide**: Ibid.

201 **More than 1,200 doctors**: "Medical Analysis of BFA Information on Kevadon Investigational Drug Recall," Frances O. Kelsey, May 31, 1962, FDA Archives.

201 **more than 240 of them**: Ibid.

Twenty-four

203 **"These drug fellows pay"**: Harris, *Real Voice*, 47.

205 **sixty-day automatic approval**: Ibid., 121–22.

206 **defend his firm's misleading ads**: Hearings Before the Subcommittee on Antitrust and Monopoly of the Committee on the Judiciary, Drug Industry Antitrust Act, U.S. Senate, Jan. 30, 1962.

206 **"I would prefer to have"**: Ibid., 3105.

206 **"price-fixing and monopolistic practices"**: Eleanor Roosevelt, "My Day," Sept. 8, 1961, *The Eleanor Roosevelt Papers Digital Edition* (2017).

206 **"hidden and serious dangers"**: Ibid.

206 **"recommend improvements in the food"**: "Annual Message to the Congress of the State of the Union," January 11, 1962.

206 **12,885 pages of documented testimony**: Harris, *Real Voice*, 136.

206 **"sincere wish"**: Ibid., 153.

206 **"stir people up"**: Ibid., 71.

207 **"This compound could have passed"**: Robert K. Plumb, "Deformed Babies Traced to a Drug," *New York Times*, April 12, 1962.

Twenty-five

209 **"I have been reviewing the files"**: Letter from Joseph Murray to Dr. von Schrader-Beielstein, Grünenthal, May 1, 1962.

210 **"I am the size"**: Author interview with Peggy Martz Smith.

211 **"The evidence is overwhelming"**: Letter from Helen Taussig to Paul White, April 3, 1962, Taussig Collection.

213 **after the March recall**: The drug was formally withdrawn March 5. Letter from Robert H. Woodward, Merrell, to Dr. H. W. v. Schrader-Beielstein, Chemie Grünenthal, March 12, 1962.

213 **some 10 to 15 percent**: June Callwood, "The Unfolding Tragedy of Drug-Deformed Babies," *Maclean's*, May 19, 1962.

213 **"difficult limitations on analysis"**: Joseph Murray to Taussig, April 30, 1962, Taussig Collection.

213 **"no simple matter"**: Ibid.

214 **"the appropriate way"**: Ibid.

214 **where Flor Van Maanen**: Van Maanen Deposition, 26.

214 **something Warkany had heard**: Letter from A. Ashley Weech to Taussig, April 24, 1962; letter from Knapp to Taussig, May 30, 1962, Taussig Collection.

214 **unduly scaring expectant mothers**: According to Taussig. See letter from Taussig to Mr. Ashley Montagu, July 20, 1962, Taussig Collection.

214 **"We can no longer afford"**: Letter from Joseph Garland, editor, *New England Journal of Medicine*, to Taussig, May 14, 1962, Taussig Collection.

215 **"inventive spirit"**: "Statement of the American Institute of Chemists," New York, May 28, 1962, submitted to Hon. Emanuel Celler, Chairman of the Committee on the Judiciary, House of Representatives, Washington, D.C.

215 **"Dr. Taussig may be"**: Goodman, "Gentle Heart," 76.

215 **3,500 babies so far**: Testimony of Helen Taussig, Hearings Before the Antitrust Subcommittee of the Committee on the Judiciary, U.S. House of Representatives, May 23, 1962.
215 **"There is a baby"**: Ibid.
216 **"normal mentalities"**: Ibid.
216 **"There is nothing you see"**: Ibid.
216 **"A drug cannot be assumed"**: Ibid.
216 **must be a factor**: Ibid.
216 **"one person in the FDA"**: Ibid.
216 **"We ought to do"**: Ibid.

Twenty-six

219 **"When I was born"**: Author interview with Darren Griggs.
220 **"It is chilling to think"**: Handwritten draft, "Commentary on 'Thoughts on Thalidomide,'" 1962, Frances Kelsey Papers.
221 **"greater therapeutic effect"**: Harris, *Real Voice*, 162.
221 **"the Wizard of Ooze"**: "Remembering Everett Dirksen," *Illinois Times*, Aug. 27, 2008.
221 **icing out Kefauver**: Harris, *Real Voice*, 164–65.
221 **"the secret meeting"**: Ibid., 164.
222 **"emasculated a bill"**: Ibid., 168.
222 **"I'm going to the floor"**: Ibid., 169.
222 **"I haven't been so shoddily"**: Ibid., 170.
222 **"Today a severe blow"**: Ibid., 171.
223 **"a mere shadow"**: Ibid., 172.
223 **"I want the people to know"**: Ibid.
223 **"king of kings"**: Ibid, 173.
223 **"He is as single purposed"**: Ibid., 178.
224 **"Don't be too sure"**: Ibid., 184.
224 **"If it hadn't been"**: Ibid.

Twenty-seven

225 **"I am desperately worried"**: Letter from Taussig to Dr. Charles Lowe, June 19, 1962, Taussig Collection.
227 **single out Mintz**: Charles Lewis, *935 Lies: The Future of Truth and the Decline of America's Moral Integrity* (New York: PublicAffairs, 2014), 116.
228 **Her care in a private facility**: Speech presented before the Mental Health Committee of the Missouri Senate, Hotel Mayfair, St. Louis, June 19, 1954, Morton Mintz Personal Archive.
228 **"This little girl of ours"**: Ibid.
229 **"basic rights of humane justice"**: Ibid.
229 **"backwardness and neglect"**: Ibid.
230 **Fishbein had decided**: Author interview with Morton Mintz.

Twenty-eight

231 **"WEARS NO MAKEUP"**: "Dr. Kelsey Would Prefer to Retain Anonymity," *Boston Globe*, Aug. 5, 1962.
232 **"When will our real Mommy be back?"**: Susan Kelsey Duffield, private diary, shared with author.
233 **"Heroine at FDA"**: "Heroine at FDA Keeps Bad Drug Off Market," *Washington Post*, July 15, 1962.

234 **"History is being made"**: Ann G. Sjoerdsma, *Starting With Serotonin* (Silver Spring, Md.: Improbable Books, 2008), 5.

234 **"courage in fighting off"**: Letter from the Dunlaps, Hollywood, California, to Frances Kelsey, July 21, 1962, Frances Kelsey Papers.

234 **"true, honest, integrity"**: Kenneth Luchs, Maryland, to Frances Kelsey, July 15, 1962, Frances Kelsey Papers.

234 **"corruption of public figures"**: Letter from Mrs. Charles L. G., Cleveland, Ohio, to Frances Kelsey, undated, Frances Kelsey Papers.

234 **"heartwarming to know"**: Ibid.

234 **"protect the citizens"**: Ibid.

234 **"IF our civilization survives"**: Letter from Mrs. Dorothy D. L., Washington, D.C., to Frances Kelsey, July 22, 1962, Frances Kelsey Papers.

234 **"big, selfish interests"**: V. B. Dingledine, Oakland, California, to Frances Kelsey, July 30, 1962, Frances Kelsey Papers.

235 **"show Congress how important"**: Mrs. Frances B., Brooklyn, New York, Aug. 2, 1962, Frances Kelsey Papers.

235 **"vote of thanks"**: Morton Mintz, "'Heroine' of FDA Keeps Bad Drug Off Market," *Washington Post*, July 15, 1962.

235 **Kefauver planned to get hold:** Senator Estes Kefauver to Commissioner Larrick, July 18, 1962, FDA Archives.

PART FOUR: THE COST
Twenty-nine

239 **"nerves"**: "The Drug That Left a Trail of Heartbreak," *Life*, Aug. 10, 1962.

239 **"HAVE PATIENT"**: Western Union Telefax to Helen B. Taussig from Edward Sattenspeil, MD, July 24, 1962, Taussig Collection.

239 **"I would strongly recommend"**: Jay Mathews, "25 Years After the Abortion," *Washington Post*, Apr. 27, 1987.

240 **52 percent:** Ibid.

240 **"a crime"**: Ibid.

241 **"abnormal growth"**: Ibid.

241 **"still mere speculation"**: Letter from Carl A. Bunde, Merrell, to Hon. Emanuel Celler, Chairman, Antitrust Subcommittee, June 11, 1962, FDA Archives.

241 **at least eighty-one doctors:** Office of Commissioner, report detailing "number of investigators by state," July 30, 1962, FDA Archives.

241 **"typical phocomelia"**: Frances Kelsey Report on Conversation with Doctor Edith Potter of the Chicago Lying-In Hospital, May 15, 1962, Frances Kelsey Papers.

242 **"no women of childbearing years"**: Arthur Ogden, MD, to Thomas Jones, July 20, 1962, Frances Kelsey Papers.

242 **77 trials in New York:** Office of Commissioner, Bureau of Field Adminstration, "The number of investigators by state . . . ," July 30, 1962, FDA Archives.

242 **"federal red tape"**: "City Seeks Doctors Who Received Drug," *New York World Telegram and Sun*, July 26, 1962.

242 **"because of inquiries"**: Memorandum of Telephone Conversation, July 18, 1962, FDA Archives.

242 **"never sold"**: Press release, William S. Merrell Company, July 20, 1962, FDA Archives.

242 *Cincinnati Enquirer*'s **nearly word-for-word:** "Merrell Firm Clarifies Position on Thalidomide," *Cincinnati Enquirer*, July 29, 1962.

243 **Vick had, in fact:** Memorandum of Telephone Conversation, July 25, 1962, FDA Archives.

243 "actively investigating": "Merrell's Chronology of Kevadon Developments," letter filed with House Antitrust Subcommittee, June 11, 1962, Frances Kelsey Papers.

243 signature thalidomide limb damage: Letter to John Lear of the *Saturday Review*, Sept. 19, 1962; letter from Taussig to Colonel Thomas Inmon, Taussig Collection.

243 at least fifty-six doctors: Memo, "Regarding Dr. Jacobzinger's letter of June 12, 1962," July 6, 1962, FDA Archives.

243 more than five thousand birth malformations: Memorandum of Telephone Conversation between Jerome Trichter, City of New York Health Department, and Charles Orr, Division of Federal and State Relations, July 19, 1962, FDA Archives.

243 SKF had shipped the sedative: Letter from Walter A. Munns, SKF, to Commissioner Larrick, July 31, 1962, FDA Archives.

244 SKF told Commissioner Larrick: Ibid.

244 the story that Merrell had 1,200: Harris, *Real Voice*, 188.

244 In Philadelphia, nearly one hundred: Memo from Philadelphia District to Bureau of Field Administration, Aug. 6, 1962, FDA0120, FDA Archives.

244 "doses of thalidomide": Memo of telephone conversation, July 30, 1962, FDA Archives.

244 "a great deal of pressure": Memo of telephone conversation, July 31, 1962, FDA Archives.

244 no abnormal births: "Abnormal Birth Probe Heartens Celebrezze: No Evidence Found Yet of Ill Effects in America from Drug Thalidomide," *Pittsburgh Post-Gazette*, Aug. 8, 1962.

245 "deformed": "Baby Deformed by Thalidomide Born in New York," Associated Press, July 31, 1962.

245 Merrell's widespread Kevadon trials: "Baby Deformed by Thalidomide Born in New York: Drug Samples in 39 States," *Beckley Post-Herald* (Beckley, West Virginia), via the Associated Press, July 31, 1962.

245 "at the appropriate time": Edmund R. Beckwith Jr. to Commissioner Larrick, report of telegram to Department of Health, City of New York, July 26, 1962, Frances Kelsey Papers.

245 "no causal relationship": "Dear Doctor" letter from Thomas Jones of Merrell, March 20, 1962, FDA Archives.

245 they could keep dispensing: Letter from Joseph Murray to Frances Kelsey, April 25, 1962, FDA Archives.

245 "intensive effort": The firm's "intensive effort recall and follow up" noted in Western Union Telegram from Edmund R. Beckwith Jr. to Commissioner George P. Larrick, July 26, 1962, FDA0181, FDA Archives.

246 "In view of the great public": "Inspection Assignment," Fred Lovsfold, District Director, July 31, 1962, FDA Archives.

Thirty

247 "DRUG MAN DOUBTS DANGER": *Washington Post*, July 29, 1962.

248 "There are people whose opinions": Testimony of Commissioner Larrick and Frances Kelsey cited is reprinted in the *Interagency Coordination in Drug Research and Regulation*, report for the Senate Subcommittee on Reorganizations and International Organizations of the Committee on Government Operations, Aug. 1 and 9, 1962.

250 "the skin of its teeth": Ibid.

250 "Later": Ibid.

250 "We are now checking": Ibid.

250 "In 1959 my wife": Ibid.
251 forty-four hospitals had been enlisted: Ibid.
251 more than six thousand hospitals nationwide: Ibid.
251 "the commercial distribution of thalidomide": Ibid.
251 Fifty-six physicians in New York: Ibid.
252 "This is a loophole": Ibid.
252 "I think the firm proceeded": Ibid.
252 "We rarely have": Ibid.
252 "I think we do, yes": Ibid. (Larrick acknowledged, however, that within the past few days, the FDA had discovered stray thalidomide on the market.)
253 "My understanding was": Ibid.
253 "the clear-cut authority": Ibid.
253 "an expert qualified": Ibid.
254 "Yes": Ibid.
254 "fine South Dakotan": Ibid.
254 "the drug was given": Ibid

Thirty-one

257 MERRELL WINS CLEARANCE: "Merrell Wins Clearance in Thalidomide Inquiry," *Cincinnati Enquirer*, Aug. 2, 1962.
258 "It was determined": James Nakada Oral History, FDA Oral History Interview, June 16, 1982, 8.
259 half of the listed investigators: Memorandum on "Recall of Thalidomide," Buffalo District to Bureau of Field Administration, Aug. 1, 1962, FDA Archives.
259 where eighty-eight doctors: U.S. Government Memorandum, Chicago District to Bureau of Field Administration, Aug. 1, 1962, FDA Archives.
260 several hundred pills to pregnant women: U.S. Government Memorandum, Seattle District to Administration, Aug. 2, 1962, FDA Archives.
260 "charity out-patients": Ibid.
260 "a cursory examination": Memo from Director, Baltimore District, to Inspector L. M. Carter, Raleigh, North Carolina, Aug. 30, 1962, FDA Archives.
260 "born without arms and legs": Memo from Baltimore District to Bureau of Field Administration, Aug. 2, 1962, FDA Archives.
260 one of his six subjects: FDA Report of interview with Dr. Trent Busby, July 31, 1962, Frances Kelsey Papers.
260 "under the circumstances": Report by Donald A. Schiemann, Inspector, Atlanta District, FDA, Aug. 9, 1962, Frances Kelsey Papers.
260 FDA representatives made contact: "U.S. Finds 67 More Doctors with Supplies of Thalidomide," *New York Times*, Aug. 3, 1962.
260 Sixty-seven of them still: Ibid.
261 "none have been traced": "Man Humbled by Thalidomide Fiasco," *Cincinnati Enquirer*, Aug. 5, 1962.
261 "absolved of blame": Ibid.
261 The unnamed doctor: Handwritten memo notes Ray Nulsen as being the doctor referenced in the *Cincinnati Enquirer* article. FDA Archives.
261 eighty-one women in the third trimester: Memorandum, Cincinnati District to Bureau of Field Administration, Aug. 21, 1962, FDA Archives.
261 denied giving the drug: "Confidential Administrative," memo of telephone conversation between Richard E. Williams, Merrell, and T. C. Maraviglia, Director, Cincinnati District, Aug. 17, 1962, FDA Archives.
261 "ulterior motives": Handwritten memo, Tom Rice to Beckwith, ca. Aug. 1962, FDA Archives.

261 **"aggressive"**: "Confidential Administrative," Cincinnati District to Bureau of Field Administration, Aug. 16, 1962, FDA1378, FDA Archives.

261 **they were interrupted:** Memorandum describing visit to the mother, Aug. 16, 1962, FDA Archives.

262 **"used the drug"**: "Confidential Administrative," memo of telephone conversation, Aug. 17, 1962, FDA Archives.

262 **he'd given thalidomide:** Memorandum, Cincinnati District to Bureau of Field Administration, Aug. 21, 1962, FDA Archives.

262 **"strange things"**: Memorandum, Cincinnati District to Bureau of Field Administration, Aug. 21, 1962, FDA Archives.

262 **"very emphatic"**: Ibid.

262 **"Cincinnati Baby's Death"**: *Cincinnati Post and Times-Star*, Aug. 21, 1961.

262 **"extremely frank"**: Ibid.

263 **207 pregnant women:** Ibid.

263 **Larrick acknowledged:** Memo of telephone conversation between Pat Boyso, Station WKRC, Cincinnati, and T. C. Maraviglia, Director, Cincinnati District, Aug. 10, 1962, FDA Archives.

263 **eight hundred tablets:** Memo of telephone conversation between Sharon Maloney, *Cincinnati Post and Times-Star*, and George Meeks, Assistant to the Director, Cincinnati District, Aug. 9, 1962, FDA Archives.

263 **"when a physician stated"**: "Thalidomide," Memo from A. T. Rayfield to George Larrick, Sept. 20, 1962, FDA Archives.

263 **"What a terrible thing"**: Author interview with Ann Morris (pseudonym).

Thirty-two

265 **"August 9, 1962"**: Letter from Truman Felt to Director, Division of Public Information, FDA, Aug. 9, 1962, FDA Archives.

267 **"fuss and feathers"**: "Modest Heroine," *Newsmakers*, Sept. 1962, 11, Frances Kelsey Papers.

267 **"She does not use cosmetics"**: "Dr. Kelsey Receives Gold Medal from Kennedy at White House," *New York Times*, Aug. 8, 1962.

268 **"President's Amendments"**: Memo from Wilbur Cohen referring to "the adoption of the President's amendments by the full committee," April 13, 1962, transcribed in Theodore Ellenbogen Oral History, March 1974, FDA.gov.

268 **She told the committee to restore:** "Dr. Kelsey Calls for Tighter Restrictions on Drugs as Senate Hearings Open," *New York Times*, Aug. 6, 1962.

268 **"This is a very good drug bill"**: Harris, *Real Voice*, 206.

268 **"Tablets of thalidomide"**: U.S. Department of Health, Education, and Welfare, press release, Aug. 23, 1962; Congressional Record: Drug Coordination, 248.

268 **2.5 million tablets:** HEW press release, Aug. 23, 1962.

269 **"That does it, gentlemen"**: Harris, *Real Voice*, 210.

269 **"The Senator from Tennessee"**: A *Legislative History of the Federal Food, Drug, and Cosmetic Act and Its Amendments* (Washington, D.C.: Department of Health, Education and Welfare, Public Health Service, Food and Drug Administration, 1979), 350.

Thirty-three

271 **"The slender Dr. Kelsey"**: "Dr. Kelsey, Heroine," *Catholic Standard*, Aug. 10, 1962.

272 **"Our problem is this"**: Bureau of Field Administration to Dr. Glenn Slocum, London, England, Sept. 25, 1962, FDA Archives.

273 **"macerated":** FDA Report of interview with Dr. Trent Busby, July 31, 1962, Frances Kelsey Papers.

273 **they mailed him a form letter:** Ibid.

273 **Busby had leveled with:** Ibid.

274 **"What company official evaluated":** Draft of Memo to James Nakada, undated, Frances Kelsey Papers.

274 **"investigated exhaustively":** Ibid.

274 **"ten-foot pole":** FDA Report of interview with Dr. Trent Busby, July 31, 1962, Frances Kelsey Papers.

274 **No cautions had been issued:** Ibid.

274 **"an expert qualified by scientific training":** Federal Food, Drug, and Cosmetic Act, approved June 25, 1938.

275 **at least 15,000 Americans:** "Thalidomide Pills Used by 15,000 Americans," *Brockton Daily Enterprise*, Aug. 8, 1962, FDA Archives.

275 **"Some American women":** Carl A. Bunde, "A U.S. Drug Firm's Shock," *Life*, Aug. 10, 1962.

275 **only sixty-seven doctors:** Letter from Walter A. Munns, Smith, Kline, & French Laboratories, to Commissioner Larrick, July 31, 1962, FDA Archives.

275 **"for use in older patients":** Bunde, "A U.S. Drug Firm's Shock."

275 **specialized in obstetrics and gynecology:** "Medical Analysis of BFA Information on Kevadon Investigational Drug Recall," Frances O. Kelsey, May 31, 1962, FDA Archives.

275 **"Within hours":** Bunde, "A U.S. Drug Firm's Shock."

276 **Merrell's fabricated defense:** Ayer, N.W., and Son, eds., *N.W. Ayer and Son's Directory [of] Newspapers and Periodicals*, 80th ed. (Philadelphia: N. W. Ayer and Son, 1962).

276 **"Exclusive: First Photos":** *National Enquirer*, Aug. 12, 1962.

276 **vast quantities of the drug:** "For Immediate Release," Aug. 23, 1962, FDA Archives.

277 **A hospital in Texas:** "Comment: Regarding Dallas District Report August 2, 1962," Frances Kelsey to James Nakada, FDA, Sept. 17, 1962, Frances Kelsey Papers.

277 **A Nebraska doctor:** "For Immediate Release," U.S. Department of Health, Education, and Welfare, Aug. 23. 1962, FDA Archives.

277 **a Missouri doctor:** Ibid.

277 **one New York physician:** "Costs of Malpractice Insurance on Increase for Physicians Here," *New York Times*, Aug. 25, 1962.

277 **under the name "Contergan":** Letter from Miller J. Sullivan, Director of Pharmaceutical Research, National Drug Company, to Commissioner Larrick, Aug. 22, 1962, FDA Archives.

277 **National Drug had sent the drug:** "Review of File on National Drug Company Investigation of Contergan (thalidomide)—NDA 12-711," Sept. 26, 1962, FDA Archives.

277 **other Richardson-Merrell subsidiaries:** Walker Labs of Mount Vernon, New York, National Drug Company of Philadelphia, Pennsylvania, and Vick Chemical of Mount Vernon, New York, were all "subsidiaries of Richardson-Merrell and all distributed thalidomide for investigational use." J. T. Baker of Phillipsburg, New Jersey, also "a Richardson-Merrell subsidiary, manufactured the bulk of the chemical in the United States under a license from Chemie Grunenthal." Memorandum from Bureau of Field Adminstration to Dr. Glenn Slocum, Sept. 25, 1962, FDA Archives.

277 **Smith, Kline & French trials:** "Thalidomide Investigation," Memo from James Nakada, Aug. 3, 1962, FDA Archives.

277 **in different colors and dosages:** "Thalidomide Dosage Forms," attachment to letter from Frederick J. Pilgrim, Merrell, Aug. 22, 1962, FDA Archives.

277 **At least 19,822 Americans:** "For Immediate Release," U.S. Department of Health, Education, and Welfare, Aug. 23, 1962, FDA Archives.

278 **"a matter of traditional medical confidence":** "To All Physicians," letter from Frank N. Getman, President, Merrell, Aug. 10, 1962, FDA Archives.

278 **"could not in good conscience":** Ibid.

278 **"would unnecessarily alarm":** Letter from Larrick to Kefauver, Aug. (day illegible), 1962, FDA Archives.

278 **"misleading to the public":** Memorandum of Interview, Dr. E. Wayles Browne, L. Lawrence Warden, FDA, and Robert C. Brandenburg, FDA, Aug. 16, 1962, FDA Archives.

278 **She discovered that:** Memorandum from Frances Kelsey to Winton Rankin, Assistant Commissioner, Sept. 10, 1962, Frances Kelsey Papers.

278 **Nine of these:** Memo from Frederick Garfield, Sept. 24, 1962, FDA Archives.

278 **an inverted kidney:** Letter from Commissioner Larrick to Dr. Jerome Trichter, Department of Health, New York, Dec. 12, 1962, FDA Archives.

279 **Maryland Department of Health:** Letter from Dr. Muriel Wolf at Harriet Lane Home to Dr. Edward Davens, Deputy Commissioner of the Maryland State Health Department, with handwritten postscript by Taussig, Aug. 30, 1962, Frances Kelsey Papers.

279 **"no basis for action":** Memo from Bureau of Field Administration to Bureau of Medicine, Subject: "Phocomelia Case," Oct. 24, 1962, Frances Kelsey Papers.

279 **the agency refused:** Memo from Bureau of Field Administration to Frances Kelsey, Oct. 19, 1962, FDA Archives.

279 **praise Merrell had been:** An Aug. 10, 1962, mailing from Merrell president Frank Getman to "all physicians in the United States" claimed that "following the hearing, Senator Hubert Humphrey, Chairman of the Subcommittee, told the Associated Press that Merrell had acted responsibly throughout and 'complied with every regulation.'" FDA Archives.

279 **"crash program":** "Too Much Too Soon? Manual Reveals Early Plan to Push Thalidomide," *Washington Star*, Sept. 16, 1962.

280 **580 kilograms:** In "The Unfinished Story of Thalidomide," *Saturday Review*, Sept. 1, 1962, John Lear, citing the 5,300 kilograms of raw thalidomide that Merrell manufactured or imported, suggests that Merrell distributed roughly 20 million pills. But Lear did not account for the 1,462 kilograms of bulk thalidomide that Merrell had shipped to Canada and the amounts allotted to animal research. "Thalidomide," Memorandum, Aug. 1, 1962, FDA Archives.

280 **"manufacturing loss":** "Thalidomide," Memorandum, Aug. 1, 1962, FDA Archives.

280 **double the FDA public estimate:** Based on a 75–100 mg daily dose, per published studies on Kevadon.

280 **discovering stocks of thalidomide:** "U.S. Finds Stores Got Thalidomide: Says Barred Drug Reached Many Pharmacy Shelves," *New York Times*, Aug. 31, 1962.

280 **a concerned director of pharmacy:** Memo of telephone conversation between Mr. Simon, Director of Pharmacy, Lenox Hill Hospital, and T. E. Byers, Chief Chemist, New York District, Dec. 31, 1962, FDA Archives.

280 **"failed to make full disclosure":** Memo from Bureau of Field Administration to Dr. Glenn Slocum, London, England, "Thalidomide Investigation," Sept. 25, 1962, FDA Archives.

280 **missing from Merrell's offices:** Ibid.

280 **"gone over":** Ibid.

280 **interoffice memos since 1960:** ". . . an almost total absence of memoranda of telephone conversations or interoffice memoranda subsequent to 1960, while the

files had many such memoranda for the year 1969." See memo from Ralph W. Weilerstein, Associate Medical Director, to the Bureau of Medicine, Sept. 4, 1962, FDA Archives.

280 **if Merrell had broken the law:** "Priority Assignment," Bureau of Field Administration to Director of Districts, Oct. 3, 1962, FDA Archives.

280 **"false and misleading assurances":** Ibid.

280 **"The investigations will require tact":** Ibid.

281 **"catapulted unwillingly":** "Deformed Babies Still Arriving," *Cincinnati Enquirer*, Nov. 24, 1962.

281 **"The United States escaped":** "Exclusive: The Untold Story of the Thalidomide Babies," *Saturday Evening Post*, Oct. 20, 1962.

281 **"swallowed as many":** Ibid., 20.

281 **"the reputations of both":** *BusinessWeek*, Sept. 15, 1962.

Thirty-four

283 **"Q: Did you ever call":** Deposition of James Rhea, *McCarrick v. Richardson-Merrell*, Superior Court for the State of California, for the County of Los Angeles. Case No. 882,426, 29, March 4, 1971.

285 **three out of four Americans:** "What America Thinks: Stricter Drug Control Needed, Poll Reveals," *Sunday Star*, Aug. 13, 1962.

285 *Newsweek* **opinion piece:** Henry Hazlitt, "Overregulation," *Newsweek*, Sept. 10, 1962, 86.

285 **"recent flurry":** Howard A. Rusk, MD, "Drug-Test Regulations: U.S. Proposals Innocuous on Surface, but Lowering of Standards Is Feared," *New York Times*, Sept. 16, 1962.

285 **"The thalidomide incident":** Ibid.

285 **launching a save-thalidomide campaign:** "Drug Panic and Its Aftermath," *Medical Tribune*, Aug. 27, 1962.

285 **"too valuable a drug to lose":** "Scientists Fear New Drug Laws," *New York Times*, Aug. 26, 1962.

285 **"thalidomide hysteria":** Letter from Louis Lasagna to Helen Taussig, Oct. 8, 1962, Taussig Collection.

285 **"reasonable and feasible":** Ibid.

285 **"cruel":** Letter from Louis Lasagna to Helen Taussig, Oct. 8, 1962, Taussig Collection.

285 **Helen Taussig blasted:** Letter from Taussig to Dr. Louis C. Lasagna, Sept. 27, 1962, Taussig Collection.

286 **red tape would dissuade:** Letter from Dr. Howard A. Rusk to Taussig, Oct. 5, 1962, Taussig Collection.

286 **Texas doctor had notified:** Letter from Taussig to Dr. Cornelius S. Meeker, Oct. 5, 1962, Taussig Collection.

286 **"I am told that not only":** Letter from Taussig to Frances Kelsey, July 8, 1963, Taussig Collection.

286 **"Do you know whether":** Ibid.

287 **"unexplained crop":** John Lear, "The Unfinished Story of Thalidomide," *Saturday Review*, Sept. 1, 1962, 38.

287 **no special training in pharmacology:** Memo of telephone conversation, Kenneth Lennington, Oct. 8, 1962, FDA Archives.

288 **"The thalidomide scandal":** Congressman Leo O'Brien, quoted in Harris, *Real Voice*, 239–40.

288 **"You played the most important part":** Ibid., 201.

Thirty-five

289 **"My mother's doctor"**: Author interview with Tawana Williams.

291 **still advocating for follow-up**: "Thalidomide Investigation," Memo from Kenneth Lennington, Nov. 9, 1962, FDA Archives.

291 **"false and misleading"**: "Thalidomide Investigation Summary," Memorandum of Conference, Nov. 16, 1962, FDA Archives.

291 **suppressed data**: Ibid.

291 **Multiple doctors**: "Thalidomide Investigations," "Confidential Administrative," Oct. 13, 1962, and Oct. 11, 1962, FDA Archives.

292 **the firm had intervened to delay**: "Accompanying this memo is a paper on thalidomide polyneuropathy by Dr. Sidney Cohen which was submitted to the AMA. I hope we can effectively prevent publication of this until we have obtained an effective NDA." Inter-Department Memo from Thomas L. Jones to F. J. Murray, Subject: "Paper by Dr. Sidney Cohen," Oct. 31, 1961.

292 **Children's Home of Cincinnati**: "Confidential Administrative," Bureau of Field Administration, Nov. 8, 1962, FDA Archives.

292 **"I kept inquiring about it"**: Theodore C. Maraviglia and Philip Brodsky Oral History, FDA Oral History Interview, Sept. 11, 1981, 26.

292 **"the reputation of the William S. Merrell Company"**: Letter from G. S. Goldhammer, Assistant Director for Regulatory Operations, Bureau of Regulatory Compliance, to Mr. James W. Knapp, Special Attorney at the U.S. Courthouse in Washington, May 22, 1964, FDA Archives.

292 **Someone in the agency's Bureau**: Ibid.

292 **"difficulties in our enforcement work"**: Ibid.

292 **"sufficiently strong or clear"**: Letter from Herbert J. Miller, Jr., Assistant Attorney General, Criminal Division, U.S. Department of Justice, to William W. Goodrich, Assistant General Counsel, Department of Health, Education, and Welfare, Sept. 21, 1964, FDA Archives.

293 **"only to physicians"**: Ibid.

293 **"as far as is known"**: Ibid.

293 **"it would be difficult to prove"**: Ibid.

293 **Five additional cases**: Letter from John L. Harvey, Deputy Commissioner, FDA, Dec. 10, 1964, FDA Archives.

293 **at least three civil cases**: *Diamond v. William S. Merrell*, filed Oct. 4, 1962; *Blachman v. Richardson-Merrell, Inc.*, filed Nov. 28, 1962. Riechmann & Ruberg filed their suits against Ray O. Nulsen in May and September 1963, followed by suits against Merrell filed in December 1964.

293 **"obviate a recurrence"**: Letter from William W. Goodrich, Assistant General Counsel at the United States Department of Justice, to Herbert J. Miller, Jr., Assistant Attorney General, Criminal Division, Sept. 21, 1964, FDA1320, FDA Archives.

293 **"Not correct"**: Ibid.

293 **"the figures for Kevadon"**: Ibid.

294 **"inexcusably bad"**: Helen Taussig to Edward Madeira, Jr., Nov. 27, 1964, Taussig Collection.

294 **FDA field offices discussed**: "Investigation of Dr. Nulsen," Memorandum of Telephone Conversation between Mr. Maraviglia, Director, Cincinnati District, and F. R. Herron, Division of Field Operations, Oct. 26, 1964, FDA Archives.

294 **"We need evidence to show"**: "Investigation of Dr. Nulsen Re: Possible Title 18, Section 10001 Violation," Oct. 20, 1964, FDA Archives.

294 **"some 40 infants born"**: "Investigation of Dr. Nulsen," Memorandum of Telephone Conversation between Mr. Maraviglia, Director, Cincinnati District, and F. R. Herron, Division of Field Operations, Oct. 23, 1964, FDA Archives.

294 **Justice Department remained firm:** An FOIA request submitted to the DOJ in 2019 to release all and any records pertaining to the decision not to prosecute Merrell was "in process" for over two years and finally resulted in zero records.

294 **"closed hearing":** Memorandum of Phone Call between T. C. Margavalia, Director, Cincinnati District, and Jack Smith, reporter, *Cincinnati Enquirer*, April 14, 1964, FDA Archives.

294 **"been done so much harm":** Theodore C. Maraviglia and Philip Brodsky Oral History, FDA Oral History Interview, Sept. 11, 1981, 27.

295 **Fifteen hundred claims:** Fine, *Great Drug Deception*, 181.

295 **"Impossible":** American Trial Lawyers Association 1969 Midwinter Meeting. Rheingold, Paul D., and Dennis L. Kripke. American Trial Lawyers Association, 1969, Midwinter Meeting, San Francisco, California. Edited by Dennis L Runyan, The W. H. Anderson Company, 1970, 656.

295 **an official Kevadon investigator:** Charles H. Brown.

296 **"Here is a man":** Court transcript, *Diamond v. William S. Merrell Co. and Richardson-Merrell, Inc.*, Eastern District of Pennsylvania, CV 62-0032132, filed Oct. 4, 1969, 149.

296 **the firm had buried:** *Sunday Times* Insight Team, *Suffer the Children*, 175.

296 **$6,000 settlement:** This is about $50,000 today. *Sunday Times* Insight Team, *Suffer the Children*, 176.

296 **"bad, bad people":** Author interview with Michael Dan, second chair to Jim Butler in the McCarrick trial.

296 **2,700 pills:** Deposition of Isadore Weinstein, Feb. 19, 1971, *McCarrick v. Richardson-Merrell*.

297 **total of thirteen civil suits:** "Thalidomide: The American Experience," *New York Times*, April 29, 1973.

297 **"No one can be sure":** Ibid.

297 **"evidence that an 'excess' ":** Ibid.

297 **"no government charges":** David Diamond transcript, 49.

297 **"facts developed":** Memo from Van W. Smart, Bureau of Enforcement, to Cincinnati District, Dec. 11, 1962, FDA Archives.

297 **"promotional literature on Kevadon":** Letter from Van W. Smart, Bureau of Enforcement, to Mr. Nathaniel B. Richter, Lichter, Levy, Lord, Toll & Cavanaugh, Oct. 9, 1962, FDA Archives.

297 **"blue pills in an unlabeled bottle":** Letter to Frances Kelsey, sender's name redacted, received Aug. 12, 1968, FDA Archives.

297 **"not be revealed under the law":** Letter from Bernard T. Loftus, Bureau of Regulatory Compliance, recipient's name redacted, Aug. 21, 1968, FDA Archives.

298 **Eleven years of negotiations:** Morton Mintz, "She's 19, Deformed, and Family Is Suing Thalidomide Maker," *Washington Post*, Nov. 15, 1980.

298 **"McKenna is probably":** Mary McGrory, "Justice and Thalidomide," *Washington Post*, Oct. 21, 1986.

298 **the mother couldn't name:** "Findings of Fact and Conclusions of Law," Case No. 1:88CV4638, United States District Court, Northern District of Ohio, Eastern Division, Aug. 9, 1995.

298 **"legal era":** "Last Thalidomide Suits Settle to End Legal Era," *National Law Journal*, July 30, 1984.

Thirty-six

299 **"I would first like to say":** Druin Burch, *Taking the Medicine: A Short History of Medicine's Beautiful Idea, and Our Difficulty Swallowing It* (London: Random House, 2009), 211.

301 **Police raids were needed:** Harold Evans, "Thalidomide: How Men Who Blighted Lives of Thousands Evaded Justice," *The Guardian*, Nov. 14, 2014.

301 **The prosecution had assembled:** Ibid.

301 **Five thousand case histories:** Ibid.

301 **four hundred coplaintiffs:** Ibid.

302 *eight hundred* **letters:** Schulte-Hillen, "My Search," 102.

302 **"I thank you":** Ibid.

303 **coordinated gymnastics and writing lessons:** Author interview with Linde Schulte-Hillen.

303 **"Nothing matters":** Schulte-Hillen, "My Search," 101.

303 **Karl wanted the Grünenthal executives:** "The Thalidomide Generation," *Life*, July 26, 1968, 62. Karl is quoted as saying, "They should be sentenced to jail as a reminder to all other drug makers."

303 **"Higher! Faster!":** Ibid.

303 **"discontinued":** "West German Thalidomide Trial Ends; $27-Million to Go to Deformed Children," *New York Times*, Dec. 19, 1970.

304 **"conscientious and careful":** Ibid.

305 **"I hope you're not going":** Brynner and Stephens, *Dark Remedy*, 81.

305 **In fact, the British government:** "We have decided to make Distaval and Companion Products available to hospitals on request throughout the UK." "Distaval: Confidential," letter to Bill Poole, Dec. 22, 1961; "Thalidomide Still Used in U.K. Under Rigid Hospital Conditions," *Medical Tribune*, Oct. 15, 1962.

305 **"great thoroughness":** "Thalidomide Tests Showed No Sign of Danger," *Sunday Times*, Aug. 1, 1962, 6.

305 **The reporter who wrote:** Brynner and Stephens, *Dark Remedy*, 82.

306 **"legal cocoon":** Harold Evans, *My Paper Chase: True Stories of Vanished Times* (New York: Little, Brown, and Company, 2009), 360.

306 **The team purchased:** Harold Evans, *Good Times, Bad Times: The Explosive Inside Story of Rupert Murdoch* (New York: Open Road Media, 2011), 89.

306 **a pharmacologist who had access:** "During the thalidomide investigation, the *Sunday Times* received pivotal Distillers documents from a whistleblower called Dr Montague Phillips." "Interview: Harold Evans: Whistleblowers, Papers, and Why the Truth-Seekers Are Still Vital," *The Guardian*, Jan. 9, 2016.

According to Phillip Knightley: "One cheque was to Henning Sjostrom, a leading Stockholm lawyer who had approached the paper in 1967 with an offer we could not refuse. He had represented the 105 Swedish children against thalidomide's Swedish distributor and had gained access to the documents that the German authorities had seized from Chemie Grunenthal when mounting the case. No German newspaper could publish them because of contempt of court, but a British paper could. Sjostrom wanted to be paid for the documents—his agent proposed pounds 2,500.

"The other went to Dr Montagu Phillips, a consulting pharmacologist and chemical engineer who had been engaged by the solicitors representing the English families to act as a professional adviser. As part of the legal process of 'discovery' the solicitors had been able to obtain all Distillers' files on thalidomide and had passed them to Phillips. Outraged by what he read, Phillips had waited for his moment in court but the years passed and it looked as if the case would never be heard. Harold Evans hesitated, but after weighing the inevitable accusations of 'chequebook journalism' against the public interest in telling the story, he eventually offered Phillips pounds 8,000." Phillip Knightley, "A Battle Won Late: Phillip Knightley Was Part of the Celebrated *Sunday Times* Team Which Exposed the Thalidomide Scandal. His Memoirs Give a New Slant to an Old Story," *The Independent*, Aug. 24, 1997.

306 **"Our Thalidomide Children"**: "Our Thalidomide Children: A Cause for National Shame," *Sunday Times*, Sept. 24, 1972.

307 **"face up to their moral responsibilities"**: "British Dispute over Thalidomide Cases Intensifies," *New York Times*, Nov. 18, 1972.

307 **emergency company shareholder vote**: Brian Cashinella, "Distillers to Raise 20m Compensation Offer for Thalidomide Children," *Sunday Times*, Jan. 6, 1973, 6.

307 **the 62 families who had sued**: Brynner and Stephens, *Dark Remedy*, 107.

307 **Sedatives like Miltown**: Sunday Insight Team, *Suffer the Children*, 71, 77.

307 **By 1962**: "Thalidomide Toll Placed at 10,000: West German Survey Finds 5,000 Infants Still Alive," *New York Times*, Aug. 30, 1962.

307 **about half dying shortly**: Ibid.

308 **as high as 150,000**: thalidomidesociety.org/what-is-thalidomide/; Johnson, Stokes, and Arndt, *Thalidomide Catastrophe*, 30–31.

308 **Spain, which had only**: "Spain Finally Recognizes Thalidomide Victims," *British Medical Journal*, Aug. 10, 2010.

308 **Italy was similarly negligent**: *Thalidomide Catastrophe*, 180.

308 **one-time top-off**: Ben Hirschler, "Thalidomide Victims Seek Compensation, 50 Years On," Reuters, April 4, 2008.

309 **Schedule IV controlled substance**: "DEA Classifies Tramadol as a Schedule IV Controlled Substance," *Pharmacy Times*, Aug. 21, 2014.

309 **"a global leader"**: grunenthal.com, accessed Aug. 31, 2022.

309 **Grünenthal currently generates**: Grünenthal Group, "Grünenthal Agrees to Acquire European Rights to CRESTOR™ (Rosuvastatin) from AstraZeneca," Dec. 1, 2020, press release, available at www.grunenthal.com/en/press-room/press-releases/2020/gruenenthal-agrees-to-acquire-european-rights-to-crestor.

309 **"Thalidomide is and will always be"**: Scott Hensley, "Thalidomide Maker Apologizes after More Than 50 Years," NPR, Aug. 31, 2012.

310 **"Put your money"**: Ben Quinn, "Thalidomide Campaigners Dismiss Manufacturer's 'Insulting' Apology," *The Guardian*, Sept. 1, 2012.

310 **"A lie wrapped in an apology"**: Harold Evans, "Thalidomide's Big Lie Overshadows Corporate Apology," Reuters, Sept. 12, 2012.

310 **Grünenthal had secretly orchestrated**: Harold Evans, "Documents Raise Fresh Questions About Thalidomide Criminal Trial," Reuters, Nov. 14, 2013.

310 **seen "a packaging unit"**: "The management knew about the intrauterine effect of the preparation at the latest by mid-Oct. The decision to carry on selling the preparation was without any doubt motivated by profit making and criminal in my view." Ibid.

310 **"conspiracy theorists"**: Grünenthal describes a "conspiracy theory created by British activists to develop claims for compensation against the German federal government." "The History of the Thalidomide Tragedy," Grünenthal website, available at www.thalidomide-tragedy.com/en/the-history-of-the-thalidomide-tragedy.

310 **"The government and the prosecution"**: Ibid.

311 **"generally supported"**: "Our Responsibility: How Grünenthal Supports People Affected by Thalidomide," Grünenthal website, available at www.thalidomide-tragedy.com/how-grunenthal-currently-provides-support-to-thalidomide-affected-people.

311 **"Financial support programmes"**: grunenthal.com.

311 **"Thalidomide was not sold"**: "Thalidomide: The Active Substance in Contergan, and Its Consequences," Grünenthal website, available at www.thalidomide-tragedy.com/thalidomide-the-active-substance-in-contergan-and-its-consequences.

Thirty-seven

313   **"Is anyone here"**: Posted to "Stop the Tears" Facebook group, Sept. 2011.
314   **"HELLO: MY NAME IS GLENDA JOHNSON"**: Glenda Johnson comment, Aug. 24, 2010, on "Thalidomide Victims Seek $6.3 Billion," *Insurance Journal*, April 3, 2008, available at www.insurancejournal.com/news/international/2008 /04/03/88808.htm?comments#comment-168175.
315   **"I Would Choose My Life"**: Eileen Cronin-Noe, "I Would Choose My Life," *Washington Post*, June 28, 1987.
315   **"It did make its way"**: Ibid.
316   **A Dominican nun**: Author interview with Sister Mary Davyd Deerwester.
316   **"deeper coverage"**: Eileen Cronin and Michelle Botwin Raphael, "Born Without Arms or Legs: The Secret Legacy of Thalidomide," *Huffington Post*, Aug. 21, 2014.
316   **Hagens Berman had filed**: "Hagens Berman Adds Five Cases to Thalidomide Litigation," Hagens Berman website, Aug. 12, 2013, available at hbsslaw.com/press /thalidomide/hagens-berman-adds-five-cases-to-thalidomide-litigation.
318   **The lawsuit had amassed**: The final number was fifty-two. *Glenda Johnson v. Smithkline Beecham Corporation*, U.S. District Court for the Eastern District of Pennsylvania, Case No. 2:11-cv-005782-PD.
320   **"They were amazed"**: Author interview with C. Jean Grover.
320   **"I liked sex"**: Ibid.
320   **"It's a strange irony"**: Ibid.
321   **"All my life"**: Author interview with Sarah Grover.
323   **"I didn't sign anything!"**: Author interview with Gwen Riechmann.
325   **"The maternity described here"**: Ethel Roskies, *Abnormality and Normality: The Mothering of Thalidomide Children* (Ithaca, NY: Cornell University Press, 1972), xi.
326   **behavior was so unsettling**: Ibid., 58.
326   **A nun offered**: Ibid., 86.
326   **But months later**: Ibid., 53.
327   **"this weird solidifying thing"**: Author interview with Jane Gibbons.
327   **"The tribe needs me"**: Ibid.
329   **medically identify formerly unrecognized victims**: "US Lawsuit Extends Thalidomide's Reach," *Nature* 479, Nov. 9, 2011.
330   **still clearly recalls**: Author interview with Donald Firestone.
330   **In fact, the one known victim**: "Summary of Abnormal Infants Associated with Thalidomide," Sept. 19, 1962, Frances Kelsey Papers.
330   **"the cost of pursuing such a claim"**: Letter from Lopez McHugh, LLP, Attorneys and Counselors at Law, to Kimberly Arndt, Jan. 2, 2014, Kimberly Arndt Personal Papers.
331   **One woman reportedly had her computer confiscated**: Author interview with Glenda Johnson.
331   **"was done on a very casual basis"**: Deposition of Written Questions of Gordon R. Forrer, MD, Oct. 1, 2014, *Glenda Johnson, et al. v. SmithKline Beecham Corporation, et al.*, United States District Court for the Eastern District of Pennsylvania, Case No. 2:11-CV-05782-PD.
331   **"I nearly fell down"**: Ibid.
331   **Presiding judge**: "Hagens Berman: U.S. Judge Rejects Pharmaceutical Companies' Attempt to Dismiss Thalidomide Cases," *Businesswire* via *The Motley Fool*, Sept. 27, 2013.
332   **"bad faith and dishonesty"**: Lisa Ryan, "Hagens Berman Sanctioned for Bad Thalidomide Suits," Law360.com, March 9, 2015.
332   **benefited "only Hagens Berman (not its clients)"**: *Johnson v. Smithkline Beecham Corp.*, Civ. No. 11-5782 (E.D. Pa. Mar. 9, 2015).

332 **issue a reprimand:** mywsba.org/webfiles/cusdocs/000000029413-0/003.pdf.
332 **A total of six plaintiffs:** "Thalidomide Morass Deepens for Hagens Berman as More Clients Sue Firm," Reuters, Nov. 29, 2021; "Client Who Sued Hagens Berman over Failed Thalidomide Case Settles," *Pennsylvania Record*, Sept. 23, 2020.
332 **"Typically, the clock starts":** Author interview with Benjamin Zipursky.
332 **"signature injury" . . . "reasonable care":** Ibid.
333 **masses of the drug:** Merrell had sent at least ten million pills to doctors. At most, 25,000 pills were rounded up in the FDA investigation. "The Unfinished Story of Thalidomide," *Saturday Review*, Sept. 1, 1962.
333 **"do the right thing":** Author interview with Benjamin Zipursky.
333 **The agency's reported nine victims:** "Thalidomide Deformity Investigation," Sept. 24, 1962, FDA Archives.
334 **"how many were actually":** Email to author from Brittney Manchester, press officer, Office of Media Affairs, FDA, Feb. 14, 2020.
334 **To my request, the FDA replied:** FDA, Author's FOIA Request, Number: 2018-9838, 2018-9829, denied on April 1, 2019. Appealed on June 21, 2019. Appeal denied Aug. 24, 2021.
334 **"four or five months prior":** This letter suggests the attorney was asking about Merrell's Kevadon investigators in Florida, unaware the drug had also been tested since late 1956. Van W. Smart to Norman K. Rutkin, Attorney at Law, Feb. 20, 1963, FDA Archives.
334 **the agency closely guarded:** "Hagens Berman: Patients Seek to Force FDA to Release Records Showing US Distribution of Thalidomide," Nov. 17, 2011, press release accessed via PR Newswire.
337 **Frances ranked number eight:** "Mrs. Kennedy is Most Admired Woman," *Washington Post*, Dec. 26, 1962.
337 **"Frances became":** Dr. James L. Goddard, Oral Histories, U.S. Food and Drug Administration, April 30–June 19, 1969.
337 **"trouble developing if Barbara came back":** Ibid.
338 **Frances's parking spot:** Alice Dredger, "Saint Frances, Walking to Her Car," Aug. 26, 2015, blog post, available at alicedreger.com/Frances/.
338 **People trying to call:** "Erroneous Information," memorandum from Frances Kelsey to Mr. James Shipp, Chief Administrative Branch, April 22, 1965, Frances Kelsey Papers.
338 **"bare-desk" treatment:** "My desk was pretty bare for a while and my morale was quite low." "The Federal Diary: President Moves to Widen Women's Role in Government," *Washington Post*, March 9, 1967.

Epilogue

343 **"FDA does not have":** Email from Brittney Manchester, FDA press officer, to the author, Feb. 14, 2020.
344 **"May 14, 2021":** U.S. Department of Justice, Criminal Division, to author, Request No. CRM- 300779274, May 14, 2021. In 2023, the author determined that a case file may actually exist elsewhere, and is currently pursuing it.
346 **research suggested:** C. Lutwak-Mann, K. Schmid, and H. Keberle, "Thalidomide in Rabbit Semen," *Nature* 214 (1967): 1018–20.
346 **probed the drug's ability:** U.S. Government Memorandum from Ralph Weilerstein, Associate Medical Director, to Bureau of Medicine, Sept. 4, 1962, FDA Archives.
347 **NIH testing thalidomide:** Harry Grabstald and Robert Golbey, "Clinical Experiences with Thalidomide in Patients with Cancer," *Clinical Pharmacology and Therapeutics* 6 (1965): 298–302.

347 **word got out:** Terence Monmaney, "Thalidomide Reemerges as Potential 'Wonder Drug,'" *Los Angeles Times*, March 26, 1998.

347 **"It works like magic":** "Leprosy's Legacy," *Washington Post*, April 25, 1989.

347 **rattled the FDA:** "Thalidomide Distribution by Three AIDS Buyers' Clubs for Cachexia Draws FDA Warning Letter," *The Pink Sheet*, Sept. 11, 1995.

347 **the agency pressed Celgene:** "37 Years Later, a Second Chance for Thalidomide," *New York Times*, Sept. 23, 1997.

347 **"met its scientific obligation":** "FDA May Approve Use of Thalidomide," *Deseret News*, Sept. 23, 1997.

347 **"Our hope":** "37 Years Later."

348 **"off-label":** "Celgene Receives FDA Warning Letter over Thalidomide Promotion," ThePharmaLetter.com, Aug. 5, 2000; "Celgene Gets Swatted with FDA Warning About Off-Label Thalidomide Sales," TheStreet.com, April 24, 2000.

348 **FDA had not yet approved:** G. A. Bruyn, "Thalidomide Celgene Corp," *IDrugs: The Investigational Drugs Journal* 1, no. 4 (1998): 490–500.

348 **revoked its support for thalidomide:** Dr. V. Pannikar, Medical Officer, Communicable Diseases (Leprosy Group) WHO, "The Return of Thalidomide: New Uses and Renewed Concerns," *Leprosy Review*, Sept. 2003; and "No Role for Thalidomide in Leprosy," WHO Leprosy Team, World Health Organization, Geneva, Switzerland, 2003, paho.org/hq/dmdocuments/2013/No-Role-Thalidomide -Leprosy-2003-Eng.pdf

348 **thalidomide was proving too risky:** Colin L. Crawford, "No Role for Thalidomide in the Treatment of Leprosy," *Journal of Infectious Diseases*, June 15, 2006, 1743–44.

348 **country with a large leprosy population:** "No Role for Thalidomide in Leprosy."

348 **off-label use to treat:** A. Maureen Rouhi, "Thalidomide: Purpose Immunomodulator," *Chemical and Engineering News* 83, no. 25 (June 2005).

348 **multiple myeloma patients paid:** Alison Kodjak, "How a Drugmaker Gamed the System to Keep Generic Competition Away," NPR, May 17, 2018.

348 **The drug was earning:** "Celgene, Sold for $74 Billion, Leaves a Legacy of Chutzpah in Science and Drug Pricing," *Stat News*, Jan. 22, 2019.

349 **"We have seen time after time":** Hearing Before the Committee on Oversight and Reform, U.S. House of Representatives, One Hundred Sixteenth Congress, First Session, January 29, 2019.

349 **allegedly prevented competitors:** "How a Drugmaker Gamed the System to Keep Generic Competition Away."

350 **patent disputes were eventually settled:** "Celgene to Allow Another Generic of Revlimid in 2022, Settling Patent Dispute," Spglobal.com, March 29, 2019.

350 **the agreements with Celgene:** "Celgene Settles U.S. Revlimid Patent Litigation with Algoven," Celgene press release, March 29, 2019, s24.q4cdn.com/483522778 /files/doc_news/2019/03/2019-03-29-CELGENE-SE,TLES-U.S.-REVLIMID -PATENT-LITIGATION-WITH-ALVOGEN_FINALv2.pdf.

350 **myeloma patients quickly complained:** "Generic Revlimid in Myeloma: Don't Get Too Excited," myelomacrowd.org/myeloma/community/articles/generic -revlimid-in-myeloma–dont-get-too-excited.

350 **"I hope that the fact":** Author interview with Jean Grover.

350 **"I would have given it to him myself":** Ibid.

Index

About the Author

JENNIFER VANDERBES is a novelist, journalist, and screenwriter whose work has been translated into sixteen languages. Her writing has appeared in *The New York Times*, *The Wall Street Journal*, *The Washington Post*, *The Atlantic*, *Granta*, and *Best New American Voices*. She is the recipient of a Guggenheim Fellowship and was named a National Endowment for the Humanities Public Scholar for her work on *Wonder Drug*.

About the Type

This book was set in Electra, a typeface designed for Linotype by W. A. Dwiggins, the renowned type designer (1880–1956). Electra is a fluid typeface, avoiding the contrasts of thick and thin strokes that are prevalent in most modern typefaces.